Controversies in Managed Mental Health Care

Controversies in Managed Mental Health Care

Edited by
Arthur Lazarus, M.D.
Medical Director
Northwestern Institute of Psychiatry
Fort Washington, Pennsylvania;
Clinical Associate Professor of Psychiatry
Temple University School of Medicine
Philadelphia

American Psychiatric Press, Inc.
Washington, DC
London, England

Note: The authors have worked to ensure that all information in this book concerning drug dosages, schedules, and routes of administration is accurate as of the time of publication and consistent with standards set by the U.S. Food and Drug Administration and the general medical community. As medical research and practice advance, however, therapeutic standards may change. For this reason and because human and mechanical errors sometimes occur, we recommend that readers follow the advice of a physician who is directly involved in their care or the care of a member of their family.

Books published by the American Psychiatric Press, Inc., represent the views and opinions of the individual authors and do not necessarily represent the policies and opinions of the Press or the American Psychiatric Association.

Manufactured in the United States of America on acid-free paper
99 98 97 96 4 3 2 1

American Psychiatric Press, Inc.
1400 K Street, N.W., Washington, DC 20005

Library of Congress Cataloging-in-Publication Data
Controversies in managed mental health care / edited by Arthur Lazarus.
p. cm.
Includes bibliographical references and index.
ISBN 0-88048-115-3
1. Managed mental health care—United States. I. Lazarus, Arthur, 1954–
RC465.6.C66 1996
366.2'0425—dc20 95-47287
CIP

British Library Cataloguing in Publication Data
A CIP record is available from the British Library.

Contents

Contributors

Martin G. Allen, M.D.
Clinical Professor of Psychiatry, Georgetown University School of Medicine, Washington, D.C.

Carol Shaw Austad, Ph.D.
Staff Psychologist, Community Health Care Plan, Wallingford, Connecticut; Assistant Professor of Psychology, Central Connecticut State University, New Britain, Connecticut

Michael J. Bennett, M.D.
Corporate Vice President for Medical Services, Merit Behavioral Care Corporation, Burlington, Massachusetts; Clinical Associate Professor of Psychiatry, Harvard Medical School, Boston, Massachusetts

Jonathan D. Book, M.D.
Senior Vice President and Chief Medical Officer, Green Spring Health Services, Inc., Columbia, Maryland; Clinical Assistant Professor of Psychiatry, University of Maryland School of Medicine, Baltimore, Maryland

David S. Brody, M.D.
Professor of Medicine and Chief, Division of General Internal Medicine, Medical College of Pennsylvania and Hahnemann University, Philadelphia, Pennsylvania

Anthony F. Buono, Ph.D.
Research Fellow, Center for Business Ethics, Bentley College, Waltham, Massachusetts; Professor, Department of Management, Bentley College, Waltham, Massachusetts

John C. Burroughs, M.S.S., M.B.A.
Product Director, Group Health Managed Care, Intracorp, Philadelphia, Pennsylvania

Thomas Carli, M.D.
Director, Consultation and General Psychiatry Division, and Clinical Assistant Professor of Psychiatry, University of Michigan Medical Center, Ann Arbor, Michigan

Alfred Carter, M.D.
Clinical Instructor of Psychiatry, Tufts University School of Medicine, Boston, Massachusetts

Nicholas A. Cummings, Ph.D., Litt.D.
President, Foundation for Behavioral Health, Reno, Nevada; Founding Chair and CEO (Retired), American Biodyne Inc., San Francisco, California; former President, American Psychological Association

Robert A. Dorwart, M.D., M.P.H.
Chairman, Mental Health Policy Working Group, Malcolm Weiner Center for Social Policy, John F. Kennedy School of Government, Harvard University, Cambridge, Massachusetts; Associate Professor, Harvard Medical School, Boston, Massachusetts; Department of Psychiatry, The Cambridge Hospital, Cambridge, Massachusetts

William R. Dubin, M.D.
Director, Clinical Services, Belmont Behavioral Health, Philadelphia, Pennsylvania; Associate Chairman, Department of Psychiatry, Albert Einstein Medical Center, Philadelphia, Pennsylvania; Professor of Psychiatry, Temple University School of Medicine, Philadelphia, Pennsylvania

Dorothy E. Dugger, M.D.
BioBehavioral Research Institute, Chester Springs, Pennsylvania; Clinical Assistant Professor of Psychiatry, Temple University School of Medicine, Philadelphia, Pennsylvania

Paul J. Fink, M.D.
Senior Consultant, Charter Fairmount Behavioral Health System and Mustard Seed, Inc, Philadelphia, Pennsylvania; Vice President, INTERCARE Behavioral Health, Philadelphia, Pennsylvania; Professor of Psychiatry, Temple University School of Medicine, Philadelphia, Pennsylvania; former President, American Psychiatric Association

Robert J. Fox, J.D.
Director of Planning, Continuum Behavioral Healthcare Corporation, Park Ridge, New Jersey

Richard G. Frank, Ph.D.
Professor of Health Economics, Department of Health Care Policy, Harvard Medical School, Boston, Massachusetts

Ronald D. Geraty, M.D.
President, Continuum Behavioral Healthcare Corporation, Park Ridge, New Jersey

William M. Glazer, M.D.
Associate Clinical Professor of Psychiatry, Yale University School of Medicine, New Haven, Connecticut

Geoffrey V. Gray, Ph.D.
President, PsychResources Group, Inc., Hamden, Connecticut

Henry T. Harbin, M.D.
President and Chief Executive Officer, Green Spring Health Services, Inc., Columbia, Maryland; Clinical Professor of Psychiatry, University of Maryland School of Medicine, Baltimore, Maryland

William Hetznecker, M.D.
Professor of Psychiatry, Temple University School of Medicine, Philadelphia, Pennsylvania

Armin U. Kuder, LL.B.
Partner, Kuder, Smollar and Friedman, P.C., Washington, D.C.

Marcia B. F. Kuntz, J.D.
Adjunct Professor Of Law, Georgetown University, Washington, D.C.

Arthur Lazarus, M.D.
Clinical Associate Professor of Psychiatry, Temple University School of Medicine, Philadelphia, Pennsylvania; Medical Director, Northwestern Institute, Fort Washington, Pennsylvania

Benjamin Liptzin, M.D.
Chairman, Department of Psychiatry, Baystate Medical Center, Springfield, Massachusetts; Professor of Psychiatry, Tufts University School of Medicine, Boston, Massachusetts

Suzanne Lizanich-Aro, R.N., M.P.H.
Consultant, Green Spring Health Services, Inc., Columbia, Maryland

Joseph S. Lombardi, Ph.D.
Adjunct Assistant Professor, Department of Management, Bentley College, Waltham, Massachusetts

Clarissa C. Marques, Ph.D.
Senior Vice President and Chief Clinical Officer, Green Spring Health Services, Inc., Columbia, Maryland

Paul R. McCarthy, Ph.D.
BioBehavioral Research Institute, Chester Springs, Pennsylvania

Thomas G. McGuire, Ph.D.
Professor of Economics, Boston University, Boston, Massachusetts

David Mechanic, Ph.D.
Director, Institute for Health, Health Care Policy, and Aging Research, Rutgers University, New Brunswick, New Jersey; Director, Center for Research on the Organization and Financing of Care for the Severely Mentally Ill, Rutgers University, New Brunswick, New Jersey; René Dubos Professor of Behavioral Sciences and University Professor, Rutgers University, New Brunswick, New Jersey

Stephen J. O'Connor, Ph.D.
Associate Professor, School of Business Administration and Master of Science Program in Health Care Management, University of Wisconsin–Milwaukee, Milwaukee, Wisconsin

Monica E. Oss, M.A.
President, Open Minds, Gettysburg, Pennsylvania; Editor-in-Chief, Behavioral Health Management

Anthony F. Panzetta, M.D.
President, Internet Behavioral Health System, Lafayette Hill, Pennsylvania; former Chairman, Department of Psychiatry, Temple University School of Medicine, Philadelphia, Pennsylvania

Michael S. Perlman, M.D.
Clinical Instructor of Psychiatry, Tufts University School of Medicine, Boston, Massachusetts

Jay M. Pomerantz, M.D.
Clinical Instructor of Psychiatry, Tufts University School of Medicine, Boston, Massachusetts

Michelle B. Riba, M.D.
Director, Resident and Fellow Education, Clinical Assistant Professor of Psychiatry, University of Michigan Medical Center, Ann Arbor, Michigan

James E. Sabin, M.D.
Associate Director, Teaching Center, Harvard Pilgrim Health Care, Boston, Massachusetts; Associate Clinical Professor of Psychiatry, Harvard Medical School, Boston, Massachusetts

Carol A. Schreter, M.S.W., Ph.D.
Freelance writer on health and aging, based in Baltimore, Maryland

Robert K. Schreter, M.D.
Private practice in psychiatry, Baltimore, Maryland; Medical Director, Psych Services, Baltimore, Maryland; Associate Medical Director, Sheppard Pratt Health Plan, Baltimore, Maryland; Assistant Professor of Psychiatry, Johns Hopkins Medical School, Baltimore, Maryland

Chip Silverman, Ph.D., M.P.H.
Director of Chemical Dependency, Government Relations and Public Affairs, Green Spring Health Services, Inc., Columbia, Maryland; former Director of the Maryland Alcohol and Drug Abuse Administration

Christine S. Spencer, Sc.D.
Assistant Professor, Center for Child and Adolescent Mental Health Services Research, Johns Hopkins School of Hygiene and Public Health, Baltimore, Maryland

T. Scott Stroup, M.D., M.P.H.
Assistant Professor, Department of Psychiatry; Research Fellow, Cecil G. Sheps Center for Health Services Research, University of North Carolina, Chapel Hill, North Carolina

Mark Tidgewell, C.P.A.
Senior Consultant, Open Minds, Gettysburg, Pennsylvania

Preface

As you browse through this book you may wonder, "Is another book about managed care really necessary?" The answer to that question, like the answers to the 27 questions that form the centerpiece of this book, seems relatively straightforward. The question elicits a reflexive answer —perhaps a simple "yes" or "no"—but then there may be some doubt and reconsideration. The answer becomes unexpectedly elusive as it invites comment and leads to closer inspection of the question at hand.

The American Psychiatric Press has published several fine books related to managed care: a manual of quality assurance, a handbook of utilization management, a basic textbook, and even a "survival guide." *Controversies in Managed Mental Health Care*, however, is a "second-generation" book. It probes areas of uncertainty and tension in the managed care world. In conceiving this book, I deliberately selected topics that could be debated but could also be addressed with authority. The ensuing spirited discussion captures, I believe, the conflict inherent in the managed care movement.

The contributors represent a diverse group of clinicians, academicians, and managed care executives, as well as other industry leaders. My instructions to them were few. I proposed a question and asked them to answer it based on their experience, beliefs, and grasp of the literature. I presumed the authors would reach a logical conclusion derived from an examination of the issues relevant to their topics. I was less concerned about whether their essays would read as an indictment of managed care or as a tribute to its potential, although certainly there are many areas where opinions converge and readers are left with a clearer vision of managed care systems of the future.

I would caution readers not to spoil the "surprise" ending of each chapter by reading the conclusion first. The contributors have worked diligently and thoughtfully to answer their questions; their responses must not be taken out of context. They may not be managed care's Boswell, but they have certainly provided enlightening accounts in response to challenging questions in difficult times. I am grateful for all their efforts.

A debt of gratitude is also owed to Denise Taylor, whose skillful handling of the manuscript led to the timely completion of the book.

This book is dedicated to the memory of my father, Aaron, to my wife, Cheryl, and to my children, Joshua, Karen, Heather, and Aryn, who make it all worthwhile.

Arthur Lazarus, M.D.

Section I

Practice and Policy

Chapter 1

Are Psychiatrists Replaceable?

Paul J. Fink, M.D.

Throughout the past several decades the death of psychiatry has been predicted by those who believe the problems of dealing with mentally ill persons are impossible to solve. In the early days of psychiatry, when there were very few effective treatments and psychiatrists often struggled simply to keep patients alive through asylum, there may have been some rationale for such dire predictions. Recently, however, as the therapeutic armamentarium of psychiatrists has grown, and as Americans have become more acutely aware of the impact of mental illnesses on society, the psychiatric profession has emerged from the dark ages into a bright, scientifically sound era. A great deal of research has been done, and patients with serious mental and chemical dependency problems can receive expert care in a biopsychosocial framework of treatment.

Ironically, in the 1990s, we find ourselves beleaguered with many problems, not only those related to managed care but also problems emanating from the intense distrust of the various ways in which psychiatrists treat patients. Psychiatrists and their patients have become the target of stigma, ridicule, and humiliation. A number of nonmedical mental health professional groups are nipping at psychiatrists' heels to share in the "pot of gold at the end of the rainbow." However, clearly, there is no pot of gold because reimbursement policies in the mental health field have become increasingly restricted and geared to denying treatment for individuals with serious mental disorders. Compatible with this trend is a movement to replace psychiatrists with therapists whose training is less extensive and is not medically based. The philosophy of substituting nonmedical therapists for psychiatrists is manifested in comments such as "psychiatrists have lost the psychotherapy battle," "only one psychiatrist is needed for every 10,000 to 20,000 covered lives," "psychiatrists are not special," and "psychologists should have prescribing privileges." Comments such as these are voiced as often by psychiatrists as by nonmedical therapists, making it difficult to demonstrate our skills as separate and nonsynchronous with other mental health professionals who are very much a part of the American health scene.

The Emergence of Nonmedical Therapists

There are an estimated 250,000 individual mental health providers in the United States. That number includes approximately 42,000 psychiatrists, 57,000 clinical psychologists, and 82,000 clinical social workers as well as a broad array of marriage and family therapists, certified addiction counselors, and other types of therapists trained in various methods and schools throughout the United States (DeWitt 1992). As recently as 1960, the roles of psychiatrists, psychologists, and social workers were clear and distinct. Psychiatrists had the overall responsibility of patient care, conducted psychotherapy, prescribed medication and other biological forms of treatment, and supervised the hospital care of patients. Psychologists primarily conducted testing and moved gingerly into group therapy and other therapeutic modalities under the aegis of psychiatrists in institutions and hospitals. Social workers were responsible for doing comprehensive psychosocial assessments, dealing with family issues, and planning for discharge. Family therapy had not yet been "invented," so there were no family therapists as we know them today. The treatment of alcohol and drug abuse was primarily in the hands of individuals affiliated with Alcoholics Anonymous, and the only mode of treatment in which physicians became involved was generally during the period of detoxification. The mental health field was far from overcrowded.

During the 1960s, the development of the community mental health system led to an explosion in the number of mental health professionals needed to staff the planned 2,000 community mental health centers. Early in the era of community mental health, the roles of caregivers were quite diffuse. Many individuals were considered "therapists," with or without training, and there was a great effort to involve patients in treatment. At first, psychiatrists provided direct patient care, then became supervisors, and ultimately were cast out of the community mental health system because it was believed that they had served their purpose and were of little value (Panzetta 1985). In addition, psychiatrists were considered costly, and the amount of money available for community mental health treatment decreased each year.

Psychoanalysis was the psychotherapeutic treatment of choice in the 1960s and the therapeutic model around which most residency training was developed. Nonmedical therapists in the United States were severely restricted from practicing analysis, and thus the marketplace was narrow and well controlled. However, in the mid-1980s, as a result of a lawsuit brought by the American Psychological Association, psychiatrists could no longer monopolize outpatient psychotherapeutic treatment. The analytic approach, while having fallen into some disrepute, was still a major force in the training of psychiatrists and an important therapeutic tool nearly exclusive to psychiatrists practicing in the United States. Thus within a brief period of time psychiatrists found themselves yielding to nonmedical therapists in two significant areas of practice: community mental health and outpatient psychotherapy.

Stigma

The stigma attached to mental illness and to the caretakers of the mentally ill has been extensively studied and documented (Fink and Tasman 1992). Psychiatrists have provided good characters for drama and movies; there have been many films and plays that characterized psychiatrists as evil, malevolent, ludicrous, seductive, or caricatures of nonresponsive disinterested types. That mischaracterization of psychiatrists in cinema and television has undermined the public's confidence in the ability of psychiatrists and has discouraged people from seeking help when they are ill (Gabbard and Gabbard 1992). Psychotherapy has perhaps been the aspect of psychiatric treatment most maligned by the media. Nowhere has the devaluation of psychiatrists been as complete and as inexorable as in the medical profession. Most of the medical specialties engage in ridiculing psychiatrists and undermining their place as brethren within the body politic of medicine (Fink 1984). Friction between psychiatrists and their medical counterparts has created a rift so deep that psychiatrists have been unwilling to participate in medical societies and in the politics of hospitals. It is not uncommon for a family physician to say to his or her patient, "You are not *that* sick; you ought to see a psychologist." That comment stems in part from the fact that psychiatrists use medication and psychologists do not. Patients who require medication are generally seen as more "sick." However, comments such as these are also made because family practitioners may be uncomfortable relating to psychiatrists. This alienation between psychiatrists and other physicians has made it very difficult for psychiatrists to establish themselves as the preeminent caretakers of patients with mental illnesses and chemical dependency disorders. Adding to the difficulty, the

American insurance companies, unlike the Canadian health care system, reimburse all manner of nonphysicians for psychological treatment. In the past two decades, this nondiscriminatory reimbursement has increased the efforts of psychologists to gain equal status with psychiatrists even though psychologists do not have a medical degree. The most objective evidence of stigmatization among physicians is that when they or their family members develop emotional problems, they often seek out psychologists for treatment.

It seems incredible that most American citizens have failed to learn or refused to learn the differences between psychologists and psychiatrists. I believe that this is attributable in part to stigma. Although an untold number of leaflets and articles in popular magazines have clearly distinguished psychologists from psychiatrists, this information seems to be evanescent and the facts remain a mystery requiring explanation many times over. Perhaps most of the information people have about psychiatry comes from informal experiences with the profession rather than from formal education experiences. They see psychiatrists and psychologists as playing similar roles when testifying in court or intervening in a mental health crisis. Unfortunately, as pointed out earlier, the confusion is made worse because these roles are often portrayed in a negative light.

It is not at all surprising that the public doesn't understand the difference between psychiatrists and psychologists given that their differences are often not a deciding factor in their selection for many roles within the mental health profession. In the real world, psychiatrists and psychologists frequently compete for the same jobs despite their very different training and experience. In part, that competition is a result of the overlap between psychiatry and psychology, but it is also partly caused by a failure to understand real differences between the two professions.

Biopsychosocial Paradigm

The biopsychosocial model has become an important ideological approach to treatment both for mentally ill and physically ill patients. Through years of research, George Engel, M.D., has made it clear that physical illnesses require attention both to biological aspects of disease and to the psychological concerns and sociocultural milieu of the patient. For mental disorders, the biopsychosocial model of treatment assumes even greater importance. Pharmacological agents are valuable only when patients are compliant with treatment, and ensuring compliance with treatment generally requires an ongoing relationship with a psychiatrist who not only prescribes medication but also helps an individual deal with emotional trauma and problems of daily living.

The manner in which those problems are handled may inhibit or enhance an individual's capacity to grow and recover from an illness.

Under managed care, the therapeutic relationship has become increasingly complex. Therapy is often coordinated by a psychopharmacologist working in conjunction with a psychotherapist or a treatment team. Frequently the team is headed by a psychiatrist; however, it is not unusual for the team to be headed instead by a psychologist, with the psychiatrist being relegated to the role of a psychopharmacology consultant rather than an active team member.

Although the distance between psychotherapists and psychopharmacologists appears to be widening, a vast amount of research has demonstrated that combined treatment with medication and psychotherapy is generally more effective than treatment with either alone. Furthermore, it is impossible to neglect the complexity of patients with serious mental illnesses such as schizophrenia, bipolar disorder, and major depression. The patients' families, their work environment (if they are able to work), and the cultural milieu (ethnic, religious, communal) are especially important to seriously ill patients who are unable to move easily within the various dimensions of society.

The biopsychosocial paradigm has been severely undermined by a number of trends within the health care system that make it difficult for any one individual to attend to the overall needs of a patient. Likewise, there is less opportunity to develop a treatment plan to address long-term problems and goals and extend treatment beyond acute intermittent care. Schreter (1993) has discussed 10 trends in managed care that have a negative impact on the biopsychosocial model. He pointed out that mental health carve-outs appear to be dedicated to reducing the use of resources for the mentally ill. These carve-outs have created new and untested models of care that have been imposed on the psychiatric profession without consensus, thus traumatizing much of the provider community. According to Schreter (1993), an increase in the fiscal management of care at the expense of clinical management, the shifting of control from the provider to the patient, and a change in basic assumptions about treatment and outcome are by-products of the managed care era. Those changes represent serious indictments of a system that has moved away from an interest in patient care toward the conservation of dollars and resources, which are then allocated to profit or to nonpsychiatric care systems.

One managed care executive told me that the hospital should never be used for treatment, only for stabilization for the movement of patients to less restrictive settings. Another disturbing trend in managed care is that the goal of outpatient treatment has been redefined with increasing emphasis on identifying the chief complaint followed by short-term treatment. Emerging models of psychotherapy in managed care assume that the psychotherapeutic process occurs in pieces over time. This effort at symptomatic treatment has led to the training of psychiatrists with no philosophical underpinning and to the gradual disappearance of the psychodynamic model as a framework for understanding mental and cognitive functioning. Yet there is growing evidence that a significant number of patients do not benefit from short-term treatment, especially patients with major clinical syndromes complicated by severe psychopathology (Muran et al. 1994; Pierce 1994).

Another worrisome trend in managed care is the move toward lower levels of care and less intense service. These trends are not an invention of managed care. They were already under way and were embraced by managed care. Nonetheless, patients have been taken away from psychiatrists and put in the hands of poorly trained or untrained paraprofessionals for treatment in nontraditional settings such as self-help groups and halfway houses. Many other nonmedical approaches to patient care have been advanced although some of the clinicians involved are untrained, uninformed, and have no real grasp of total patient care. The biopsychosocial paradigm is further threatened by fiscal issues favoring limited forms of treatment, usually given by the least experienced and least knowledgeable agent.

The Special Treatment of Psychiatry

The American Psychiatric Association (APA) and other important organizations in the field of mental health have been active in the political arena for a significant amount of time. Important lobbying efforts have resulted in both good and bad outcomes. When the concept of diagnosis-related group (DRG) was developed, the APA was able to convince the Congress that psychiatric hospitals should be excluded from DRGs because prospective reimbursement models relying on psychiatric diagnoses have not been found to have much predictive validity (English et al. 1986; Stoskopf and Horn 1992). This led to favorable treatment for psychiatric patients even though there were built-in limitations in the Medicare system.

With the advent of resource-based relative value scale (RBRVS), there was an expectation that psychiatrists would receive preferential treatment, but at the last minute that decision was overturned by a single individual who, in unilateral fashion, left psychiatrists once again at the bottom of the heap, even though psychiatry is recognized as one of the cognitive specialties that should have been given some special accord. More recently, special treatment in psychiatry has once again led to undesirable results, particularly in the use of behavioral carve-outs by major insurance companies throughout the United States. Because policymakers do not want to be troubled with ill-defined areas of mental illness and substance abuse, insurance companies sold these portions of their portfolio to specialty companies developed and designed especially for the mentally ill. Carve-out companies vary from those that are excellent to those that are extremely egregious in their treatment of the mentally ill, budgeting limited dollars for expensive and necessary psychiatric treatment.

Managed mental health care companies began insidiously and have become an extremely powerful force in the insurance industry. They have essentially dictated the course of psychiatric treatment in the United States by establishing their own parameters for utilization review and medical necessity. Most psychiatrists and other mental health professionals have complied with managed care companies because "he who pays the piper calls the tune."

Negative Behavior of Psychiatrists

Managed care organizations are not solely to blame for the current turmoil in the psychiatric profession. Practicing psychiatrists and other professionals are equally culpable. There have been instances of serious fraud and compliance with institutions that misused patients by unnecessarily hospitalizing them. Many psychiatrists have been unwilling to change their behavior to work within managed care systems even when excellent treatment could still be provided. Most will not get up at night to see their patients, and they often refuse to abide by managed care rules. They then become indignant when they are eliminated from a network or decredentialed. Some psychiatrists have provided minimal care while billing under maximal current procedural terminology codes. They have committed a number of acts which, I believe, lead to serious ethics questions concerning the way they have cared for their patients. For example, the medical director of a managed care organization told me that a psychiatrist refused to transfer a psychotic patient from a medical service to an inpatient psychiatric unit because the psychiatrist feared that he might not be reimbursed for inpatient treatment yet he was certain he would be reimbursed as a consultant.

The inconsistency that has come to characterize the way some physicians address their Aesculapian responsibility is a sad reality contributing to the growing negative reputation of physicians in the United States. Ironically, most surveys demonstrate that patients like their own doctors but dislike most other physicians. The destructive behavior of a handful of physicians tarnishes the image of physicians (Bluestone 1993), and psychiatrists in particular, and leads to efforts to replace them by all types of allied mental health professionals. Only in this type of atmosphere could the question be asked, "Are psychiatrists replaceable?"

Changes in Practice Patterns

Because managed care companies have forced significant changes in the way psychiatric services are reimbursed, psychiatrists must be flexible and diversify their practice to survive (Fink 1994). Changes in practice need to be incorporated in ways that accentuate the skills that psychiatrists obtain during medical school and residency training. Psychiatrists in a solo practice that emphasizes individual psychotherapy will most likely find their income significantly restricted. However, those who can conduct group therapy should be able to maintain their income or perhaps increase it. There is great value in learning and conducting group therapy—better use of time, increased cost-effectiveness, and greater income potential.

Under managed care, emergency psychiatry, consultation-liaison psychiatry, and crisis intervention will become more important (Fink 1993a). Psychiatrists will need to sharpen their skills in those areas and abandon any less useful areas. The combined use of psychotherapy and pharmacotherapy will be highly valued by managed care organizations because one person (a psychiatrist) will be able to provide both a therapeutic relationship and a specific biological intervention. However, although I do not favor it, an arrangement in which psychiatrists provide the pharmacotherapy while less expensive care providers provide the bulk of the much more time-consuming psychotherapy would be considered by some to be equally valuable. Also valuable may be psychiatrists who are skilled at being team leaders. The team leader often holds the key to setting the focus and direction of treatment. The decisions made by the team leader greatly influence the various team members' level of involvement in treatment, including that of the psychiatrist.

Managed care will motivate psychiatrists to develop group practices (Brown 1993; Moran 1993). However, there must be a willingness to assign different tasks to different psychiatrists as well as to provide comprehensive on-call coverage. Groups of psychiatrists can better serve the community because they can employ subspecialists within the group yet share both the assets and expenses related to practice. In addition to traditional reasons for forming group practices—sharing call, controlling overhead, and simple relief from the isolation of solo practice—there are reasons related to managed care. A practice geared toward managed care and employer contracts must have adequate geographic coverage, comprehensive information systems, and enough psychiatrists to treat a defined population.

Another practice model gaining popularity among psychiatrists is network-based practice (Chapter 25). Networks include not only psychiatrists but also psychologists, social workers, and other therapists. It is important for psychiatrists to take a leadership role in network development (Siegler et al. 1993) or they will be relegated to signing prescriptions and taking care of patients in the hospital, after which they will be asked to relinquish patients to less costly therapists. Within networks, it may be possible for psychiatrists to carry out treatment in community agencies, schools, various clinics, and departments of government. However, psychiatrists must be prepared to share risks in capitated contracts and discount their fees to drive a large volume of referrals and have credibility in the marketplace.

Although there are many positive aspects to the development of group practices, networks, and other similar arrangements, there are some serious problems. A paradigm shift in the value system of medicine is taking place passively and perceptibly. The shift can be most clearly seen in the acceptance of giving less care to individual patients in exchange for managing the health of whole populations in the context of limited resources. The transition from private practice to practice within an organized system of care requires a change in the way physicians practice (Moran 1993). Managerial concepts such as continuous quality improvement are admirable, but they reduce the value of the physician-patient relationship and instill a corporate approach to patient care rather than a medically based approach to treatment. Regardless of the practice arrangement, physicians must relinquish autonomy to corporate entities. However, in doing so, cost-effective physicians should not be micromanaged lest the imposition of managed care methods prove to be detrimental to overall patient care.

Managed care companies must be prevented from making capricious decisions about deselecting psychiatrists by barring them from joining managed care organizations or arbitrarily terminating them from networks. There are a number of landmark situations throughout the United States in which physicians have been unjustly removed from provider panels and their patients have been moved unceremoniously to other providers with little regard for ongoing treatment, the physician-patient relationship, and interactions that have been medically therapeutic. Federal draft legislation proposed by the American Medical Association may remedy that problem by allowing all physicians in the health plan's area to apply for credentials and by offering due process appeals to physicians who are terminated from health plans without cause (McCormick 1994).

The APA Response

The APA has developed a number of programs to help psychiatrists cope with problems related to managed care. The managed care hot line, which received approximately 8,000 calls in its first 3 years of operation, is perhaps the most visible of those efforts. The most prevalent concerns of psychiatrists calling the hot line are treatment access and denial, confidentiality, and the refusal of managed care organizations to publish medical criteria. Although representatives from a few managed care companies appear to be intransigent, most have been willing to work with the APA in rectifying grievances and allowing psychiatrists to have greater input into patient care.

The APA has witnessed a high level of confrontation and conflict between managed care companies and psychiatrists. Some, but certainly not all, managed care companies have taken a bullying attitude, inciting psychiatrists and leading to altercations. These disagreements would have been much better handled had a collegial effort occurred first and had discussions focused on patients' interests. Much of the conflict with managed care companies has centered on the companies' desire to practice medicine, for example, by prescribing treatment to the attending psychiatrist and dictating services that will and will not be reimbursed. That type of disrespect and disregard has been the most annoying and humiliating aspect of the penetration of managed care companies into new communities.

In addition to the hot line, the APA's committee on managed care has developed an important strategic document, "Network Development and Practice Models for Managed Competition," to help psychiatrists comply with the rigors of managed care and work within a managed care model. The APA has instituted a series of programs throughout the United States to teach psychiatrists how to negotiate with managed care companies in a style that will avoid future acrimony. Managed care organizations have had valid concerns about psychiatrists who appear to be intractable and have refused reasonable requests consistent with good managed care practice.

Finally, the APA is in the process of developing a practice research network (see, for example, Green et al. 1984), medical-necessity criteria, and practice guidelines that, it is hoped, will be adopted nationwide.

Psychiatrists' Roles in Managed Care

There are many opportunities for psychiatrists to become involved with managed care operations (Fink 1993b; Lazarus 1994), and an increasing number of psychiatrists are moving in the direction of either part- or full-time employment in managed care systems. Typical roles of psychiatrists include those of provider, reviewer, and administrator. Psychiatrists may independently contract with managed care organizations, in which case their daily work encompasses other responsibilities, or they may work exclusively in a managed care capacity, for example, as a salaried HMO staff physician. Psychiatrists who provide direct patient care for managed care companies or HMOs will be challenged to work within the framework, policies, and procedures of the organization. Managed care is clearly the system of tightest control. For those psychiatrists who feel comfortable in that position, it may be an excellent way to work synergistically with managed care rather than being antagonistic to it.

Peer reviewers are responsible for conducting inpatient and outpatient utilization review of treatment, whether the review occurs 5 miles or 500 miles from the actual site of care. A competent reviewer will foster goodwill for the company, create harmony with the attending psychiatrist, and ensure exemplary patient care. Adversarial reviews may be handled well or poorly, depending on the interpersonal skills of both parties.

Psychiatrists who have left clinical practice to become administrators may make significant contributions to managed care companies and to patient care (Penzer 1989). Therapists generally have the type of experience and background that enables them to make astute clinical judgments, tolerate ambiguity, make difficult decisions, and deal with upset and angry individuals. Psychiatrists who work in an administrative capacity for managed care companies may also be effective in introducing organizational changes to the company and helping employees of the company understand the principles of managed care so they can be more knowledgeable about their work. Although administrative life may not be a good fit for many psychiatrists, an increasing number are considering employment in managed care systems in positions that require administrative responsibilities (Chapter 22). Further training in management theory would thus be helpful for the many psychiatrists who aspire to work as administrators in organized systems of care.

The Ethics of Double Agentry

I have written previously about the significant ethical challenges facing psychiatrists in the years to come (Fink 1989); this topic is discussed further in Chapter 9. The ethical struggles that psychiatrists have had as a result of managed care relate mainly to their loyalty to competing interests, namely, patients, hospitals, insurance companies, managed care organizations, and employers. What is the major obligation of psychiatrists and how do they balance all concerns? The task of being a double agent, that is, working in a corporate capacity and at the same time taking full responsibility for patient care, has been discussed extensively by Walsh (1987), Shortell (1991), and others (Lemieux-Charles et al. 1993). The task has become increasingly difficult given the limited resources and rationing strategies that make up much of health care today. Nonetheless, if psychiatrists maintain a keen sense of their roles as physicians, they will continue to pay critical attention to both the obvious and subtle needs of patients by making the best decisions for the greatest long-term gain.

Increasingly, as I conduct case conferences for residents and medical students, I find myself questioning the quality of care and the general state of our profession. The cases often involve patients who are victims of the "revolving door syndrome" that, in contemporary practice, has been imposed by managed care in the same way that it was imposed by the public sector 20 or 30 years ago.

There is, in fact, a moral obligation to provide high-quality care to patients. Cost-containment directives and other fiscal considerations challenge that obligation every day. Individuals in management positions have the extra burden of trying to balance available resources for the good of the patient and for the good of society. As treatment becomes increasingly prioritized, our moral mission may become increasingly difficult to fulfill. There is no easy solution to the ethical dilemma of being a double agent in the current health care system.

Conclusion

Managed care has fueled the debate regarding clinician substitutability and the belief that psychiatrists are irrelevant. Managed care has also intensified the competition between psychiatrists and psychologists and added to the desire of psychologists to prescribe medication and have full hospital privileges. The biopsychosocial model is undergoing tremendous upheaval in light of the managed care movement. Despite these changes, psychiatrists have an essential and continuing role in the health care system, and they are certainly not replaceable. Some psychiatrists, however, may not survive the problems that currently face them in this new practice environment. These problems relate not only to managed care but also to stigma, negativity, low pay, and ethical dilemmas.

Psychiatrists can position themselves favorably in the new health system if they keep pace with training imperatives and practice patterns demanded by managed care. But there must also be changes in the way managed care companies operate and changes in the way the public, government, and other professionals (medical and nonmedical) view psychiatry. Ideally, the following principles would guide all treatment in organized systems of care (England and Goff 1993):

- Base quality on an understanding of the needs and expectations of consumers and payers.
- Continually attend to specification of treatment for measurable improvement.
- Involve everyone in the system in improvement and reinforce the notion that everything can be improved.

Those are the challenges that face us in ensuring that psychiatrists are not replaced and that they flourish and remain vital to the American health care system.

References

Bluestone N: The bottom line. JAMA 269:2580, 1993

Brown SJ: Psychiatric group practice builds a "corridor" to better income, less risk in managed care. Clinical Psychiatry News, August 1993, pp 3, 20

DeWitt PM: The psyche market. American Demographics, September 1992, pp 62–65

England MJ, Goff VV: Health reform and organized systems of care, in Managed Mental Health Care. Edited by Goldman W, Feldman S. San Francisco, CA, Jossey-Bass, 1993, pp 5–12

English JR, Sharfstein SS, Scherl DJ, et al: Diagnosis-related groups and general hospital psychiatry. Am J Psychiatry 143:131-139, 1986

Fink PJ: You are the only sane psychiatrist I know. JAMA 251:611, 1984

Fink PJ: Presidential address: on being ethical in an unethical world. Am J Psychiatry 146:1097-1104, 1989

Fink PJ: Earning a living in psychiatry: tomorrow's picture. Psychiatric News, January 1, 1993a, p 14

Fink PJ: Psychiatrists' roles in managed care programs. Hosp Community Psychiatry 44:723–724, 1993b

Fink PJ: Adapting your practice to changes in the mental health field. Directions in Psychiatry 14 (suppl 8):1–4, 1994

Fink PJ, Tasman A (eds): Stigma and Mental Illness. Washington, DC, American Psychiatric Press, 1992

Gabbard GO, Gabbard K: Cinematic stereotypes contributing to the stigmatization of psychiatrists, in Stigma and Mental Illness. Edited by Fink PF, Tasman A. Washington, DC, American Psychiatric Press, 1992, pp 113–126

Green LA, Wood M, Becker L, et al: The ambulatory sentinel practice network: purpose, methods, and policies. J Fam Pract 18:275–280, 1984

Lazarus A: Opportunities for psychiatrists in managed care organizations. Hosp Community Psychiatry 45:1206–1210, 1994

Lemieux-Charles L, Meslin EM, Aird C, et al: Ethical issues faced by clinician/managers in resource-allocation decisions. Hosp Health Serv Adm 38:267–285, 1993

McCormick B: Managed care and medicine in "fairness" fight. Am Med News, May 9, 1994, pp 1, 34

Moran M: Psychiatrists in group practices. Psychiatric News, July 16, 1993, pp 10–11

Muran JC, Segal ZV, Samstag LW, et al: Patient pretreatment interpersonal problems and therapeutic alliance in short-term cognitive therapy. J Consult Clin Psychol 62:185–190, 1994

Panzetta AF: Whatever happened to community mental health? Hosp Community Psychiatry 36:1174–1179, 1985

Penzer WN: Clinician turned administrator: drawing upon clinical experience for managerial expertise. Administration and Policy in Mental Health 17:105–109, 1989

Pierce C: "A marriage made in hell": managed care and personality disorders. Clinical Psychiatry News, July 1994, p 7

Schreter RK: Ten trends in managed care and their impact on the biopsychosocial model. Hosp Community Psychiatry 44:325–327, 1993

Shortell SM: Effective Hospital-Physician Relationships. Ann Arbor, MI, Health Administration Press, 1991

Siegler JE, Axelband M, Isikoff J: Psychiatry: taking a leadership role in managed health care. Psychiatric Times, July 1993, p 32

Stoskopf C, Horn SD: Predicting length of stay for patients with psychoses. Health Serv Res 26:743–766, 1992

Walsh DC: Corporate Physicians: Between Medicine and Management. New Haven, CT, Yale University Press, 1987

Chapter 2

Is Private Practice Compatible With Managed Care?

Jay M. Pomerantz, M.D.
Benjamin Liptzin, M.D.
Alfred Carter, M.D.
Michael S. Perlman, M.D.

In this chapter we describe a new multidisciplinary, private practice model called a professional affiliation group (PAG). Our multidisciplinary organization of 15 PAGs has been in operation in Western Massachusetts since 1992. It offers provider-managed mental health and substance abuse treatment to 63,000 members of an independent practice association (IPA) health maintenance organization (HMO).

In the first part of the chapter, we discuss and illustrate the dynamics and role relationships within an individual PAG. In the second part we focus on the combining of PAGs to form a provider–managed care network, or what may be described as a *behavioral group practice without walls.* We offer the PAG as a model of treatment that uses managed care concepts and is readily adaptable to private practice.

Roles Within the PAG

The PAG is by definition a small group of three to eight fully licensed independently practicing mental health professionals of different disciplines. It includes at least one psychiatrist who functions as the PAG leader for reasons we will elaborate on later. Each psychologist, psychiatric social worker, psychiatric nurse, and psychiatrist maintains an office, autonomy, and full responsibility for his or her patients. Each professional bills for services independently. The PAG meets regularly, approximately every 2 weeks, to discuss problem cases, coordinate treatment, and clear up any problems with the allocation of sessions in managed care situations. Because the PAG is only advisory, legal responsibility continues to reside with the treating professional(s).

As a first principle, already alluded to above, each mental health professional maintains clinical responsibility for patients, as in solo private practice. All must arrange for 24-hour availability for their patients in emergency situations. Belonging to a PAG in no way dilutes individual clinical responsibility, nor is it a substitute for it. Clear boundaries avoid many problems (Gutheil and Gabbard 1993). While away on vacation, professionals of the same discipline may cover for one another, as is the custom in individual private practice.

Cotreatment

Once responsibility continues to be fixed on the individual professional, innovative combinations can arise. For example, medication is an increasingly useful part of modern mental health treatment. Patients need not be limited to a psychiatrist as their primary therapist to be assured of proper psychopharmacological help. Within a PAG system, a nonpsychiatrist therapist can simply request that the psychiatrist see the patient, first providing a summary of the case and possible indication for medication. Part of the mutual understanding is that the psychiatrist will make every attempt to see the patient in a timely manner. Emergency situations will get a quick response, although there is always the option of referral to an emergency department or crisis team (if one exists in the area). The advantage of regular meetings between the psychiatrist and a limited number of nonpsychiatrist primary therapists is obvious. The result is genuine cotreatment rather than isolated and fragmented medication management.

In the cotreatment situation, both the nonpsychiatrist and the psychiatrist gain from a closer working relationship than usually exists in private practice. Each comes to know the other's style of working and accommodates it. If problems emerge, there is a forum of concerned, experienced professionals who know both of them to resolve any dispute. The PAG meetings make certain that the rules for information interchange and the like are reasonable and acceptable to all. Although psychiatrists have some extra power in that they have the prescription pad and medical expertise, the psychiatrist is, by the PAG's composition, clearly outnumbered and impinged on by group pressure. The way a PAG operates in a clinical situation is illustrated by the following case example.

Case 1. Mr. A, a 64-year-old retired man, was discharged from a general hospital psychiatric unit in Florida and moved to New England. He joined an HMO shortly thereafter. The central intake of the HMO agreed to refer Mr. A to a psychologist who had previously successfully treated his niece. The patient's antidepressant medication would be monitored by the PAG psychiatrist. Indeed, within a few days of the psychologist's initial evaluation, the PAG psychiatrist saw the patient and had access to the hospital records and the psychologist's impression and treatment plan. The patient's depression occurred shortly after his wife suffered a minor stroke. The psychologist planned to work weekly with the patient, probably short-term, about health concerns. The patient appeared to be doing well; therefore, the psychiatrist continued the antidepressant at the previous dose level. A week later, the day after the second visit with the psychologist, the patient made a serious suicide attempt with a butcher knife attack on himself. He required hospitalization both for surgical treatment and subsequent psychiatric care. The case came up for discussion at the next PAG meeting, where in the presence of all six mental health professionals, the notes and impressions of both the psychologist and PAG psychiatrist were reviewed. It was striking how similar the man's presentation had been. The conclusion, by both professionals, that he was not an imminent threat to himself seemed warranted. Nor was anything in the previous hospital records predictive of the dramatic suicide attempt. Naturally, both professionals felt better after the discussion. At least they were together on the case. The PAG's conclusion, subsequently borne out by the patient, was that something new happened. It turned out that the patient had discovered his wife bleeding on urination. He panicked, felt she was bleeding to death, didn't want to face life alone, and took the knife to himself. It was an impulsive act, not something he planned.

It is entirely speculative what might have happened in a situation where medication management is more divorced from the psychotherapy. In this case, both psychiatrist and psychologist had continuing rapport. They survived a critical incident without blaming one another. The PAG as a whole faced the issue of how difficult it can be to predict patients' self-destructive actions.

In this kind of cotreatment situation, as in any situation where two professionals both see an individual patient, an untoward result such as suicide might easily result in a malpractice tort being brought against one, or more likely, both of them (Appelbaum 1991). That possibility is not increased by the existence of a PAG. In fact, the PAG arrangement might work in both professionals' favor. There was ongoing consultation and information interchange between them as there should have been for optimal treatment.

Consultation

Another role relationship that arises within a PAG is that of consultation. In this situation, any member serves as a consultant to any other. Difficult cases are reviewed by the entire PAG, which has within it expertise greater than that of any individual member.

Case 2. At a routine PAG meeting, a psychiatric social worker asked for some help with possibly medicating an 11-year-old boy who had been school phobic for 3 months. She felt that medication, or even hospitalization, was in order because all of her efforts with the mother and boy had failed. The patient would simply cry and get the teacher to send him home. Not being a child psychiatrist, the PAG psychiatrist had little to offer, but two of the PAG psychologists did treat children. One maintained a consultative role with the school in question and volunteered that the guidance counselor at the school was very adept at this kind of problem. The other psychologist suggested that the father might be of more help than the mother and that firmness and the resolve of the family and the therapist might work better than any medication. At the next PAG meeting, no one was surprised to find the boy in school without much fuss.

In this kind of situation, the psychiatric social worker benefited from the ideas and support of other PAG members. In addition, she was able to note in her records the consultative help. In the event of an untoward result, she would be in a better legal position than if she had not sought aid. The other members of the PAG are not exposed to liability for merely rendering their advice. None saw the patient or family, nor did any of them have a professional obligation toward the patient or family. The possibility of one PAG member bringing suit against another for poor advice is moot, because the advice is not binding. This is a consultative rather than a supervisory relationship among fully licensed, individual professionals. There was nothing stopping the psychiatric social worker from disregarding the PAG's advice.

The failure to appreciate the power of consultation has kept mental health professionals apart. Each jealously guards autonomy and fears supervision, the predominant modality of training. *Supervision* is an infantilizing term for the supervisee, and it carries legal peril for the supervisors, who become liable for a treatment they are not giving (Woodward et al. 1993). The consultative model we employ differentiates our program from other previous attempts at interdisciplinary coordination of outpatient treatment (Burt et al. 1992). Hierarchical groupings also risk mashing together techniques or what Leston Havens (1973) termed "homogeniz[ing] complexities" (p. 330). Experienced therapists function best on their own, not when they are obliged to apply unfamiliar therapeutic strategies at the behest of a supervisor.

Coordination

Individual patients are often not the only members of their family with problems. Many times the spouse and one or more children are in treatment with other therapists. Sometimes, one or more of them has a psychiatrist prescribing medication and another professional doing the psychotherapy. These multiproblem families are sometimes best treated together in family therapy but at other times are best treated separately. Yet, if there is no coordination between the various therapists, there is great potential for working at cross purposes. Obviously, each patient must sign a permission form for the therapists to coordinate care. It is also our experience that an ongoing conversation between therapists who know and trust one another, as in a PAG, works best. We illustrate this with the following example.

Case 3. Mrs. B is a 29-year-old married mother of two children, ages 4 and 1. She suffered a severe postpartum depression after delivering the youngest child. Shortly after the delivery, she was transferred to the psychiatric inpatient unit where she was eventually treated with ECT (electroconvulsive therapy) for a psychotic depression and incapacitating obsessive-compulsive behavior. She chose to continue with her previous therapist, a psychologist, after discharge from the hospital. Because she had to continue her antidepressant medication, the PAG psychiatrist was brought into the case. The 4-year-old son was also in treatment; he was being treated by with another psychologist who specializes in child work. The psychiatrist knew less about this patient than either of the other treating professionals but heeded their advice about not lowering the woman's medication (she was distressed about weight gain from clomipramine) because of a clear description from each therapist about Mrs. B's capacity for denial. The 4-year-old was completely out of control in the psychologist's office. Mrs. B seemed, even on medication, too preoccupied with her daily rituals to set limits. Instead of less medication, the situation called for continuing the present dose or increasing it. If the situation did not improve, a family meeting including the husband (whom no one knew) might be in order. It was helpful that the various treating professionals worked together in a PAG within a self-managed system. In another system, the attempt to explain the situation to a distant case manager would entail countless phone calls, no doubt resulting in confusion and, most likely, inappropriate care.

Cost-Effectiveness

The third area of relationship between members of a PAG involves managing care so that it is cost-effective. The system we have instituted requires the PAG psychiatrist to become the coordinator of the effort to control costs. Every new patient in the system gets approval on the telephone for up to five visits for evaluation or short-term treatment or both. If the patient and therapist feel additional sessions are necessary, the therapist obtains the patient's written permission to fill out a treatment plan form requesting additional sessions. The therapist follows a systemwide protocol (based on multiple parameters including diagnosis, global assessment of functioning, possibility of harm to self or others, presence and severity of substance abuse, and likelihood of imminent psychiatric hospitalization) to request the appropriate number of additional sessions. If the psychiatrist agrees that the treatment form complies with the protocol, the psychiatrist signs off on the request. There is no additional review. In the unusual situation in which there is a disagreement about the appropriateness of the request for a given number of sessions, the matter is taken up at the next meeting of the PAG. A further possibility is for another member of the PAG, usually the psychiatrist, to personally see the patient to evaluate the case. In actual practice, the more difficult cases requiring extensive treatment are already known to the psychiatrist in the role of medication prescriber. This dual responsibility of the psychiatrist, as manager of treatment allocation and potential or actual clinical cotreater, makes for responsible decision making. With the possibility of an interview by another PAG professional at any time, there is no room for the exaggeration of the patient's difficulty on the part of the primary therapist. So, too, there is little room for the denial of needed treatment when the patient may then fall apart, requiring the same psychiatrist to take on cotreatment and legal responsibility. Furthermore, the discussion about the appropriateness of a request for additional sessions takes place in person, among practicing clinicians, with no one benefiting from the arbitrary denial of care. Still, budgets do have to be met, so there is motivation for all the PAG members to be cost-effective. The details of the overall financial arrangements for a PAG network can vary widely, and we will elaborate on them in the second part of this chapter. We subscribe to the ethical rule of thumb proposed by Sabin (1989, p. 11): "If a clinician is not prepared to describe the terms under which he is treating the patient, including financial incentives and restrictions on referrals, the system in which he is working is not ethical."

There is some potential liability for the PAG psychiatrist in this role of allocator of treatment resources not dissimilar from that of the case manager for an insurance company or managed care carve-out (Sederer 1992). The likelihood of problems is far less in a PAG system because of the close collaboration and final agreement between the PAG psychiatrist and therapist. It is basically a nonadversarial system, in contrast with many managed care situations. Still, we would advise insurance coverage for this essentially administrative duty. That coverage can usually be obtained free of charge by the inclusion of all PAG psychiatrists in the administrative liability policy maintained by any organization that a PAG system would contract with. For example, in the situation of a PAG network operating within an IPA/HMO, coverage is obtained by including the PAG psychiatrists in the patient care assessment committee, thereby covering the PAG psychiatrists for any suits brought against them in their role as managers of the session allocation process. It is quite appropriate in our view to have "medical necessity" determined in each case by the patient's therapist and confirmed by a physician specialist in that area. That is in marked contrast with the usual arrangements in managed care companies.

Although the administrative role of the PAG psychiatrist in approving treatment plans requesting further sessions is a potential source of conflict, we have found that this method is so superior to existing managed care that everyone is quite happy with it. The trade-off for the nonpsychiatrists is that they have a colleague, available in crises with difficult patients, able to skillfully prescribe psychotropic medication. Further support and dispute resolution are available from the PAG as a whole. For psychiatrists there is a new role, cotreatment rather than traditional medication management. They also retain their own psychotherapy cases and avoid the hassle of distant managed care companies controlling their every action. The arrangements may also include, as we have, a contingent management fee for the PAG psychiatrist. The other mental health professionals also receive contingent compensation for the time spent at PAG meetings. We may be the only managed care organization paying treating professionals for the considerable time spent justifying utilization. This money is available because there are no management company profits to pay, no toll-free numbers to maintain, and no outside case managers to support.

Combining PAGs for a Network

The strength of the PAG concept comes into its own when a number of PAGs combine to form a network or what is termed a behavioral group practice without walls. The arrangement in our existing network, formed to manage the mental health and substance abuse care for an IPA/HMO, has been described elsewhere (Pomerantz et al. 1994). The mental health component of the HMO (Health New England) was reconfigured so that its

100 outpatient providers were divided into 15 PAGs, each coordinated by a managing psychiatrist. All the providers continued on a fee-for-service basis, but the entire program, including the affiliated inpatient units, was joined by a common target budget. There was a 15% withhold deducted from all payments and held in reserve against any potential cost overrun for the year. A limited contingent management fee was available if the program came in under budget. The program is now in its third year of operation and by all measures is extremely successful. It has always come in under the target budget, received a 94% satisfaction rating from patients on an anonymous survey, and won the allegiance of all providers.

This kind of arrangement might be summarized as modified group capitation. Each individual provider is allocated a portion of the total budget by a fee-for-service calculation. This arrangement balances out the desire for individual providers to maximize their income by providing treatment services against the constraints of an overall mental health–substance abuse budget limit. There is continuing oversight by peers and, in particular, the PAG psychiatrist. Each provider periodically receives a printout of his or her statistics vis-à-vis all other providers in the system. The number of patients seen, number of visits per patient, and average cost per patient during the time period are all spelled out. Everyone knows that the return of the sizable withhold depends on meeting the target budget. Also, any management fees are contingent on total expenditures coming in under the target budget. Every provider in the system is both at risk for cost overruns and, to a certain extent, rewarded for cost-effective care. The contingent management fee is capped at 50 cents per member per month and divided up by a complicated formula. The net effect is a balance of forces. Medical necessity drives care, rather than economics. The criteria for medical necessity, both for inpatient and outpatient services, are written down and freely available to all providers in the system. Periodic systemwide meetings supplement PAG meetings for the discussion of administrative issues.

Another way of looking at our current structure is to call it a "virtual" behavioral group practice (Pomerantz et al. 1995). The lack of a corporate entity (with a single tax identification number and centralized billing) is by design and has certain advantages. The arrangement is transparent to patients. It limits professional and legal responsibility to the treating mental health professional(s). Billing and copayment collection proceed in an efficient and personal way, resulting in less overhead and fewer complaints; hospitals and clinics can participate along with private practitioners; and the network is easy to form and does not require capital or entrepreneurial skills.

The downside to the system is that it is different. Purchasing organizations expect to deal with a formal organization. Although there is disadvantage in the current marketplace for an amorphous organization such as ours, it is clearly too early to predict what lies ahead. We may have developed the prototype of a flexible, coordinated, individual practitioner network, or the PAG system may represent a transitional stage along the way to a large incorporated group practice (see, for example, Lazarus 1995). Other scenarios are also possible.

The arrangement currently in vogue is physician-hospital organizations (PHOs). This type of arrangement contracts for the total health care needs of a population by offering a complete package at a fixed price, or capitation. Alternatively, it can work out arrangements for fee-for-service with some risk sharing on the part of the PHO. The opportunity is clearly there for a PAG network to work within such a PHO. An offer of local, organized, multidisciplinary treatment for a fixed fee is an attractive alternative to distant managed care companies. The local mental health professionals can offer as low a price as anyone else, but they might advocate for a more complete package of services costing perhaps a bit more. The issue should be quality, not just price. Satisfied and healthier patients may cost a medical plan less in the long run. This "medical offset" argument is real (Chapter 15), but it may need special intervention strategies and better measurement before it is generally accepted. For example, a PAG model might conceivably include primary care physicians in the mental health PAGs. In short, the carve-out is an invitation to divided and diffuse responsibility, whereas a PAG system for mental health treatment fits well with the PHO concept of total, integrated, coordinated care.

There will be other arrangements as well. Recently, a statewide group of psychiatrists incorporated to form a preferred provider organization. Such a group would be well advised to adopt a multidisciplinary PAG-type model if it is to sell its services to large employers or insurance companies. The marketplace tells us that not all patients require or accept going to a psychiatrist. It is also quite obvious that costs will be lower in any organization that can use relatively low-cost providers as well as high-priced ones (when the clinical situation permits such flexibility). The PAG model safely extends cost-effective multidisciplinary outpatient treatment even to patients requiring medication and allows close collaboration between the psychiatrist and primary psychotherapist.

In addition, by working together at the clinical level, political turf battles may subside. We may see the end of attempts by psychologists to legislate a right to prescribe medication or psychiatrists giving and interpreting projective tests. This fractionation of the field may have invited the mental health carve-out phenomenon. The mental health managed care companies, to their credit, do apportion care among the specialties and force collaboration when necessary.

PAGs can be a useful idea even in the absence of a network. At a minimum, a single PAG (or several PAGs) can join an outside managed care company as a group. The advantages of cotreatment, consultation, coordination, and availability to new patients continue in any context.

Conclusion

Many experts have predicted the demise of private mental health practice because of the rise of managed care. On the contrary, we believe that managed care will revitalize solo practice and that the PAG—a behavioral group practice without walls--will emerge as a viable model of interdisciplinary mental health care delivery in the managed care era. Although other treatment models will likely operate and even compete with the PAG within a managed care framework, we view the PAG as possibly the most contemporary and cost-effective form of private practice.

References

Appelbaum PS: General guidelines for psychiatrists who prescribe medication for patients treated by nonmedical psychotherapists. Hosp Community Psychiatry 42:281–282, 1991

Burt VK, Summit P, Yager J: Outpatient management teams. Acad Psychiatry 16:24–28, 1992

Gutheil TG, Gabbard GO: The concept of boundaries in clinical practice: theoretical and risk-management dimensions. Am J Psychiatry 150:188–196, 1993

Havens LL: Approaches to the Mind: Movement of the Psychiatric Schools from Sects Toward Science. Boston, MA, Little Brown, 1973

Lazarus A: A business plan for starting a behavioral group practice. Behavioral Healthcare Tomorrow 4(4):29–32, 1995

Pomerantz JM, Liptzin B, Carter AH, et al: The professional affiliation group: a new model for managed mental health care. Hosp Community Psychiatry 45:308–310, 1994

Pomerantz JM, Liptzin B, Carter A, et al: Development and management of a "virtual" group practice: behavioral clinicians and organizations linked by a capitation contract with an HMO. Psychiatric Annals 25:504–508, 1995

Sabin JE: Psychiatrists face tough ethical questions in managed care settings. Psychiatric Times, September 1989, pp 10–12

Sederer LI: Judicial and legislative responses to cost containment. Am J Psychiatry 149:1157–1161, 1992

Woodward B, Duckworth KS, Gutheil TG: The pharmacotherapist-psychotherapist collaboration, in American Psychiatric Press Review of Psychiatry, Vol 12. Edited by Oldham JM, Riba MB, Tasman A. Washington, DC, American Psychiatric Press, 1993, pp 631–649

Chapter 3

What Is the Role of the Primary Care Physician in Managed Mental Health Care?

David S. Brody, M.D.

Primary care physicians are important providers of mental health care. An estimated 25% of the patients they see have one or more diagnosable mental disorders (Barrett et al. 1988; Hoeper et al. 1979; Kessler et al. 1987; Von Korff et al. 1987), and another 13% appear to have subthreshold mental disorders (Spitzer 1995). In fact, more than 50% of patients with mental health problems are seen only in the general medical sector (Kamerow et al. 1986; Regier et al. 1978; Shapiro et al. 1984), and there are more visits to primary care physicians for psychotropic medications than there are to psychiatrists (Beardsley et al. 1988).

In the medical setting, mental disorders have a substantial impact on mortality, morbidity, dysfunction, and the use of health care services (Frasure-Smith et al. 1993; Houpt et al. 1980; Katon and Sullivan 1990; Ladwig et al. 1994; Rodin and Voshart 1987; Wells et al. 1989). It has been shown that patients with mental disorders receive twice as much general health care as those without these disorders (Hankin et al. 1982; Houpt et al. 1980). Proper treatment of their mental disorders appears to reduce the use of health care services by these patients (Borus et al. 1985; Mumford et al. 1984).

Unfortunately, it has been well documented that primary care physicians frequently fail to recognize the presence of common mental disorders such as anxiety and depression among their patients (Brody 1980; Goldberg et al. 1982; Jencks 1985; Schulberg et al. 1985). Even when these disorders are identified accurately, primary care physicians appear to use counseling techniques less often than would be beneficial (Johnson 1973; Shepherd 1973) and often use psychotropic medications inappropriately (Johnson 1974; Kamerow et al. 1986; Schurman et al. 1985).

On the basis of this data, it is clear that although mental disorders are common and important problems in the primary care setting, primary care physicians have not demonstrated that they are consistently able to recognize and appropriately manage these problems.

Thus, it is not surprising that there is great variability in the extent to which individual primary care physicians participate in the mental health care of their patients. Although some physicians feel quite comfortable counseling patients and prescribing a variety of psychotropic medications, other primary care physicians see their role as being limited to recognizing patients who might have a mental disorder and referring them to a mental health specialist (Orleans et al. 1985). The challenge for managed care is to develop a system or systems of mental health care that effectively integrate primary care physicians and mental health specialists.

Potential Roles of Primary Care Physicians

Within that system there are a variety of roles that primary care physicians might play. They might be involved in identifying patients with symptoms suggestive of a mental disorder, evaluating those symptoms, and establishing a diagnosis. Primary care physicians might be involved in educating patients about their mental disorders and negotiating how they will be managed. They might be involved in managing the mental disorder either as the primary provider or in a more supportive role. They might also be involved in monitoring the outcomes of care by periodically evaluating the patient's clinical status and identifying relapses and recurrences. Finally, primary care physicians might be involved in efforts to prevent mental disorders.

Managed care systems will have to decide which of these roles they wish to encourage primary care physicians to play. In arriving at these decisions, it is important to recognize the unique opportunities as well as the barriers that affect the ability of primary care physicians to provide effective mental health care. On the positive side, the continuity of care that exists in the primary care setting affords primary care physicians the opportunity to establish therapeutic relationships with their patients over time. The trust and confidence that develop within the context of that relationship enable primary care physicians to effectively influence patient behavior. For example, most studies have shown that when primary care physicians simply communicate a smoking cessation message to patients, about 5% of patients will quit (Russel et al. 1979; Stewart and Rosser 1982; Wilson et al. 1982). It is important to realize that the overall effect the primary care physicians have is actually much greater because they generally have multiple opportunities to help modify perceptions and behaviors as they follow their patients over time.

The long-term continuous relationship that characterizes primary care also makes primary care physicians ideally situated to monitor the clinical course of their patients' mental disorders and identify patients who have relapsed or experienced recurrences, thereby facilitating earlier interventions for symptomatic patients.

Primary care physicians are also well situated to reassure patients who manifest their emotional distress by complaining of somatic symptoms, as well as patients whose mental health symptoms are caused or exacerbated by concerns about their physical well-being. These patients may be experiencing subthreshold or mild mental disorders primarily on the basis of their concerns about their illness. Reducing those concerns has been shown to alleviate symptoms of emotional distress and possibly prevent a more full-blown mental disorder (Brody et al. 1991).

Finally, it must be realized that some patients will prefer to have their mental disorders treated by their primary care physicians (Orleans et al. 1985). This preference may result from either the confidence they have in their primary care physician or the concerns they have about being treated by mental health specialists. It may also be caused by financial considerations because patients may be less likely to have insurance coverage for services provided by mental health specialists than for services provided by primary care physicians.

Barriers to Treatment

On the negative side, there are numerous barriers to effective mental health care by primary care physicians that must be overcome. These barriers relate to the primary care physicians themselves, to their patients, and to the system in which the care takes place.

Many primary care physicians lack sufficient knowledge and skills to effectively care for patients with mental disorders. In part, these deficiencies result from a lack of training, and in part they reflect the absence of well-defined management strategies and interventions that can be realistically and effectively provided by primary care physicians. There has been a tendency to focus primary care physicians' training in the management of mental disorders almost exclusively on the development of skills (e.g., interviewing skills, communication skills) without specifically delineating how and when these skills should be applied. That strategy has created an impression that managing mental disorders is an art form—a process that is inconsistent with the way primary care physicians are taught to manage other types of medical disorders.

In addition to deficits in knowledge and skills, the attitudes of some primary care physicians regarding mental disorders and their management may be a barrier to overcome. These practitioners may perceive mental health problems as irrelevant to their objectives for the medical visit or as being beyond their capacity to address effectively. When a patient with a potential mental health problem is encountered in the medical setting, the physician may consider some or all of the following questions: 1) How important is it for me to address this mental health problem? 2) Is there something I can reasonably do for the patient with this problem? 3) How effective is the care I can provide likely to be? If the physician does not perceive the mental problem to be significant or if he or she feels incapable of contributing to effective management, the problem will likely be ignored.

Primary care patients with mental disorders present unique challenges. These patients will commonly have somatic symptoms rather than symptoms that are more specific to their mental disorder (Zung et al. 1993). Once the mental disorder has been identified and diagnosed, they may be reluctant to accept the diagnosis and the physician's treatment recommendations. This reluctance may result from concerns about the meaning of the disorder (e.g., I must be crazy), the cause of the disorder (e.g., I am weak and not capable of dealing with my problems), the treatment of the disorder (e.g., it will last a long time, be embarrassing, and be very expensive), and the prognosis of the disorder (e.g., it will not get better). Those types of concerns are generally less common among patients who see mental health specialists than they are among primary care patients with mental disorders.

In addition to physician- and patient-related barriers to good care, the system in which the care takes place may not facilitate optimal mental health care. Most managed care systems make it difficult for primary care physicians to provide mental health care simply because of time constraints. Primary care physicians are expected to see large numbers of patients, especially when they function as gatekeepers, and they are therefore able to devote only 10 to 15 minutes for a typical office visit. If they spend more time counseling a depressed patient, they are not likely to receive additional compensation. Some fee-for-service insurance companies do not provide any reimbursement to primary care physicians for mental health care.

Managed health care systems may also impede access to mental health specialists by requiring that patients first obtain a mental health referral from their primary care physician. That approach places an additional obstacle in the path of obtaining mental health services, especially emergency services (Lazarus 1993); some patients may feel uncomfortable revealing their perceived frailties to physicians on whom they depend for their general medical care. Although the approach can increase primary care physicians' awareness of their patients' mental disorders, this information can also be provided through better communication from the mental health specialists to these primary care physicians.

Improving Primary Care Physicians' Mental Health Skills

Primary care physicians' role in managed mental health care in large part will depend on how the treatment barriers are addressed. A variety of approaches have been used to train primary care physicians to provide more effective mental health care. These approaches have usually focused on developing certain skills, such as interviewing or communication skills. Although it has been shown that these approaches can improve the short-term performance of the desired skills, there are few data indicating that the approaches actually improve long-term outcomes (Brody and Larson 1992). Teaching these types of skills to primary care physicians may, therefore, not be sufficient to consistently improve the care and outcomes of primary care patients with mental disorders.

Clear guidelines for identifying, evaluating, diagnosing, and managing primary care patients with mental disorders are also needed, and these guidelines must be specific to the primary care setting, relatively easy to learn, and feasible to implement within the time constraints of primary care. Guidelines for the detection, diagnosis, and treatment of depression by primary care physicians have recently been developed by the Agency for Health Care Policy and Research (Depression Guideline Panel 1993a and 1993b). Although these guidelines have generated considerable controversy (Munoz et al. 1994), the process used to develop them should serve as a model for other mental disorders commonly encountered in primary care settings.

Strategies are needed to help implement the guidelines when the primary care physician encounters a patient with a mental disorder. Several recently developed approaches could be of great benefit in this regard. The identification and diagnosis of mental disorder could be facilitated by a system such as PRIME-MD (Spitzer 1995). This system, which consists of a self-administered screening questionnaire for patients, a Clinician Evaluation Guide (CEG), and an instruction manual, enables primary care physicians to identify and diagnose patients with the following five types of mental disorders: 1) mood disorders, 2) anxiety disorders, 3) eating disorders, 4) somatoform disorders, and 5) alcohol abuse. Patients complete the questionnaire before seeing their physician. The CEG, a structured interview with decision rules for arriving at diagnoses consistent with DSM-IV (American Psychiatric Association 1994), is used to follow up on positive responses to the screening questionnaire. PRIME-MD is being modified so that it will be consistent with DSM-IV criteria.

PRIME-MD has been tested in 1,000 patients seen in four primary care sites. Spitzer and colleagues (1995) found that primary care physicians using PRIME-MD were able to diagnose at least one mental disorder in 39% of these patients. There was good agreement between primary care physicians' diagnoses using PRIME-MD and the blended diagnoses of a mental health professional. The CEG takes about 8–10 minutes to administer.

The further evaluation of patients with mental disorders can be facilitated by a self-administered feedback questionnaire completed by patients before their medical visit. A recent study evaluated the effect of providing medical residents with feedback on the following: 1) the presence of a mental health problem, 2) the impact of this problem on patient functioning, 3) the situational sources of the problem, 4) the patient's desire for help with the problem, and 5) the specific types of mental health interventions the patient desires (Brody et al. 1990). When compared with control patients who completed the same set of questionnaires , patients seen by physicians who had received this feedback reported that they were more satisfied with their physicians and that the counseling they had received from the physician was more effective. Patients in the feedback group also reported greater decreases in the amount of overall stress experienced and greater increases in their perceived control over this stress after the medical visit when compared with control group patients, whose physicians did not receive the feedback.

The management of mental disorders may be facilitated when a psychiatrist provides specific management guidelines to primary care physicians after a consultation. In a study of patients with somatoform disorders, Smith and associates (1986) compared the efficacy of treatment provided by primary care physicians who had received management guidelines following a psychiatric consultation with treatment provided by practitioners who did not receive guidelines after a psychiatric consultation. The use of management guidelines was associated with a 53% reduction in average quarterly total health care charges but did not produce significant changes in functional health status or patient satisfaction.

Integrating Mental Health Providers Into the Primary Care Setting

Improving the link between mental health specialists and primary care physicians can also facilitate the identification, evaluation, and management of primary care patients with mental disorders. Integrating mental health specialists into primary care practices can reduce the physician- and patient-related barriers to consultation. It can improve communication and ultimately lead to more effective collaboration between primary care physicians and mental health specialists (Strathdee 1987). In this collaboration, the mental health specialist's role could range from simply providing advice and guidance to primary care physicians (who would be the direct providers of mental health care) to being primarily responsible for identifying and managing patients with mental disorders at the primary care site. The most common and probably most effective models of collaboration are ones in which primary care physicians identify and refer patients with mental disorders to mental health specialists. The specialists perform a consultation and then either advise the primary care physician about how to manage the patient or provide treatment themselves, in which case primary care physicians play a more supportive role. In the latter model, the mental health specialist typically might assume primary responsibility for the management of the mental disorder during the acute phase and then gradually shift more responsibility to the primary care physician for continuing care and long-term follow-up.

The opportunity to work in a collaborative relationship with a mental health specialist should improve primary care physicians' ability to diagnose and manage mental disorders. It is therefore likely that over time primary care physicians who work in an integrated system will be capable of assuming more responsibility for the management of mental disorders.

Organizational Challenges

The design and operation of managed care programs may have a significant effect on the way primary care physicians are used in mental health treatment. For example, in carve-out programs, in which behavioral treatment is segregated from medical treatment, it is often more difficult to achieve integration and continuity of care (Blackwell 1994). On the other hand, most managed care programs employ gatekeeping mechanisms, thereby tethering primary care physicians to mental health providers through referral and feedback loops.

Managed care programs, like community mental health centers, encourage the treatment of patients by psychiatrists and psychotherapists working as a team. This type of shared arrangement has occasionally been a source of confusion for primary care physicians in terms of referral lines and lines of clinical accountability. Which clinician should primary care physicians designate as the *point person* for mental health treatment—the psychiatrist or the psychologist? Lazarus (1995) made several useful suggestions for primary care physicians who are confronted with that dilemma. Optimal practice will require that all providers cooperate with each other and openly discuss their roles and responsibilities in patient care, including on-call scheduling, emergency coverage, and clinical supervision.

Reimbursement policies may be an important factor in determining primary care physicians' willingness to evaluate and manage mental disorders. Primary care physicians generally devote little time to that aspect of care. If they are expected to spend considerably more time identifying and managing mental disorders, their compensation should be adjusted to reflect this effort. The adjustment can be made through increasing capitation rates or through separate fee-for-service payments. Before it can be done, however, a system of quality assurance must be developed to ensure that the care being provided and reimbursed is truly effective. The essential components of a quality assurance system should include an evaluation of the primary care physician's ability to detect patients with mental disorders, the type of treatments the physicians provide, and the effectiveness of those treatments.

Conclusion

It is clear that mental disorders are commonly seen in the primary are setting and that these disorders contribute not only to morbidity and dysfunction but also to excessive use of health care services. Unfortunately, primary care physicians have thus far not been very successful in diagnosing and treating these problems. Consequently, their role in the management of mental disorders has not been well defined. A variety of barriers must be overcome if primary care physicians are to be more successfully integrated into the mental health care process. Guidelines for the identification, evaluation, and treatment of specific types of mental disorders that are most frequently seen in primary care settings should be developed. The guidelines must be feasible given the limited training and available time of primary care physicians.

In this chapter, I described several tools and techniques that have been developed to facilitate the identification and management of mental disorders by primary care physicians. Neither these methods nor practice guidelines will effectively improve mental health care unless the system of care is also modified. The system must create greater links between primary care physicians and mental health specialists, perhaps by locating these two types of providers in the same office. Primary care physicians must be adequately compensated for the mental health care they provide, and systems of quality assurance must be developed to monitor the effectiveness of their care and provide them with feedback on their performance.

References

American Psychiatric Association: Diagnostic and Statistical Manual of Mental Disorders, 4th Edition. Washington, DC, American Psychiatric Association, 1994

Barrett JE, Barrett JA, Oxman TE, et al: The prevalence of psychiatric disorders in a primary care practice. Arch Gen Psychiatry 45:1100–1106, 1988

Beardsley RS, Gardocki GJ, Larson DB, et al: Prescribing of psychotropic medication by primary care physicians and psychiatrists. Arch Gen Psychiatry 45:1117–1119, 1988

Blackwell B: No margin, no mission. JAMA 271:1466, 1994

Borus JF, Olendzki MC, Kessler L, et al: The "offset effect" of mental health treatment on ambulatory medical care utilization and charges. Arch Gen Psychiatry 42:573–580, 1985

Brody DS: Physician recognition of behavioral, psychological, and social aspects of medical care. Arch Intern Med 140:1286–1289, 1980

Brody DS, Larson DB: The role of primary care physicians in managing depression. J Gen Intern Med 7:243–247, 1992

Brody DS, Lerman CE, Wolfson HG, et al: Improvement in physicians' counseling of patients with mental health problems. Arch Intern Med 150:993–998, 1990

Brody DS, Miller SM, Caputo GC: Patient attitudes and recovery from mental health disorders. Presented at the Fifth Annual NIMH International Research Conference on the Classification, Recognition and Treatment of Mental Disorders in General Medical Settings, Bethesda, MD, September 1991

Depression Guideline Panel: Depression in Primary Care, Vol 1: Detection and Diagnosis (AHCPR Publ No 93-0550). Rockville, MD, U.S. Department of Health and Human Services, Agency for Health Care Policy and Research, April 1993a

Depression Guideline Panel: Depression in Primary Care, Vol 2: Treatment of Major Depression (AHCPR Publ No 93-0551). Rockville, MD, U.S. Department of Health and Human Services, Agency for Health Care Policy and Research, April 1993b

Frasure-Smith N, Lesperance F, Talajic M: Depression following myocardial infarction: impact on 6-month survival. JAMA 271:1819–1825, 1993

Goldberg D, Steele JJ, Johnson A, et al: Ability of primary care physicians to make accurate ratings of psychiatric symptoms. Arch Gen Psychiatry 39:829–833, 1982

Hankin J, Steinwachs DM, Regier DA, et al: Use of general medical care services by persons with mental disorders. Arch Gen Psychiatry 39:225–231, 1982

Hoeper EW, Nycz GR, Turner RW, et al: Estimated prevalence of RDC mental disorder in primary medical care. International Journal of Mental Health 8:6–15, 1979

Houpt JL, Orleans CS, George LK, et al: The role of psychiatric and behavioral factors in the practice of medicine. Am J Psychiatry 137:37–47, 1980

Jencks SF: Recognition of mental distress and diagnosis of mental disorder in primary care. JAMA 253:1903–1907, 1985

Johnson DAW: Treatment of depression in general practice. Br Med J 2:18–20, 1973

Johnson DAW: A study of the use of antidepressant medication in general practices. Br J Psychiatry 125:186–192, 1974

Kamerow DB, Pincus HA, Macdonald DI: Alcohol abuse, other drug abuse, and mental disorders in medical practice: prevalence, costs, recognition, and treatment. JAMA 255:2054–2057, 1986.

Katon W, Sullivan MD: Depression and chronic medical illness. J Clin Psychiatry 51 (suppl 6):3–11, 1990

Kessler LG, Burns BJ, Shapiro S, et al: Psychiatric diagnoses of medical service users: evidence from the Epidemiological Catchment Area Program. Am J Public Health 77:18–24, 1987

Ladwig KH, Roll G, Breithardt G, et al: Post-infarction depression and incomplete recovery 6 months after acute myocardial infarction. Lancet 343:20–23, 1994

Lazarus A: Managed competition and access to emergency psychiatric care. Hosp Community Psychiatry 44:1134–1136, 1993

Lazarus A: The role of primary care physicians in managed mental health care. Psychiatric Services 46:343–345, 1995

Mumford E, Schlesinger HJ, Glass GV, et al: A new look at evidence about reduced cost of medical utilization following mental health treatment. Am J Psychiatry 141:1145–1156, 1984

Munoz RF, Hollon SD, McGrath E, et al: On the AHCPR Depression in Primary Care guidelines: further considerations for practitioners. Am Psychol 49:42–61, 1994

Orleans CT, George LK, Houpt JL, et al: How primary care physicians treat psychiatric disorders: a national survey of family practitioners. Am J Psychiatry 142:52–57, 1985

Regier DA, Goldberg ID, Taube CA, et al: The de facto US mental health services system. Arch Gen Psychiatry 35:685–693, 1978

Rodin G, Voshart K: Depressive symptoms and functional impairment in the medically ill. Gen Hosp Psychiatry 9:251–258, 1987

Russel MAH, Wilson C, Taylor C, et al: Effect of general practitioners' advice against smoking. Br Med J 2:231–234, 1979

Schulberg H, Saul M, McClelland M, et al: Assessing depression in primary medical and psychiatric practices. Arch Gen Psychiatry 42:1164–1170, 1985

Schurman RA, Kramer PD, Mitchell JB: The hidden mental health network. Arch Gen Psychiatry 42:89–94, 1985

Shapiro S, Skinner EA, Kessler LG, et al: Utilization of health and mental health services. Arch Gen Psychiatry 41:971–978, 1984

Shepherd M: The general practice research unit at the Institute of Psychiatry. Psychol Med 3:525–529, 1973

Smith GR, Monson RA, Ray DC: Psychiatric consultation in somatization disorder: a randomized controlled study. N Engl J Med 314:1407–1413, 1986

Spitzer RL, Williams JBW, Kroenke K, et al: Utility of a new procedure for diagnosing mental disorders in primary care: the PRIME-MD 1000 study. JAMA 272:1749–1756, 1995

Stewart PJ, Rosser WW: The impact of routine advice on smoking cessation from family physicians. Can Med Assoc J 126:1051–1054, 1982

Strathdee G: Primary care–psychiatry interaction: a British perspective. Gen Hosp Psychiatry 9:102–110, 1987

Von Korff M, Shapiro S, Burke JD, et al: Anxiety and depression in a primary care clinic: comparison of Diagnostic Interview Schedule, General Health Questionnaire, and practitioner assessments. Arch Gen Psychiatry 44:152–156, 1987

Wells KB, Stewart A, Hays RD, et al: The functioning and well-being of depressed patients: results from the Medical Outcomes Study. JAMA 262:914–919, 1989

Wilson D, Wood G, Johnston N, et al: Randomized clinical trial of supportive follow-up for cigarette smokers in a family practice. Can Med Assoc J 126:127–129, 1982

Zung WWK, Broadhead WE, Roth ME: Prevalence of depressive symptoms in primary care. J Fam Practi 37:337–344, 1993

Chapter 4

Are Practice Guidelines Useful in Managed Care?

William Hetznecker, M.D.

Large social movements often induce significant changes in small social systems such as medical care, gender relationships, buyer-seller transactions, and the use of resources. At least two major movements have fueled health care reform: consumerism in all its forms and the dawning realization across all segments of society that resources of every kind are limited.

Health care has been scrutinized primarily because of spiraling costs related to medical treatment in the 1970s and 1980s. The rapid escalation of costs related to health care spending has, in fact, threatened the economic balance and well-being of United States citizens.

Managed care in its various permutations has become a significant mechanism to reduce the cost of medical treatment. *Managed care* is a term applied to a range of financial, administrative, oversight, and monitoring activities and to the delivery of clinical services. All activities are designed to influence the behavior of consumers, providers, and payers of health care services to obtain a balance between two general purposes: containment or reduction of health care costs and promotion and maintenance of high-quality care. The activities employed to accomplish these goals include, but are not limited to, reducing, restructuring, or restricting health benefits; increasing consumer financial responsibility—by requiring co-payments, for example; utilization review; case management; preferred provider or exclusive provider contracting; increasing patient enrollment in health maintenance organizations (HMOs); establishing self-insurance programs for large businesses; and instituting quality improvement programs.

Focus on Quality

Both cost control devices and quality improvement mechanisms will shape future medical delivery and educational policies relevant to the training of health care workers. Quality as a central concern in the delivery of health care is part of a larger movement spreading from the production to the service sectors. *Quality assurance, continuing quality improvement*, and *total quality improvement* are terms used to characterize practices and procedures based largely on the Deming (1986) method of management. Quality improvement initiatives have been implemented with varying degrees of intensity and systematization. The longer-term results of these efforts are yet to be measured. Payers who are interested in quality have usually expressed their concerns in more muted, reverential terms compared with the language of cost-containment.

Concerns about quality in health care do not begin with managed care. Medical and health educators, editors of professional journals, and scientific investigators have espoused and promoted quality as a perjuring goal. The belief that accurate information in the form of scientific results will improve the quality of medical practice has been an essential tenet of the health care field. The unanswered question regarding this belief is whether quality can be scientifically validated. Attempts to define and measure the quality of specific interventions promise to be a major focus of managed care activities.

Another development influencing the attainment of quality is the consumer movement. Patients are no longer merely passive recipients of diagnostic tests and treatment interventions. They have become proactive and now demand answers to basic questions. Do my doctors know what they are doing? Are they providing state-of-the-art care for my condition? As a result of attempting to answer questions like those, practice guidelines have been created and have come center stage. Society is asking physicians to "take off your clothes and expose yourself so that I (patient/payer) can examine you." Stated less metaphorically: "Doctor, please make explicit the thinking that guides your judgment in arriving at your diagnosis and treatment. Please demonstrate to me whether your conclusions are supported by contemporary research and the informed judgment of your peers."

One of the goals of practice guidelines is to establish rational and systematic approaches to the diagnosis and treatment of specific disorders. Practice guidelines tend to set explicit (not rigid) boundaries on treatment variation as exemplified in phrases like *practicing quality medicine* and *delivering quality care*. Practice guidelines, however, are only one of a set of requirements for achieving quality care. Another important dimension of quality is related to interpersonal skills. Because practice guidelines are primarily cognitive in nature, their implementation may be influenced by stylistic differences between physicians and differences in the communication abilities of physicians.

In this chapter, I use the term *practice guideline* to connote an indication or outline of policy and conduct. I use the word *criteria* in reference to the propositions of utilization review organizations and other types of managed care firms. The word *algorithm* is used when describing the technique of applying a decision tree to graphically demonstrate the step-by-step procedure of a guideline. The term *practice parameter* is used by the American Medical Association and American Academy of Child and Adolescent Psychiatry as the identifying term for its practice guidelines. *Standards* are recommendations that should be followed in almost all cases; justification should be provided when they are not followed.

Purpose and Development of Practice Guidelines

Practice guidelines are designed to delineate an approach to the diagnosis, treatment, and management of medical disorders. The content of a guideline is usually determined by scientific evidence and the consensus of experts. The goals of practice guidelines are to ensure quality health care, reduce variability in the delivery of health care, and ensure that treatment is cost-effective.

Guidelines may also be used to identify uncontrolled variation in medical practice. Berwick (1992, p. 175) stated, "To learn we must systematize variation and that leads us to guidelines." Clinton and associates (1994) have summarized the method used by the Agency for Health Care Policy and Research (AHCPR) in developing guidelines. The agency may form panels of experts and consumers or award contracts on a competitive basis to nonprofit and public bidders. The contractors, in turn, are required to form a panel of experts and consumers. The panel is the basic vehicle for the development of guidelines. Criteria used by AHCPR to select areas for guideline development include the adequacy of available scientific evidence, the magnitude of the clinical problem, the potential to prevent future occurrences of the disorder, the estimated effect of the guideline in reducing variation, the needs of indigent and the elderly persons, and the cost to payers.

In creating guidelines, the following characteristics are included: validity, reliability, clinical applicability, flexibility, and clarity. Guidelines are developed in a multidisciplinary manner with careful documentation of assumptions, actual evidence, and the method of making decisions. Once developed, guidelines are assigned a scheduled review date by AHCPR.

The methodology used by AHCPR in developing guidelines has been summarized by Clinton and colleagues (1994) as follows:

- The clinical condition is chosen based on previously identified criteria.
- The condition is clearly defined.
- Scientific literature is critically reviewed for appropriateness and effectiveness.
- Estimates of outcome for the target population are reviewed.
- Identified benefits and harms are reviewed.
- Health outcomes are reviewed.
- Current and potential costs are reviewed when cost data are available and considered reliable to provide alternative strategies for the prevention, diagnosis, and treatment of the condition.
- Information and comments on the guideline topic are solicited from professional and consumer organizations and manufacturers to be presented in open panel or in writing.
- Guidelines are drafted.
- External peer review of guidelines is implemented.
- Draft guidelines are revised based on analysis of pretesting and comments received from external peer reviewers.

The Harvard Community Health Plan developed guidelines in the form of clinical algorithms (Gottlieb et al. 1993). In addition to reviewing the literature, consensus is obtained from physicians and other clinicians in the health plan. Consensus is arrived at through the use of a nominal group process and the Delphi method. These techniques are relatively formal and elicit input from many individuals in a timely fashion. Fink and associates (1984) described a similar approach for arriving at a consensus, but it is one that relies more on quantitative methods.

The critical issue in developing practice guidelines is whether they will be useful and have a desired effect. The task of implementing guidelines, even in relatively small organizational settings, is daunting. An intensive effort is required to install guidelines and make them easily available and usable (Gottlieb et al. 1993).

Practice guidelines must be integrally linked to the total quality management system of the health care organization for which they are developed. Consequently, the only valid assessment of the effectiveness and the appropriateness of practice guidelines is well-designed outcome studies that incorporate clinical data and cost data as part of the measured outcomes. Installing and using guidelines effectively in an organization has ramifications for every aspect of that organization.

Guidelines and Utilization Review Criteria

Utilization review (UR) criteria, sometimes referred to as UR guidelines, describe severity-of-illness characteristics and intensity-of-treatment requirements. UR criteria are used to arrive at decisions regarding admission to or continuance of care at a particular level of treatment. UR criteria are used to support decisions to approve or deny certification of treatment. Technically, a decision not to certify treatment is distinct from an administrative decision not to reimburse care.

UR criteria tend to be more abstract and less prescriptive than practice guidelines. Also, because UR decisions are made for the purpose of authorizing or certifying insurance coverage, they do not determine whether medical care is given or withheld. That decision is the primary and sole responsibility of the attending physician or clinician of record.

The data, symptoms, and behavior specified in practice guidelines are similar to those in UR criteria. The viewpoint of practice guidelines, however, is that of the provider, whereas UR criteria are designed by the managed care organization and thus may be more cost-conscious. Dr. John McIntyre (Pierce 1992), past president of the American Psychiatric Association (APA) and current chairman of the APA's steering committee on guidelines, contended that the development of practice guidelines is useful in that managed care firms may be encouraged to use the guidelines in developing their own UR criteria. He hopes that outcome will result in clinically sound treatment as well as cost-efficient decisions.

Two examples illustrate differences between clinical practice guidelines and UR criteria. A practice guideline in narrative form might be worded as follows:

Suicidal risk: If a patient's recent behavior indicates a high risk of lethality, admit the patient to the hospital immediately.

In algorithm form, it may appear as follows:

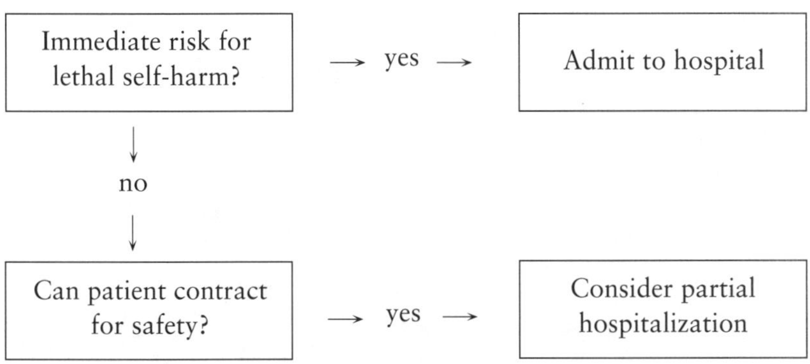

UR criteria might read narratively as follows:

1. Patient has a valid DSM-IV diagnosis (American Psychiatric Association 1994).
2. Patient manifests immediate risk for lethal self-harm.

These two criteria would meet the necessary and sufficient conditions for certifying insurance coverage in an inpatient psychiatric unit.

Types of Guidelines

The American Medical Association (AMA 1995) publishes a yearly directory of practice parameters. The 1995 edition contains approximately 1,800 listings. These parameters are developed and published by national medical specialty societies, the federal government, and research organizations. In the field of mental health and substance abuse, there are several types of guidelines (Table 4–1). Disorder-specific guidelines provide detailed information related to the diagnosis and treatment of specific DSM-IV diagnostic entities. Behavioral-specific guidelines are aimed at particular behaviors not necessarily subsumed under a specific diagnostic entity. Such behaviors may be observed or reported as part of the clinical condition in a variety of DSM-IV Axis I or II disorders, for example, suicidal behavior or guidelines related to the treatment of victims of sexual abuse.

Program guidelines constitute an important and rapidly growing area of guideline development. Some program guidelines have been developed in unique practice settings to facilitate the proper utilization of specialists and certain services, for example, electroconvulsive therapy and neuropsychological testing. Guidelines for partial hospitalization have been published by the American Association of Partial Hospitals. The APA has published guidelines related to the roles and expectations of psychiatrists practicing in staff-model HMOs and community mental health centers.

Practice guidelines that address the diagnosis and treatment of a particular disorder often have multiple origins. Guidelines related to depression are a notable example. Two national organizations—the Agency for Health Care Policy and Research (AHCPR) and the APA—have developed guidelines for depression. In addition, the Harvard Community Health Plan and the Albert Einstein Medical Center/ Belmont Center for Comprehensive Treatment have also developed practice guidelines for depression. These guidelines have a good deal in common because they are based on the general medical literature. However, the length and content of these documents vary considerably. The AHCPR guidelines are contained in two volumes with two additional short pamphlets (a patient's guide and a quick reference guide for clinicians). The guidelines were written primarily for primary care physicians (Depression Guideline Panel 1993). The APA document contains 26 pages and was written mainly for psychiatrists (American Psychiatric Association 1993).

Practice guidelines are truly in their infancy. Competition and rivalry between guidelines abound. Will various professional organizations vie with each other to promote their own "brand" of guidelines? For example, a spokesperson for the American Psychological Association criticized the APA's 1993 guideline for depression, citing its overemphasis on psychopharmacological treatment (Oberman 1993). Will guidelines be subject to the same cottage industry competition that has characterized the domain of assessment instruments, rating scales, symptom checklists, and other tools? Many types of instruments exist for depression alone. The lack of standardization of methodology limits the usefulness of comparing studies of the same disorder. At this stage of development, promoting or imposing a single set of guidelines for each disorder is premature. Yet the goal of conducting reliable and valid outcome studies requires standardized and generally applicable practice guidelines.

In comparison to the degree of development of guidelines for medical and surgical conditions, those for psychiatric and substance abuse disorders are clearly in their infancy. Medical-surgical guidelines have been developed over a number of years and from many sources, including specialty groups and specially constituted bodies such as the Agency for Health Care Policy and Research. The clear advantage medical-surgical guidelines have over the present state of guidelines for psychiatric and substance abuse disorders is that there are many more objective measures for determining the status of medical-surgical conditions, from both a diagnostic and a therapeutic perspective.

In addition, the number and the sophistication of medical case-controlled studies with randomly assigned treatment interventions are far advanced compared with studies in the psychiatric field. The available outcome knowledge is more refined. Acknowledging those realities, however, does not constitute sufficient reason to despair or avoid developing practice guidelines for psychiatric and substance abuse disorders. A start must be made. Although there are diverse theories about the origin and treatment of behavioral disorders, this diversity does not set them uniquely apart from medical-surgical disorders.

One need only look at guidelines for treating prostate cancer to recognize significant differences of opinion regarding the assessment and treatment of this condition (Goldfinger et al. 1994). The salient point is that it is time for practitioners, academicians, and professional leaders to actively

Table 4–1. Guidelines in psychiatry

Type of guideline	Topic	Organization	Date published
I. Practice guidelines[a]			
	Depression in Primary Care	AHCPR	1993
	Eating Disorders	APA	1993
	Major Depressive Disorders	APA	1993
	Bipolar Disorder	APA	1994
	Substance Use Disorders	APA	1995
	Schizophrenia	APA	UD
	Anxiety and Panic Disorder	APA	UD
	Delirium	APA	UD
	Geriatric Care	APA	UD
	Mental Retardation	APA	UD
	Alzheimer's & Related Dementias	APA	UD
	Psychiatric Evaluation of Adults	APA	1995
	Nicotine Dependence	APA	UD
	Attention-Deficit/Hyperactivity Disorder	AACAP	1991
	Conduct Disorders	AACAP	1992
	Anxiety Disorders	AACAP	1993
	Childhood Schizophrenia	AACAP	1994
	Depression	AACAP	UD
	Bipolar Disorder	AACAP	UD
	Sexual Abuse Evaluation/Forensics	AACAP	UD
	Obsessive-Compulsive Disorder	AACAP	UD
	Substance Abuse Disorders	AACAP	UD

II. Program guidelines			
	Standards and Guidelines for Partial Hospitalization	AAPH	NS
	Standards and Guidelines for Child and Adolescent Partial Hospitalization	AAPH	NS
III. Miscellaneous guidelines			
	Guidelines for Psychiatrists in Consultative, Supervisory, or Collaborative Relationships with Nonmedical Therapists	APA	1981
	Guidelines on Confidentiality	APA	1987
	Guidelines for Psychiatric Practice in Community Mental Health Centers	APA	1987
	Guidelines for Psychiatric Practice in Staff-Model HMOs	APA	1989
	Guidelines Regarding Psychiatrists' Signatures	APA	1989
	Guidelines for Appropriate Transfer of Managed Care Plan Subscribers	Colorado Medical Society	1991
	Guidelines for Psychiatric Practice in Public Sector Psychiatric Inpatient Facilities	APA	1994

Note. AACAP = American Academy of Child and Adolescent Psychiatry. AAPH = American Association for Partial Hospitalization, Inc. AHCPR = Agency for Health Care Policy and Research. APA = American Psychiatric Association. NS = not specified. UD = under development.

[a]American Academy of Child and Adolescent Psychiatry uses the term *Practice Parameters*.

begin developing guidelines. Guidelines require clinical testing, revision and refinement, and implementation. The goal is to reach a broadly accepted consensus on the most appropriate guideline(s) for assessing and treating a wide range of disorders in the behavioral spectrum.

Guidelines and Clinical Judgment

One of the inviolate maxims of treatment is that all clinical decisions ultimately rest with the professional judgment of the attending physician. No one who does not have this direct responsibility to the patient can subsume treatment or presume to dictate treatment to the clinician of record. The same rule should apply to the use of practice guidelines (Johnson 1993). In fact, such a statement accompanies all APA practice guidelines.

The practice of medicine, psychiatry in particular, requires more than a set of dicta or simply applying certain formulae. The process of rendering psychiatric treatment is by nature interactional. As such, it retains a degree of ambiguity and unpredictability. Although guidelines attempt to reduce clinical variability, "one should plan to build guidelines that are approximations or bounds on the fully prescriptive ideal for complex matters . . . . Practice guidelines serve as guardrails to *practice decisions* rather than cookbooks" (McDonald and Overhage 1994, p. 872).

Guidelines do not and cannot capture important nuances, variations, and shadings of mood and affect as communicated by paraverbal means. These means include pace and tone of voice, inflection, facial expression, gesture, and body posture and movements. Data from those sources are essential in forming diagnostic impressions. The reciprocal paraverbal interactions between the psychiatrist and the patient are equally essential to the development and maintenance of the psychiatrist-patient relationship. That is true whether the focus of interaction is on the patient's response to medication or to specific psychotherapeutic techniques.

Guidelines cannot and should not be expected to provide precise rules to distinguish patients who are excessively cautious from those who are hypervigilant and oversuspicious from those who are overtly paranoid. Those distinctions are a matter of on-the-spot clinical judgment. In fact, each of those behaviors may be present at different times or exist simultaneously, emerging over the course of an evaluation.

Practice guidelines focus attention on data for the purpose of ruling in or ruling out certain courses of action. This is not to imply that multiple symptoms, comorbid conditions, or a multimodal approach to treatment is ruled out by the form or content of practice guidelines. Guidelines, especially those in algorithm or decision tree formats, tend to encourage binary thinking. However, human life, medicine in general, and psychiatry especially deal with shadings, gray areas, and ambivalence. Love and hate of the same person, instantaneous vacillation between choices, conflicting feelings and emotions—these are experiences common to all individuals and an essential component of psychiatric practice that computer logic cannot address.

Advantages and Disadvantages of Practice Guidelines

Advantages and disadvantages of practice guidelines are a matter of speculation given their inchoate state of development. There are no well-designed outcome studies using practice guidelines in the field of psychiatry or chemical dependency. The possible advantages of guidelines, some of which have been mentioned in previous sections, are listed below:

- Guidelines may provide a way to reduce unexplained variation in practice.
- Guidelines could be used to achieve more scientifically driven or consensus-based practice. Approaches to treatment would be more consistent and uniform but not rigid.
- Guidelines can contribute to an improvement in the quality of treatment.
- Guidelines may increase personal efficiency and decrease unnecessary interventions, thus contributing to a reduction of health care costs.
- Guidelines, particularly during their development, can sharpen and improve the clarity of clinical thinking.
- Guidelines could support the development of integrated networks insofar as optimal treatment depends on a system of integrated care that may not exist in certain parts of the country.
- Guidelines could help educate health care providers.
- Guidelines could clarify the relevance and importance of certain data in treatment decisions.

There are also potential disadvantages to using practice guidelines:

- Guidelines may be used as manacles and unduly constrain the judgment of physicians.
- Guidelines may be followed slavishly without regard to "real-time" treatment.
- Guidelines may be used in litigation against physicians who, in turn, may resort to using guidelines merely as a defensive strategy.
- Guidelines may generate antagonism and outright revolt on the part of physicians if they become regulatory instruments.
- Guidelines have the potential to dampen and discourage innovations in treatment.

- Guidelines may foster incorrect or oversimplistic notions of patient management.
- Guidelines may increase interdisciplinary divisiveness.
- Guidelines run the risk of becoming the pet products of academicians, researchers, quality improvement specialists, payers, and politicians.
- Guidelines can be interpreted as a simple fix for a complex set of clinical problems.

Resistance to Practice Guidelines

Barriers to implementing guidelines must be identified and overcome. They can include physician disagreement, ineffective dissemination of guidelines, and fear of recrimination in a malpractice suit in the event that guidelines become cast in stone. Alternatively, guidelines may be written so broadly as to offer no advantage over a well-written review article.

Resistance to practice guidelines must be placed in the larger sociopolitical context of health care. Physicians have been faced with a significant number of changes in the past 15 years that have affected everything from their decisions about patient care to revisions in payment schedules and the emergence of managed care and other cost-containment measures. Most of these changes have been imposed externally by government and regulatory agencies. Clearly, this is reason enough for most physicians to resist using guidelines and view them as another example of the "hassle factor."

The magnitude of the changes in the practice of medicine and psychiatry during the past 15 years is bound to induce fear and strong negative reactions among physicians and professional organizations representing them. Accommodation to external mandates affecting the psychiatric profession has been evident only during the past several years. It is noteworthy that the American Academy of Child and Adolescent Psychiatry initially assumed a more constructive posture to outside regulation than did the APA. The early response of the APA to managed care was characterized by bellicosity accompanied by whining and hand wringing. The academy became proactive in the mid-1980s and established a work group on consumer issues and a work group on quality issues. Later it established task forces in managed care and universal access to health care. The managed care task force was established in 1989. The committee contained members of the academy and representatives of managed care companies. An information letter, *Managed Care Report*, has been published quarterly since 1992. The American Academy of Child and Adolescent Psychiatry has also published several practice parameters, beginning in 1991 with the publication of the first practice parameter on attention-deficit/hyperactivity disorder.

The backing of senior mentors and respected leaders in psychiatry is critical to the acceptance of practice guidelines. Involving psychiatrists at both national and local levels will ensure that guidelines are used properly in the day-to-day management of patients (Greco and Eisenberg 1993).

Conclusion

The development of practice guidelines to shape treatment and the birth of managed care to shape health care delivery are two distinct but clearly related phenomena. If managed care had not yet come into existence, the value of guidelines would still be evident. Their value lies in their ability to clarify treatment approaches, reduce practice variation, and provide a building block for total quality improvement endeavors. Because guidelines are often lumped with managed care activities, resistance to them is greater than if they had emerged in an environment free of managed care.

That practice guidelines have emerged together with managed care may actually benefit patients. Synergy created by these two developments may empower physicians and other clinicians in the delivery of health care, especially in managed care settings where clinical autonomy has decreased. However, without physician input at every stage of guideline development, guidelines will most likely be ineffective and unused.

Practice guidelines developed with physician participation can also counter the tendency of some managed care companies to act in an arbitrary manner. Guidelines will require managed care organizations to seriously consider the complexities and clinical realities presented by each individual patient. Enhancing the provision of quality care as well as managing costs will be a likely by-product of using practice guidelines correctly.

References

American Medical Association: Directory of Practice Parameters: Titles, Sources and Update, 1995 Edition. Chicago, IL, American Medical Association, 1995

American Psychiatric Association: Practice guideline for major depressive disorder in adults. Am J Psychiatry 150 (suppl):1–26, 1993

American Psychiatric Association: Diagnostic and Statistical Manual of Mental Disorders, 4th Edition. Washington, DC, American Psychiatric Association, 1994

Berwick DM: Practice guidelines: promise or threat. HMO Practice 5:174–177, 1992

Clinton JJ, McCormick K, Besteman J: Enhancing clinical practice: the role of practice guidelines. Am Psychol 49:30–33, 1994

Deming WE: Out of the Crisis. Cambridge, MA, Massachusetts Institute of Technology Center for Advanced Engineering Study, 1986

Depression Guideline Panel: Depression in Primary Care: Vol 2: Treatment of Major Depression (AHCPR Publ No 93-0551). Rockville, MD, U.S. Department of Health and Human Services, Public Health Service, Agency for Health Care Policy and Research, April 1993

Fink A, Kosecoff M, Chessin MR, et al: Consensus methods: characteristics and guidelines for use. Am J Public Health 74:979–983, 1984

Goldfinger S, Garnett LR, Gillyatt P (eds): A Special Report: Prostate Diseases. Boston, MA, Harvard Medical School Health Publication Group, 1994

Gottlieb LK, Sokol HN, Murrey KO, et al: Algorithm-based quality improvement clinical guidelines and continuous quality improvement. HMO Practice 6:5–12, 1993

Greco P, Eisenberg JM: Changing physicians' practices. JAMA 329:1271–1273, 1993

Johnson RE: Practice guidelines: efficacy and implementation in HMOs. HMO Practice 7:119–121, 1993

McDonald CJ, Overhage JM: Guidelines you can follow and you can trust. JAMA 271:872–873, 1994

Oberman L: Groups differ over government guideline. Am Med News, May 17, 1993, p 6

Pierce C: APA Ready to Launch Practice Guideline Era. Clinical Psychiatry News, June 1992, p 22

Section II

Clinical Issues

Chapter 5

Can Managed Care Improve Mental Health Outcomes for Children and Adolescents?

Ronald D. Geraty, M.D.
Robert J. Fox, J.D.

Although there is general agreement that the unique mental health needs of children and adolescents require tailored treatment and service delivery systems, considerable work remains in the development and evaluation of treatment modalities and optimal systems for the delivery of care. There have been encouraging programs and innovative approaches in addressing the needs of children and adolescents (England and Cole 1992; Friedman and Kutash 1992), yet changes in the cultural environment have further complicated and heightened the urgency to improve the delivery of care (Friedman 1992).

Epidemiological studies during the past decade have estimated the overall prevalence of moderate and severe psychiatric disorders in children and adolescents at 14%–22% (Brandenburg et al. 1990; Costello 1989). These estimates are significantly higher than the median prevalence of 11.8% estimated by earlier studies (Gould et al. 1980). The more recent estimates may evidence more sophisticated techniques for identifying disorders or, in fact, may reflect more widespread problems for youth as enhanced risks of violence and substance abuse are compounded by a weakening of family support systems in current society. In any event, the extent of treatment needs is formidable.

Mental health and substance abuse treatment for youth is more complex than treatment for adults. Because of a higher degree of dependence on their family members and their environment, children and adolescents are more vulnerable to mental stresses created when support factors in the family, school, and community are compromised. A variety of environmental factors, such as poverty, parental psychopathology, maltreatment, sexual abuse, neglect, physical development difficulties, familial disorganization, and homelessness, may initiate or compound childhood disorders (Saxe et al. 1988). Therefore, treatment must address environmental and familial variables and dynamics, as well as the child's intraindividual difficulties.

Benefit-Driven Treatment

In light of the diverse range of potential environmental risks, it would seem almost self-evident that a system of interaction between an array of treatment and community service providers and agencies would afford the most appropriate intervention milieu. However, traditional approaches to the provision and reimbursement of care have helped to perpetuate a system of care that frustrates the unique mental health needs of children and adolescents. Health benefit designs popularized during the 1970s and continued into the 1980s favored reimbursement for inpatient hospitalization and curtailed the financial viability of outpatient care and other treatment provided in less intensive settings. This *benefit-driven* bias toward inpatient care brought about a tremendous growth in the development and utilization of private psychiatric treatment facilities in the past decade. In the absence of more coordinated care systems, public health programs also lacked the capacity and mechanisms to integrate comprehensive ranges of services.

Thus, given the practical financial considerations of responsible parties seeking treatment services, health benefit structures drove a system of care placing a primary emphasis on costly and intensive hospitalization, irrespective of the appropriateness of treatment setting and modality. In the early to mid-1980s, studies demonstrated that there had been an enormous increase in the number of admissions of children to private psychiatric facilities and that the average length of stay for children and adolescents was 50% longer than that for adults (Friedman and Kutash 1992). Beyond the obvious detriments in terms of cost, benefit-driven systems have run the constant risk of disrupting the clinical decision-making process through a minimization of environmental covariants involved in the psychiatric disorder. The singularity of this approach isolates the treatment of the individual from crucial interaction within the family and community and de-emphasizes individualized approaches to care aimed at understanding stress in the patient's daily activities.

Integrated Treatment Systems

In recognition of the need for interactive and integrated systems of care, there have been several positive developments in the public and private sectors in recent years. Through a system of grants and assistance, the Child and Adolescent Service System Program (CASSP) administered by the National Institute of Mental Health (NIMH) has promoted more coordinated systems of care for chronically mentally ill patients. Since 1984, CASSP has funded the development of community-based systems of care for children and adolescents and their families. Under these interactive systems, a range of community-based services are offered through the cooperative efforts of providers and service agencies. Systems of care under CASSP are based on individualized and flexible efforts to maintain the family intact and to provide care in the least restrictive setting that is clinically appropriate (Friedman and Kutash 1992).

In the private sector, the Robert Wood Johnson Foundation has funded a Mental Health Services Program for Youth through which grants have been awarded to a number of states. The goal of the project implementation is to develop systems of care for mentally ill children and adolescents that coordinate the services of child welfare, mental health, public health education, and juvenile justice agencies with those of mental health care providers in the private sector. The program is grounded in three basic assumptions:

1. The best treatment occurs in the natural setting of the child's family and community.
2. Intensive care is possible in normal settings (home, school, work, playground), and structured treatment can be provided through a highly individualized and complex package of services "wrapped around" the child and family. Structured treatment can take place in environments other than institutional settings.
3. Service delivery must be organized to respond consistently to the ever-changing needs of young patients who are growing and developing (England and Cole 1992).

A key House subcommittee supported an amendment to the Clinton administration's proposed Health Security Act that would have emphasized the use of community-based and outpatient treatment consistent with medically necessary care. Specifically, the amendment, offered by Congressman George Miller of California, would have expanded mental illness and substance abuse benefits to include intensive community services of 180 days per year for individuals under age 22 years. Furthermore, it would have required that mental illness and substance abuse services be furnished through organized systems of care for children who have serious emotional disturbances or substance abuse disorders and who are, or are likely to be, involved with a public child-serving agency. An organized system of care was described in the amendment as a community-based service delivery network that provides for the participation and coordination of agencies and providers serving eligible children, the involvement of families in the planning of treatment and delivery of services, the development and management of individualized treatment plans, and the delivery and coordination of multiple services. The amendment would have also established funding for comprehensive state-developed managed mental health and substance abuse programs that would be required to promote the integration of the delivery of services by public and private providers and to promote the link of mental health and substance abuse services with primary and preventive health care services (Miller 1994).

The developmental initiatives referenced above provide excellent examples of opportunities for the public demonstration, examination, and assessment of more sophisticated approaches to individualized case management within systems of integrated interagency or provider care delivery. On the face of it, implementation of integrated systems of care does not alter the fundamental elements of treatment (i.e., the initial diagnostic assessment and treatment plan). Rather, the immediate benefit lies in the *delivery* of care in a manner that encourages participation in the therapeutic process, as appropriate, by all sectors of the environmental support system. However, an equally important result of the movement toward integrated delivery systems is the creation of a greater potential for more varied opportunities to examine the effectiveness and efficiency of treatment modalities and settings. With the removal of traditional barriers to the maintenance of the patient's daily activities in home-based and community environments, a greater pool of experience in less restrictive settings makes possible a more thorough examination of the effects of treatment techniques and settings on outcomes.

As encouraging as developmental funding programs are, the question remains: Will the full potential of integrated and interactive systems of care be realized? Furthermore, can managed care systems play a leading role in the realization of that potential? Are managed behavioral health care paradigms suited to the interactive, integrated, and cooperative systems of care needed to optimally serve the treatment needs of children and adolescents?

An assessment of the systemic ills to be remedied and the challenges faced in creating better care delivery systems lends insight.

Goals of Treatment

Initiatives such as CASSP were created and implemented after repeated findings that in the absence of coordinated systems of care, individual programs designed to assist mentally ill children frequently were not accessed (Dougherty 1988). Although progress has been made, multidimensional needs too often remain unserved as the health care system struggles to deliver effective care.

As has been detailed elsewhere (Friedman 1992; Friedman and Kutash 1992), several basic challenges face child and adolescent mental health care. To summarize, the mental health and substance abuse field must

- Reorient delivery systems in a manner that accommodates the diverse needs of children and adolescents and addresses interrelated problems in mental health, substance abuse, juvenile justice, education, vocational settings, and the family unit.
- Provide care delivery and financing systems that are flexible enough to support a continuum of treatment settings and community-based care, while counteracting overutilization of hospital-based care.
- Provide protection so that children and adolescents are admitted for inpatient treatment based on clinical need rather than reimbursement incentives.
- Forge public-private partnerships that can successfully coordinate and use diverse resources in creating healthier community and family environments.
- Strengthen quality control and increase accountability for effectiveness.
- Provide better research on the effectiveness of care.

In addition, surveys have shown that, similar to the adult population, large numbers of mentally disturbed children receive treatment in family practitioners' offices (Saxe et al. 1988). Effective systems of care must foster a higher degree of involvement of pediatricians and family practitioners with other loci of service provision for youth.

Managed Behavioral Health Care Systems

Has the managed care industry developed methods not only to manage psychiatric and chemical dependency treatment delivery, but also to remove the traditional systemic hurdles that stand in the way of effective and appropriate treatment? Specialty managed behavioral health care companies have many years of experience in managing psychiatric and chemical dependency health care delivery systems and now manage the care for approximately 100 million people. The typical operating characteristics of managed behavioral health care companies include precepts, mechanisms, and techniques fundamental to successfully integrated delivery systems. Geraty et al. (1994) noted that the features of a well-designed managed behavioral health care program include the following:

- Individualized case management
- Early intervention
- Development of specialty networks with a continuum of care and access to a full range of disciplines
- Quality management approaches
- A consumer orientation
- Innovation

Through the clinical approach of individualized case management, multidisciplinary case management teams using developed criteria enhance clinical value for each patient by advocating for the most appropriate and most specific treatment. This approach stands in sharp contrast to the shortcomings and inequities of benefit-driven systems under which reimbursement biases have provided incentives for the overuse of inpatient institutional care.

By stressing early intervention, managed behavioral health care systems further support the goal of enhancing access to appropriate care by affording the opportunity to address needs at an early stage in less intensive treatment settings. Such early intervention is made possible through specialty networks consisting of a broad range of provider disciplines and a full continuum of treatment settings, including inpatient, residential, partial hospital, day treatment, intensive outpatient, outpatient, and home-based care. Another feature of managed behavioral health care systems is quality management geared to improving the clinical process for individual patients from initial assessment to treatment plan implementation to the monitoring of outcomes.

Through a strong consumer orientation, individual patients and their families remain informed about methods of accessing treatment and about treatment itself. The flow of information to those seeking the benefits of treatment is fundamental to successful individualized case management. Furthermore, managed behavioral health care companies have shown great promise in working with professional organizations and academic centers in improving the clinical and administrative knowledge bases.

The consumer-oriented, individualized case management methods of managed behavioral health care companies also help to structure links with community-based support groups and other resources as components of the overall delivery matrix (Marques et al. 1994). Integrating the efforts and expertise of service organizations and a full range of providers establishes a ready capability to serve the diverse needs of children and adolescents. In particular, the managed behavioral health care industry has demonstrated its ability to integrate services with primary care physicians in the medical-surgical delivery system through improved referral procedures, patient matching and patient advocacy, integrated communication, and mechanisms to avoid cost-shifting and to benefit from the advantages of medical cost offset. Increasingly, accountability for the efficacy of managed behavioral health care techniques is being ensured through the assumption of financial risk by managed care companies under capitation and price guarantee arrangements.

Typically, managed behavioral health care systems use problem-focused, goal-oriented therapy techniques that, in appropriate cases, reduce the need for lengthy hospitalization and facilitate the effective use of less restrictive treatment settings. These techniques have helped to contain runaway costs and reverse adverse fiscal incentives; enhanced the possibilities of integrated, community-based care systems; and provided the basis for research that indicates there are positive clinical effects resulting from less restrictive care settings (Barglow et al. 1992). In fact, there is no evidence that inpatient hospitalization in general is more effective than treatments available in intensive community-based settings, and there are many demonstrations of effective service delivery for youth outside the hospital (Friedman 1992). However, it must be recognized that much work remains to be performed in the clarification of the best methods for coordinating the provision of care within integrated delivery systems. Integrated delivery systems are not unique in their need to refine the clinical approach toward even more positive outcomes, but the fact that they have built comprehensive, organized frameworks for such improvements is more than noteworthy.

Outcomes Management

Currently, there is a broad array of research supporting the efficacy of behavioral treatment for children and adolescents (Casey and Berman 1985; Weisz et al. 1987). Yet there is still a great need for multivariable studies of treatment effects for significant numbers of patients in terms of disorder types, treatment settings, provider disciplines, timing of intervention, familial and community context, and length of treatment. With programs that manage treatment for extensive patient populations within the full spectrum of treatment settings, the managed care industry has the experience necessary for raising the level of sophistication in outcome research. Moreover, managed behavioral health care programs afford the additional research advantage of managing outcome data from care administered under a variety of public and private benefit plans. Such data will provide an important basis for graduating beyond the simple measurement of treatment outcomes to organized outcomes management within diverse delivery systems. As more experience becomes interactive, cooperative service environments can be achieved and more specialized outcome data can be generated. These data will be crucial to the evaluation and refinement of the daily interactions between mental health care providers and public and private community organizations in delivering effectively integrated services to children and adolescents.

Specifically, outcomes management data will continue to allow integrated mental health care delivery systems to positively affect care delivery at several levels:

- Data from multiple treatment and service settings will help influence provider practice patterns across the continuum of care and will help optimize the application of timely community-based services.
- As the knowledge base increases, programmatic needs of overall care systems will be identified and thus will help set the direction for new developmental programs to build on established successes.
- Outcomes data will provide the foundation for improved clinical training for those professionals serving the needs of children and adolescents. Stronger ties will develop between the private sector and academic centers as the clinical and administrative benefits of coordinating treatment, education, and service provision within integrated systems become more obvious. As a result, the opportunities for more extensive academic and professional training on the specifics of integrated care delivery systems and the broad continuum of treatment and service settings will be realized.
- The availability of more sophisticated and broader-based outcomes data will enhance the ability of public policymakers to make informed decisions on funding for mental illness and substance abuse benefits and research.

As has been stated elsewhere:

> Clinical and research findings in the mental health and substance abuse field are critical not only for serving individual children and families, or for establishing improved service delivery systems. They are also

> critical for examining broader public policy changes that are necessary to prevent problems in children and families and the entire country. (Friedman 1992, pp. 175–176)

Health Reform

Congress and the executive branch continue to formulate health care reform packages to remedy many of the shortcomings of the current health care system (see Chapter 23). The political environment presented by this reform activity holds great potential for achieving tremendous strides in the establishment and promotion of more progressive systemic approaches to the care of our nation's youth.

Largely in response to the health care reform policy activities, a group of leading companies in the managed behavioral health care industry formed the American Managed Behavioral Healthcare Association (AMBHA) at the end of 1993. With the desire to help formulate a clinically sound and affordable national health plan, AMBHA developed Principles on Healthcare Reform, a set of seven principles that support the use of individualized case management within integrated care delivery systems as the best means of accomplishing the goals of improved access, cost-effectiveness, and quality. Especially pertinent to the need to further establish and evaluate integrated, community-based care systems, the principles include the following tenet:

> The encouragement of public and private funding for research and training in new treatment approaches which are based upon the knowledge, expertise and cooperative efforts of public and private delivery systems, and the further refinement of outcome measurements and health services delivery will be key elements in improving future treatment of mental illness and chemical dependency, particularly the care of those people with serious and persistent mental illness. (Geraty et al. 1994, p. 4)

The necessity of promoting greater cooperation between public and private programs is readily apparent—particularly in the context of child and adolescent care and at a time of health care reform. Toward that end, AMBHA and the National Association of State Mental Health Program Directors (NASMHPD) sponsored a study completed in May 1994 that examined the costs of providing comprehensive, nondiscriminatory, and affordable mental health and substance abuse benefits for both privately insured populations and those within the publicly financed system of care (Melek 1994). The study is especially significant because it is the first effort to assess the cost implications of a managed care, public-private integrated system of behavioral health care. It was found that the cost of providing comprehensive, nondiscriminatory mental benefits was considerably less than earlier administration estimates. The study concluded that the widespread use of managed care approaches and the state-level integration of public and private mental health systems would be two critical factors in achieving lower costs.

Managed care is being increasingly accepted as the viable approach to high-quality, cost-effective treatment. In April 1994, a group of seven national organizations representing consumers, public and private sector providers, and managed care organizations entered into a cooperative effort to advocate for a comprehensive mental health and substance abuse benefit that is managed. The group included the National Association of Psychiatric Treatment Centers for Children, the National Community Mental Healthcare Council, the American Association for Partial Hospitalization, the National Association of Psychiatric Health Systems, the National Mental Health Association, AMBHA, and NASMHPD.

In a letter to members of Congress dated April 19, 1994, this diverse group explicitly supported a managed mental health and substance abuse benefit that must

- Offer a range of comprehensive services with a full range of community-based services. The inclusion of this continuum of services ensures the availability of the most clinically effective and least intensive service appropriate to the needs of the individual.
- Focus on quality. This goal can be achieved through, among other measures, the ongoing definition and improvement of standards of what constitutes medically necessary care, patient advocacy programs, and clinical outcomes information.

Conclusion

The answer to the question "Can managed care improve mental health outcomes for children and adolescents?" is an unequivocal "Yes!" In fact, it is hard to imagine that significant progress could be made outside of present and future efforts conducted within managed integrated delivery systems. Of course, the new path of outcome research and management will be neither short nor simple. As integrated delivery systems adapt in the evolving community-based environments of care delivery, new avenues of learning will be paved and novel approaches to effective treatment and delivery will arise.

Fortunately, accomplishing these aims will not require the invention of entirely new methods. The experience of managed behavioral health care systems in developing high-quality treatment delivery techniques has produced the operating principles and infrastructure that will yield the essential outcome research data of the future. These data will be the base on which the mental health community can construct efficient mental health and substance abuse delivery systems for the provision of effective care.

References

Barglow P, Chandler S, Molitor N, et al: Managed psychiatric care for adolescents: problems and possibilities, in Managed Mental Health Care: Administrative and Clinical Issues. Edited by Feldman JL, Fitzpatrick RJ. Washington, DC, American Psychiatric Press, 1992, pp 261–271

Brandenburg NA, Friedman RM, Silver SE: The epidemiology of childhood psychiatric disorders: prevalence findings from recent studies. J Am Acad Child Adolesc Psychiatry 29:76–83, 1990

Casey RJ, Berman JS: The outcome of psychotherapy with children. Psychol Bull 98:388–400, 1985

Costello EJ: Developments in child psychiatric epidemiology. J Am Acad Child Adolesc Psychiatry 28:836–841, 1989

Dougherty D: Children's mental health problems and services: current federal efforts and policy implications. Am Psychol 43:808–812, 1988

England MJ, Cole RF: Building systems of care for youth with serious mental illness. Hosp Community Psychiatry 43:630–633, 1992

Friedman RM: Mental health and substance abuse services for adolescents: clinical and service systems issues. Administration and Policy in Mental Health 19:159–178, 1992

Friedman RM, Kutash K: Challenges for child and adolescent mental health. Health Aff 11(3):125–136, 1992

Geraty RD, Bartlett J, Hill E, et al: The Impact of Managed Behavioral Healthcare on the Costs of Psychiatric and Chemical Dependency Treatment. Alexandria, VA, American Managed Behavioral Healthcare Association, 1994

Gould MS, Wunsch-Hitzig R, Dohrenwend BP: Formulation of hypotheses about the prevalence, treatment and prognostic significance of psychiatric disorders in children in the United States, in Mental Illness in the United States. Edited by Dohrenwend BP, Dohrenwend BS, Gould MS, et al. New York, Praeger, 1980, pp 9–44

Lipsey MW, Wilson DB: The efficacy of psychological, educational, and behavioral treatment: confirmation from meta-analysis. Am Psychol 48:1181–1209, 1993

Marques C, Geraty RD, Bartlett J, et al: Quality and Access in the Managed Behavioral Healthcare Industry. Alexandria, VA, American Managed Behavioral Healthcare Association, 1994

Melek SP: Managed Behavioral Healthcare Cost Report for the Commercial Insured and Uninsured Populations. Chicago, IL, Milliman & Robertson, 1994

Miller G: Amendment to H.R. 3600, House Education and Labor Committee, Labor-Management Subcommittee, May 17, 1994

Saxe L, Cross T, Silverman N: Children's mental health: the gap between what we know and what we do. Am Psychol 43:800–807, 1988

Weisz JR, Weiss B, Alicke MD, et al: Effectiveness of psychotherapy with children and adolescents: a meta-analysis for clinicians. J Consult Clin Psychol 55:542–549, 1987

Chapter 6

Is Public Behavioral Health Care Manageable?

Anthony F. Panzetta, M.D.

The managed care momentum has increasingly been recognized by public payers of medical benefits, particularly financially strapped Medicaid plans. Many states have turned or will turn to managed care for assistance. When it is recognized that managed care will inevitably play a large role in the general health care environment, then it can be seen that managed care in the public sector is also inevitable. The public sector obligation for health care is especially significant in the areas of mental health and substance abuse. Beyond providing Medicaid coverage, states have traditionally been responsible for providing mental health care to indigent persons and to those whose health insurance has been exhausted.

In pondering the shape managed care will take in the future with respect to the public sector, certain questions arise:

- How rigorously will managed care be implemented? Will it be applied so loosely or casually that its power and value are lost?
- Who will primarily benefit from public sector managed care initiatives—service recipients, providers, payers, the public, or managed care companies?
- How will states design and implement managed care activities? Will they attempt to build in-house capacity or form partnerships with leading managed care organizations?

- Why should public sector behavioral health care systems consider partnering with private sector organizations in pursuing managed care initiatives? Will public sector agencies attempt to apply managed care without the benefit of expertise developed in the private sector regarding utilization management, decision support, information technology, total quality management, and financial risk management?
- How can managed care partnering between the public and private sector be synergistic? What are the mutual benefits that will advance state-of-the-art services and systems in both sectors?

The Four Phases of Managed Care

One of the issues confounding managed care is the inconsistent definition applied to this movement. In my view, there are at least four phases in the evolution of managed care. The first three coexist in today's marketplace, and the fourth is yet to emerge in any substantial way. These phases apply to both the private sector marketplace and the public sector.

The most primitive phase was *utilization review*. That is how managed care made its debut. Although health maintenance organizations (HMOs) had been around for some time before the appearance of utilization review, most of medicine had been able to ignore this phenomenon and so it seemed relevant only to a small proportion of patients and physicians. However, utilization review focused on the fee-for-service industry and primarily on the traditional indemnity insurance market, so both physicians and patients were forced to acknowledge this phase of managed care. Because utilization review was intrusive and threatening, it is no surprise that this first phase of managed care resulted in physician and patient resentment and suspicion.

The second phase of managed care was the development of *selective contracting* between payers (or their managed care agents) and providers. Better known as *preferred provider systems,* selective contracting resulted in indirect competition between providers. Some providers were in networks and others were not. Some providers chose not to participate in this phase of managed care because discounted fees were usually paid to selected providers. Because of these discounts, and the imposition of externally developed standards of care, the second phase of managed care has also resulted in provider suspicion and hostility toward managed care organizations.

The third phase of managed care was the development of *provider risk*. Capitation (prepaid) payments, characteristic of HMOs, entered the marketplace on the heels of selective contracting, thereby further splintering the provider communities into managed care players and nonplayers. This phase of managed care largely removed the need for externally imposed utilization management because providers had significant incentive to develop their own systems internally. As providers entered into capitation arrangements, they became more integrally involved in the managed care industry. From hostile participant to consenting partner—that is the dramatic shift that has occurred as managed care has moved from utilization review to provider risk.

The fourth phase of managed care is just beginning to crystallize and will most likely have a dramatic effect on the managed care environment and provider community. This is the phase of *technology transfer*. As some providers find themselves assuming increasing risk for medical services, they will begin to import the technology of utilization management into their own organizations. That will be particularly true for large provider organizations. As this technology transfer occurs, the need for intermediary organizations will be reduced. There will be less of a role for middlemen when payers and providers find that they can face one another across the negotiating table without the need for other parties.

The fourth phase of managed care is important to consider when looking at the role of managed mental health care organizations in the public sector.

A Public Behavioral System Partnership

The provider systems in the public sector have largely operated independent of managed care. In some areas, there has been limited experience with forms of utilization review; however, the first phase of managed care has done little to prepare the public provider community for the demands of full-throttle managed care.

It is my opinion that partnerships between public and private systems hold the most promise over the short term both for the regular recipients of public mental health services and for severely mentally ill persons (Panzetta 1994). Rather than replace existing public sector delivery systems, as in thorough privatization, a strategic partnership between private managed care companies and selected components of the public sector could provide a new model to contrast with other models of managed care that are developed over time.

This strategy is based on the assumption that the essential ingredients for a managed behavioral health care program for Medicaid recipients already exist in the current public health delivery system. This partnership will bring the community mental health centers and other publicly funded programs into a direct and vital role in the new managed care marketplace. Additionally, this proposal acknowledges that the logical locus of control for such programs is at the county level. Where applicable, such a strategy would have administrators from county offices of mental health and drug and alcohol programs serving as full partners.

I believe that a partnership model can best serve the needs of Medicaid recipients and accomplish the goals of 1) upgrading the existing delivery system through rigorous quality management, 2) providing a training component so that all providers in the system become informed about the essentials of managed care, 3) taking into account the special needs of chronically and severely mentally ill persons, 4) integrating and coordinating mental health and substance abuse treatment with general health and surgical treatment, 5) integrating all funding sources leading to *single-stream funding*, and 6) achieving cost-effectiveness, with savings reinvested into the delivery system programs or returned to general funds.

The strategic and operating plans developed by such partnerships would be county or region specific and would be developed with the participation of all the strategic partners. Risk would be assumed by the managed care company and could be shared by the strategic partners according to their ability to assume risk. In some instances, the strategic partners might assume all the risk. Savings that may accrue as a result of this strategic partnership would be distributed to the partners according to formulae that take into account factors such as level of risk assumed by the partner and contributions to operations.

The obvious alternative to a partnership approach is one in which attempts are made to build managed care into existing public programs. In this strategy, the state attempts to create its own managed care expertise and turn this capacity inward to its existing programs. This do-it-yourself strategy will have unfortunate consequences. The expertise required to create and maintain quality managed care is not easily attained; it comes from an evolutionary experience developed over years of trial and error and is not simply the application of technical ideas. Quality managed care comes from the development of an entire system of professionals, steeped in the technical ideas and experienced enough to know how to accommodate those ideas to different circumstances in the real world. Without adequate technical and actuarial knowledge, without advanced information and decision support systems that take full advantage of the newest computer technology, and without true managed care experience, the difficulties many states will encounter not only will adversely affect their organizations and service recipients but also will provoke unwarranted criticisms because what could have been achieved with properly designed and rigorously implemented managed care approaches will not be realized.

Key Objectives of a Managed Care Strategy for Public Systems

Integrated Funding and Coordinated Services

A problem in many public mental health systems is the fragmentation and lack of coordination among inpatient, community support, and clinic services. Likewise, clinicians and mental health workers are frustrated by bureaucratic, disjointed, or bifurcated funding sources. There are separate line-item budgets for inpatient and community services, as well as state general funds versus Medicaid and other federal sources. A managed care approach must begin by taking the multiple funding sources and creating an integrated funding and service design that addresses clients' needs. This task is fraught with political and historical difficulties as each funding source (e.g., Medicaid, state mental health programs, state substance abuse programs, federal agencies) strives to maintain its jurisdiction, power, prerogatives, priorities, and separate vision. The implementation of the change from fragmentation to integration of funding is a central objective of any managed care strategy that has a chance to work in the public sector. With the current interest in managed care by Medicaid, there is a window of opportunity for developing an integrated single-stream funding mechanism. Because private managed care companies lie outside of the traditional government health systems, they can play the role of intermediary between these often disjointed governmental agencies. By developing strategic partnerships with Medicaid, with offices of mental health, with offices of drug and alcohol programs, and with other significant entities like Medicaid-oriented HMOs, the integrated focusing of funding sources does not seem as unlikely as it did before the health financing crisis brought managed care to the table.

Outcome Management

Another key objective of managed care programs is to implement outcome-guided service system design. Many public and private sector behavioral health care systems have gradually turned their attention from the traditional concerns with staff mix, therapeutic approaches, and retrospective audits of processes toward output measures. Few, however, have grasped the fundamental difference that managed care *starts* with desired outcomes and then flexibly and creatively works *backward* to identify and apply the most essential (and perhaps the fewest) economical and effective actions to achieve those desired outcomes. Outcome-based service system design is the wave of the future, but it is also the most challenging task facing managed care systems and health systems in general.

Standardization

Managed care must make explicit what has often been implicit in the past. That is, managed care operates best when standards are developed that reflect the best current state of scientific and clinical knowledge. Rather than allowing a large behavioral health care system to function according to the whims or biases of its providers, managed care approaches determine the standards and the expectations in advance and then monitor adherence to standards for those who work in the system. These standards must be public and defensible and carry the approbation of the health and social sciences.

Cost Control and Savings

Managed care concentrates on creating value for the least possible cost. All sectors, public and private, have that goal as a burning imperative. That is the promise of managed care, and that is what has focused so much attention on managed care. Saving money carries with it, however, the intriguing questions: Who shall benefit from this saving? Will those monies go to shareholders of for-profit managed care companies? Will the money saved be reinvested in the health care delivery system so that more can be achieved for less? Will those monies be returned to governmental general funds? There is no set answer to those questions, although the issue is discussed further in Chapter 19.

The important point to make is that economies clearly can be achieved with the use of a managed care approach, particularly in the public sector. The disposition of those savings is a subject for negotiation. Some payers want to share in the savings. Some want to pour back a portion of the savings into the health care system. Some want to reduce their up-front risk or eliminate it entirely and so are not part of the distribution of savings just as they are not subject to the financial risk. There are many permutations, and they need to be made explicit at the outset so that future disputes regarding the disposition of savings can be avoided.

Special Needs of Public Recipients of Managed Care

There are special circumstances that exist in the public sector that must be addressed by a managed care organization. Because most managed care companies have developed within the private sector, many of these companies do not recognize those special needs. They may go forward in the public sector only to discover later that their efforts are failing and the financial projections they had made are woefully incorrect—to the detriment of patients, payers, providers, the general public, and themselves.

Some of these special needs can be subsumed under the general rubric of *community support*. Beyond the delivery of more traditional medically oriented services, there exists the need for ancillary services such as intensive case management, habilitation and rehabilitation programs, housing, social services, mobile outreach, and long-term support programs for seriously mentally ill persons (Dangerfield and Betit 1993; Mechanic 1992). Failure to provide those measures in the public sector will result in the inability of the basic medical services to affect utilization and quality. Unfortunately, as stated, few managed care organizations fully understand this dimension. These needs have been addressed, sometimes well and sometimes poorly, by the community mental health systems developed since federal enabling legislation of the mid-1960s. It would be foolhardy for any managed care entity to ignore this enormous resource; hence, there exists a potential for strategic partnerships between managed care companies and community mental health organizations.

The flip side of this situation calls for the existing community mental health systems to recognize that their service delivery systems must be reinvented (Panzetta 1985). The technology of managed care is not simply community mental health revisited. My own simplification is to think of the community mental health system as an array of extraordinarily comprehensive service providers and the managed care company as the utilization managing, quality assuring, outcome measuring, and complementing strategic partner. Together one plus one can equal four. In other words, the result of strategic alliances can be greater than the sum of the parts (see Chapter 24).

Nowhere is this possibility more obvious than in the care of chronically and seriously mentally ill persons. These individuals require services that go well beyond the traditional array of mental health services. The community mental health centers have a long and often distinguished history of providing care to chronically mentally ill persons. Some authorities feel that these populations should be carved out of the managed care purview and entrusted to the special efforts of experienced providers, such as community mental health centers (Gerson 1994). In some areas this will no doubt be the model that is followed. However, there is nothing implicit in the managed care approach suggesting that severely impaired individuals cannot benefit from managed care (Christianson et al. 1992; Leadholm and Kerzner

1993). If the plan advocated above is followed, then managed care companies will be forging strategic partnerships with the same community mental health centers that have experience with such populations.

Implementation Issues

The implementation of managed behavioral health care in the public sector is complicated by significant conflicts around 1) expansive versus restrictive benefits, 2) competing or disjointed governmental agency disputes, 3) risk assumption and the disposition of savings dollars, and 4) public health's concern with prevention and health promotion.

Expansive Versus Restrictive Benefits

It is important to recognize that in the public sector, especially in the Medicaid arena, mental health services are generally significantly more expansive than in the private sector. For many years, the public sector has provided the care of last resort for many persons suffering from mental disorders. Generally, the community mental health system provided care as budgets have allowed, and during lean times community programs became increasingly creative as they strove to meet enormous patient needs. Perhaps more than in the private sector, the mind-set of the community mental health system is based on an *entitlement* orientation rather than on a *benefit* orientation.

Treatment in the public sector is rarely thought of as drawing down on an established and discrete set of benefits. A patient does not generally run out of benefits in the public sector. If something runs out, it is program support dollars, not individual benefits. Caseloads may suffer because the funds to support caseload activity are strained, but the suffering is spread throughout the caseload and is not differentially experienced by the high user. A patient in the private sector would use up his or her benefit insofar as in private sector managed care each person has a specified benefit as set forth by the plan in which the subscriber holds coverage.

The differences between public and private coverage of mental illnesses are enormously important. Over the years, the public mental health establishment has fought battle after battle to increase its funding sources. These battles have resulted in a kaleidoscope of reimbursable services in the public sector. When compared with the narrow benefits for mental illness in the private sector, it is easy to understand why the public sector fears that privatization through managed care will destroy this fragile and hard-won set of supportive and therapeutic services.

These problems highlight the fact that we need increasing specificity regarding benefits. One of the hallmarks of managed care is its use of explicit standards in management activities. If benefits or entitlements are not thoroughly delineated at the outset, then efforts to manage them will be marked by conflicts among managers, providers, patients, advocacy groups, subscribers, and payers. Given the issues of chronicity, serious mental illness, concomitant mental retardation, separate or coexisting substance abuse, legislatively mandated services, and other expectations, the need for up-front clarity is crucial. There is no reason that a partnership cannot be effective in the public sector if these requirements for explicitness are met.

Competing Government Agencies

The problem of jurisdictional control between state agencies is a difficult hurdle in the task of implementing managed care in the public sector. In Pennsylvania, Medicaid originates in the Department of Public Welfare. As the state attempts to move its recipients into managed care, it has contracted with various HMOs to provide comprehensive care (including mental health and substance abuse services) to Medicaid recipients. There is no coordination between Medicaid dollars and those dollars that come from the Department of Mental Health for the program support of seriously mentally ill individuals. A typical community mental health center will receive monies directly from Medicaid for fee-for-service activities provided to Medicaid recipients and program funds from the Office of Mental Health (OMH) for the treatment of patients who may or may not be Medicaid recipients. HMO Medicaid recipients may or may not have access to those program support dollars, and this access may be determined by the policy decisions of OMH administrators. Additionally, OMH falls ultimately under the jurisdiction of the Department of Public Welfare, whereas substance abuse activities fall under the Department of Health. This bifurcation between mental health and substance abuse funding further impedes the movement of both areas into comprehensive managed care programs such as HMOs.

Other states have other arrangements, but the general point is that managed care works best when there is single-stream funding for public sector mental health and substance abuse services. Where there is not such single-stream funding, as in Pennsylvania, the road to implementation requires the development of alliances or partnerships. Bringing the disparate agencies together through contractual arrangements with managed care companies could create the equivalent of single-stream funding and maximize managed care effectiveness (Taube et al. 1990).

Risk Assumption and the Disposition of Savings Dollars

After discovering a way to save money, the new irony is the concern now being expressed in many quarters about too much money being saved. When windfall profits are discovered, the natural first reaction is that these profits (savings) are the result of overaggressive management of utilization. However, the first questions to be answered are the questions about quality of care: Are savings the result of denying access to treatment? The result of inferior care? The result of an inappropriate interpretation of benefits?

If the savings occur and quality has been ensured, then concern is shifted toward the disposition of the savings. In the early years of transition from a traditional public sector strategy to a managed care strategy, windfall savings can occur. Many pricing strategies at the beginning of a managed care contract are based on the managed care organization's being paid some of the documented costs for the preceding year(s). If the managed care company receives 90% of the costs of a public sector population and if those costs occurred in a nonmanaged environment (as is likely), then the early savings can be quite impressive. These windfalls are likely to be short-lived, however, because subsequent negotiations between government and managed care organizations will start at a new baseline.

The same correction process should take place if there are losses that go beyond what might be considered reasonable. The risk component of such public sector contracts should be subject to either stop-loss insurance strategies or limited contract lengths (perhaps 1 year) or both so that price corrections can take place as new levels of utilization emerge over time. Long-term contracts become increasingly possible as the uncertainties about utilization rates are reduced.

A further issue emerges as the nonprofit public sector is confronted with managed care organizations that may be operating as for-profit companies. The idea of public sector savings going to shareholders is provocative. However, these concerns are all manageable if the payer and vendor cover all the potential outcomes in their negotiations and reach mutually acceptable terms. There could be an explicit shared risk arrangement between payer and vendor and therefore shared access to savings (profits). Savings could be returned to the delivery system for enhancements, or they could be returned to the general fund for overall budget relief. There is no reason that a for-profit company should prove to be less desirable than a nonprofit organization if the contract spells out mutually acceptable terms.

Prevention and Health Promotion

The prevention of disease and promotion of health have been largely the responsibility of public health advocates, most prominently government. Although there are many calls for the implementation of preventive practices, these calls tend to be largely rhetorical. The competition for scarce dollars has resulted in strong priorities for direct services to impaired persons. Although prevention and health promotion have a long-term salutary effect on health care costs, it is rare to see this long-term approach chosen, particularly if such a choice results in reduction in already strained direct care support. The potential of HMO-oriented managed care in the area of prevention is great. The original motivation for HMOs was largely based on the expectation that prevention and health promotion would play large roles. The financial rewards underlying the HMO encourage reduced utilization of care. The promise of the HMO was that it could effect such reduction by investing in prevention and health promotion. A countering charge is that this promise has been distorted. The charge is that utilization is being controlled and reduced by denying care, not by preventing disease.

The point is that there are strong financial incentives for managed care organizations to practice preventive medicine. The key is in the development of increasingly more sophisticated quality oversight systems that monitor managed care activities. These systems are already reshaping the practices of managed care companies; therefore, these traditional concerns of public health advocates can be incorporated into the practices of managed care companies.

Conclusion

There should only be one final bottom line to the management of public behavioral health care: Can managed care improve quality while reducing costs? The promise is that with an effective, open partnership with key public agencies, it can. The question cannot be answered through debate. Recent experience suggests that the promise can be fulfilled. The mental health and substance abuse areas of the public sector are complicated but not beyond the capacity of managed care. Innovative strategic partnerships between managed care companies and public organizations in partnership target areas can raise the outcome to exciting new levels. There is no blueprint that will work in all circumstances. Each county, each municipality, and each sector has its own peculiar forces to be addressed, but the promise is so compelling and the national attention is so riveted on managed competition that this process will not be stopped by parochial timidity or self-interest. Such a partnership approach takes advantage of what each stakeholder has to offer and allows for rapid and effective participation in the managed care marketplace. As experience warrants, I would expect that the public sector would also migrate to the fourth phase of managed care.

References

Christianson JB, Lurie N, Finch M, et al: Use of community-based mental health programs by HMOs: evidence from a Medicaid demonstration. Am J Public Health 82:790–796, 1992

Dangerfield D, Betit RL: Managed mental health care in the public sector, in Managed Mental Health Care. Edited by Goldman W, Feldman S. San Francisco, CA, Jossey-Bass, 1993, pp 67–80

Gerson SN: When should managed care firms terminate private benefits for chronically mentally ill patients? Behavioral Healthcare Tomorrow 3(2):31–35, 1994

Leadholm BA, Kerzner JP: Implementing a system of public managed care: the Massachusetts experience. Behavioral Healthcare Tomorrow 2(4):36–38, 1993

Mechanic D: Editorial: managed care for the seriously mentally ill. Am J Public Health 82:788–789, 1992

Panzetta AF: Whatever happened to community mental health: portents for corporate medicine. Hosp Community Psychiatry 36:1174–1179, 1985

Panzetta AF: For a public-private system partnership. Behavioral Healthcare Tomorrow 3(2):41–46, 1994

Taube CA, Goldman HH, Salkever D: Medicaid coverage for mental illness: balancing access and costs. Health Aff 9(1):5–18, 1990

Chapter 7

Will Academic Psychiatry Survive Managed Care?

Michelle B. Riba, M.D.
Thomas Carli, M.D.

At a recent department of psychiatry faculty meeting, it was announced that the department had just won its first managed care contract. Congratulations were bestowed on the head of the outpatient psychiatry clinic and the administrator, both of whom had spent much of their time in the past several weeks negotiating this contract. The clinic director had no previous experience negotiating this type of business deal but, by necessity, she learned how to do it quickly. Her other academic deadlines were necessarily put off during this time—writing manuscripts, implementing new pharmaceutical protocols, teaching, and so forth.

As the reality of the contract set in, questions arose regarding the number of covered lives, how many patients were currently in treatment, the preapproval process required by the managed care company, the multiple forms and treatment plan data that would be required, and an estimate of the number of participating faculty (residents could not bill unless a faculty member was directly involved in the treatment of the patient).

The department was already in the process of reorganizing care on the inpatient units because the residency program did not "match" and these units would soon be functioning with fewer trainees. The medical student education coordinator asked whether students' rotations would be affected by the contract and whether the contract was compatible with the medical school's mission to offer more outpatient experiences for third-year clerks. The researchers in the room were wondering whether this new arrangement would affect present and future clinical trials.

The full spectrum of issues regarding the managed care contract began to unfold quickly.

The resources required for this university department of psychiatry to be a successful competitor in the managed care world are directly related to its survival. In this chapter we provide an overview of some of the challenges, opportunities, and problems that await academic medical centers and departments of psychiatry in the era of managed care. Specific issues that we address include the transition from inpatient treatment to outpatient care, faculty morale and development, conducting and funding research, and educating and training medical students and residents.

Academic Medical Centers

The fate of academic psychiatry departments in the managed care arena is intimately tied to the fate of academic medical centers (AMCs) in the same environment. It is important to distinguish AMCs from teaching hospitals. There are 126 American medical schools. There are 61 university-owned teaching hospitals, and perhaps less than half of these can be considered research intensive. Most medical school education and postgraduate residency training takes place in nonuniversity public and private hospitals. Almost 20% of the hospitals in the United States manage at least one residency program (Iglehart 1993). In this chapter's discussion about academic psychiatry, the emphasis will be on the 61 university-owned teaching hospitals and their departments of psychiatry. The other public and private hospitals providing training programs in psychiatry will most likely share some, but not all, of the concerns of AMCs.

There are a number of differences that distinguish AMCs from other health care organizations. AMCs are located predominately in urban areas with populations of more than 1 million people (Iglehart 1993), yet they account for only 20% of the hospital beds; provide 50% of the uncompensated care in this country (Bulger 1993); and have markedly higher costs, less than half of which can be accounted for by the fact that they treat more severely ill patients (Iexxoni et al. 1990). However, higher costs, urban settings, and large amounts of uncompensated care are only a part of what distinguishes AMCs from other health care systems. The most important distinguishing feature is the requirement to balance the tripartite mission of providing education, research, and clinical services. Each of these areas is in the throes of enormous change. Changes in one area are often at odds with changes in the other. How these changes intersect, compete, and achieve synthesis will determine the fate of AMCs and their component parts, including departments of psychiatry.

If we begin by examining the changes in clinical service delivery that AMCs must confront, perhaps the most profound change is that they must now operate in a competitive marketplace. In the past, the steady flow of patients to an AMC could accommodate its tripartite mission. Even if there was a disproportionate share of indigent patients, occupancy rates were high, relatively long lengths of stay accommodated research and teaching, and patient referrals flowed in. As patterns of care have shifted from individuals to populations and *covered lives,* AMCs suddenly find themselves competing in the managed care marketplace with many other health care entities. Along with this competition, the traditionally superior attitude of some AMCs, the "Mecca-mentality," has been harshly challenged. One challenge has been to demonstrate that the high costs of AMCs are correlated with improved patient satisfaction and outcomes. A more fundamental challenge has been to demonstrate that teaching, research, and patient care must necessarily go together (Blumenthal and Meyer 1993). Clinical services within AMCs must now respond to the same forces affecting other health care institutions. A fundamental transformation of the very structure of AMCs is needed if they are to maintain clinical leadership in the new marketplace (Blumenthal and Meyer 1993). These changes in clinical service require briefer treatments with proven efficacy, a major shift from inpatient to outpatient care, and a heightened responsiveness to the needs of patients and purchasers of health care. This transformation of clinical services is bringing into sharp focus the tensions and conflicts that have been inherent in AMCs.

AMCs have traditionally required a cooperative alliance between the medical school and the teaching hospital. This historical alliance is being severely tested. The hospital director must now steer a massive, high-cost service delivery system into a streamlined, cost-efficient, and clinically coordinated integrated system of care. Medical school deans must increasingly fight for the preservation of teaching and research within that same newly integrated system. For example, should the new multimillion-dollar patient-friendly outpatient building accommodate students and clinical research? Both the medical school and hospital are also part of the larger system of the university, and the tensions within AMCs have not escaped the attention of university presidents and regents. AMCs are major sources of costs and revenues for universities. A financially viable AMC is of critical interest to these parent universities. As survival in the clinical marketplace becomes a question, financial bottom lines increasingly take priority over more academic interests.

Although AMCs are important primary care sites for indigent patients, the identity of AMCs has focused on the delivery of tertiary care. As health care reform prioritizes primary care, AMCs will be significantly affected. There are two responses to this change in priority. One is the reallocation of faculty positions from tenured track to primary care and clinical track. The other strategy is the development of networks between AMCs and other public and private hospital systems that have been more exclusively devoted to primary care. Both of these strategies involve a fundamental shift in the way academic medicine views itself. Specialty departments must downsize, a truly difficult task within the constraints of tenured positions and the lack of mandatory retirement age rules. The formal and informal caste system that has always placed physician-researchers above clinical-track faculty is being challenged and perhaps turned on its head. AMC specialists must now become the grateful and responsive recipients of referrals from primary care physicians in the community.

AMCs have traditionally been organized around specialties, with individual departments the equivalent of self-contained fiefdoms or principalities. Chairpersons of departments, chosen by and aligned with deans of medical schools, have often been uneasy partners with hospital administrators. Chairpersons are usually appointed because of success in research and other scholarly endeavors. Redesigning service delivery systems often conflicts with the values that elevated them to their positions. Like any other leader, chairpersons must fight for the survival of their organization or group. Yet AMCs cannot compete in the world of managed care with autonomous departments that answer only to deans. The decentralized structure of AMCs works reasonably well in a fee-for-service environment, but it is antithetical to a managed care world (Blumenthal and Meyer 1993). AMC faculty prefer to be "soloists," but health maintenance organizations (HMOs) seek "highly coordinated symphonies" (Wasserman and Fox 1993). When the direction of change is toward multispecialty groups providing care under programs or "product lines" such as primary care, cancer, geriatrics, women's health, and so on, what is the role of individual departments? It is possible that the days of departmental fiefdoms are coming to an end. The AMC of the future will need to have large, central clinical programs that have overarching control of numerous departments. Capitated funding will require that these new programs also be *cost centers* with commingling of funds that have traditionally been categorized along departmental lines.

The tensions inherent in AMCs also exist at the level of individual faculty members, who face the same forces that private practitioners face with respect to managed care and health care reform. In addition, the identity of academic physicians may be threatened more than that of their nonacademic counterparts. Although many academic physicians enjoy and perhaps even excel in providing clinical service, academic medicine was chosen because of its unique emphasis on research and the pursuit of knowledge linked to teaching. Are these activities compatible with an environment that increasingly emphasizes the primacy of clinical service delivery? Faculty members in many AMCs must now generate up to 80% of their salary either through clinical revenue or research funding. With research dollars harder to attain and service requirements consuming considerable time, what are the benefits of remaining in academia? This problem is a crisis for the group of junior physicians who are under the "tenure clock." They have 5 to 7 years to secure a research path, establish external funding, and publish 20 or more papers. With promotion committees still operating under rules, values, and reward systems that haven't adjusted to the clinical and fiscal urgencies of managed care, the survival of junior faculty may be precarious.

Although the discussion thus far has been about AMCs, the issues apply equally to departments of psychiatry within these centers. We now turn to the unique challenges facing academic psychiatry as well as to the unique resources we consider essential to meeting those challenges.

Departmental Strategies for Change

Psychiatry and mental health service delivery systems have, in many ways, been leaders in managed care. Psychiatry has been dealing with cost constraints, limited benefits, case management, utilization review, and capitation longer than many other specialties. Academic psychiatry departments, perhaps spurred by accounts of fellow departments that failed to make the managed care transition in a timely way, often have been leaders within AMCs in adapting to the new marketplace. It may not be coincidental that an increasing number of medical school deans and managed care executives are former chairpersons of psychiatry departments. Academic psychiatry departments are transforming themselves by becoming active and competitive forces in managed mental health care, and they are doing so in ways that capitalize on their unique skills and attributes.

Departments of psychiatry are actively "capturing populations." For example, some universities and AMCs have formed their own HMOs. The exact relationship between the department and the HMO's mental health carve-out program varies. Often the department and the managed care program are administratively and financially separate. Some faculty may work in both settings, and trainees may rotate for periods under the managed care program. The department's inpatient units and subspecialty programs are part of the HMO's closed panel of providers. Mostly, however, these parallel universes are kept separate. Fitting trainees into the HMO is often problematic for a number of reasons having to do with patient preference, lack of experience in time-limited treatments, and costly teaching time. Many departmental faculty members are too research focused or subspecialized to fit into a managed care setting. Moreover, it is not desirable to include every faculty member in managed care activities.

This parallel relationship between the academic department and HMO is a compromise solution and a way to balance competing values and priorities. It also allows for the growth of the HMO staff (as more patient groups are added) during a time when academic departments are largely in a no-growth financial position. The disadvantage of this type of parallel arrangement is that it can foster an illusion that the department can carry on business as usual and that major changes in service delivery that managed care requires are in the province of the HMO. It may be best to view this parallel arrangement between departments and the HMO as an interim solution or hybrid attempt that will give way to more integrated models in the near future.

Another way that departments of psychiatry are capturing populations is through direct or strategic contracting as part of a larger medical center contract or directly between the department and purchaser of care. The majority of care is often provided by the department, perhaps using its separate managed care program. A major innovation of this model involves proposals to place the department "further up the food chain" and have the academic department manage a network of providers, some internal and many external to the department. Clearly, managing the network allows the department to set the clinical standards and make a profit. The unique ability of academic psychiatry departments to provide state-of-the-art diagnosis and delineate treatment guidelines makes this pivotal role in managing a network of providers very attractive. The network could include courtesy faculty (who in return for trainee supervision benefit by being on a closed panel of providers), or it could include other mental health service systems throughout the region or even the state. This model of developing networks promises to be a major vehicle for AMCs and departments of psychiatry and is in line with the larger business patterns of "growing and shrinking at the same time" and "collaborating with competitors" (Naisbitt 1993).

Competing for mental health contracts in the current health care environment is not easy for academic departments. However, there are two relatively neglected areas that show promise. One area is the public sector. AMCs have traditionally served the Medicaid and Medicare populations disproportionately compared with nonacademic settings. State governments often have a large investment in general funds to AMCs. As states move to managed Medicaid, AMCs become an important potential provider (Hillman et al. 1991). The interest and expertise of academic departments of psychiatry in treating severely mentally ill patients (both child and adult) makes them especially attractive to managed Medicaid planners. Contracts between psychiatry departments and community mental health centers will take on increasing importance. It may be the only way these departments can keep their beds filled. The academic–public sector alliance is thus seen as a key strategy for survival.

A second and frequently neglected area of networking for psychiatry departments is surprisingly close at hand—the medical center itself. The largest pool of potential patients for psychiatry departments is actually those patients currently being seen in other medical and surgical programs in the medical center. Most academic departments of psychiatry, with the exception of their usually small inpatient consultation-liaison programs, have historically neglected the mental health needs of patients in the medical center at large. Some medical departments have responded by hiring their own behavioral psychologists and social workers to meet those needs. Assuming that the larger AMC system secures managed care contracts, serving the mental health and psychiatric needs of these medical and surgical patients is potentially the largest source of patient flow for departments of psychiatry. Here, too, the network model can be used. In addition to reallocating resources of the psychiatry department so that more faculty and more of its services are targeted to the medical center, the existing providers of mental health care in the medical center who are outside the psychiatry department (such as social workers) can be included in the closed panel of providers. If and when AMCs move to large cost center programs and deemphasize the role of individual departments as discussed above, then departments of psychiatry would be uniquely positioned to become mental health and substance abuse providers for entire medical centers. The organizing umbrella program for this arrangement could be the outpatient consultation-liaison psychiatry service (Gonzales 1993).

Clinical Services

It is not sufficient for departments of psychiatry to capture populations and win contracts. No matter how far up the food chain their networking takes them, they still must deliver clinical care and to deliver that care will involve a massive transformation of the way services are organized. The shift from predominately inpatient care to outpatient care is reshaping all service systems. In academic psychiatry, it means additionally that the former site of most research activity and the dominant site of training is becoming less able to accommodate these needs. Many of today's academic psychiatrists were trained at a time when patients could be evaluated drug free for the first 2 weeks of inpatient treatment. They also learned the fundamentals of psychodynamic psychotherapy with patients who may have been treated on the inpatient unit for 6 months or longer. With average lengths of stay now less than 2 weeks and continuing to decrease, it seems clear that research and education must move to outpatient settings. The key elements to service restructuring involve rapid access to evaluation and treatment and the development of a continuum of care ranging from inpatient programs to standard outpatient and long-term maintenance therapy.

Although these basic ingredients of the new service system are difficult for every provider organization to implement, it is especially problematic in academia. Even if the wake-up call has been heard loud and clear, changing service systems is a slow and tedious process. No matter how powerful and convincing the leader, rapid change is anathema to academia. Balancing this relative inertia are some unique strengths of academic psychiatry that bode well for its ability to move ahead. One major strength is its central leadership role in defining standards of treatment and differential therapeutics. A related strength is the ability of psychiatry departments to do meaningful outcomes research.

One additional impediment to redesigning service systems in academic psychiatry merits special consideration. It is probably impossible for a faculty member to gain tenure by an exclusive focus on general psychiatry, particularly in research-intensive departments. Currently, subspecialization is the rule. Yet managed care systems require a strong primary care presence (i.e., primary mental health care or general psychiatry). It is therefore likely that departments of the future will consider strategically positioning non–tenure-track or clinical faculty in these general programs (as well as perhaps the intensive care inpatient units).

Even if academic psychiatry departments have the courage and wisdom to transform their service delivery systems to fit the paradigm of new managed care and even if they are able to gather managed care contracts, their survival is still not guaranteed. The other two components of the tripartite academic mission—research and education—are also undergoing fundamental changes that require new adaptations for survival.

Research

The clinical investigator in academic medicine is an example of an endangered species (Wyngaarden 1979). Funding for research is becoming much more difficult to obtain. In 1975, 40% of new investigator-initiated applications to the

National Institutes of Health (NIH) were funded. In 1990, that rate had dropped to 14.2% (Cadman 1994). Resubmitted grant applications had a success rate of 70% in 1975 but only 35% in 1990 (Cadman 1994). It is estimated that an investigator must submit six grant applications to get one funded and that obtaining stable funding from NIH requires writing a grant application every 8 months (Cadman 1994). During the past 20 years federal support for health research as a percentage of national health care expenditures has dropped by more than one-half (DeBakey 1993).

Shrinking research dollars and increasing competition for existing dollars are only part of the academic psychiatrist's problems. Two other factors are relevant. Academic psychiatrists must spend more time in service delivery. In the 1960s, 40% of a medical school's revenues came from research. In 1990 this percentage was only 17%. At the same time, medical school revenues from clinical service have grown from 15.6% in 1980 to between 30% (Cadman 1994) and 45% (DeBakey 1993) currently. Generating salary, especially that portion defined as *incentive* under faculty practice plans, takes up an increasing part of faculty members' work week. Research time, still the key to tenure-track survival, must be guarded with a vengeance.

As if shrinking dollars and increasing requirements for clinical service were not enough, the academic psychiatrist is also buffeted by a major change in the ground rules of what is fundable research. The majority of research-intensive psychiatry departments have focused on either molecular psychiatry (psychobiology) or descriptive and epidemiological research. Americans and the federal government are now calling for outcomes research. Pressure to conduct research on outcomes management (Ellwood 1988) is causing changes in funding patterns. The National Institute of Mental Health, the National Institute on Drug Abuse, and the National Institute on Alcohol Abuse and Alcoholism must now devote up to 15% of their total budgets to services research (American Psychiatric Association 1993). The Agency for Health Care Policy and Research has become a major funding source, and although no one doubts the need for outcomes research in all fields of medicine, there is a serious paucity of trained researchers in medicine. With so few mentors, junior tenure-track faculty are reluctant to retool their research trajectory in the limited years they are allotted. Senior tenured faculty would have to make a major shift in their area of research interests. Changes in funding sources, however, do have a powerful way of shaping research foci. This pressure, coupled with academic psychiatry's past expertise in the area of clinical trials, strongly suggests that the research mission of the future will be in outcomes and services research. With that shift, we will see less discrepancy between the molecular psychiatrist's research and his or her clinical duties. Health care reform will be closely followed by *managed scholarship* (Huxtable 1994).

Education and Training

Many of the important issues concerning graduate and postgraduate psychiatric education are related to economics and the health care reform movement (Borus 1994). At the 1994 annual meetings of some of the leading educational groups, such themes as "Maintaining Educational Quality in a Changing Environment" (American Association of Directors of Psychiatric Residency Training) and "Enhancing Professional Development in a Time of Change" (Association for Academic Psychiatry) reflected this concern. At the same time, options for maintaining programmatic control over educational and professional endeavors were explored.

The decreasing number of American-trained medical students who are choosing psychiatry as a career (Weissman et al. 1994) has evoked much consternation. In the 1994 resident match, internal medicine, pediatrics, and family practice all had a higher proportion of positions filled by United States graduates compared with 1993 and with 1990, whereas psychiatry recruitment continued to decline compared with 1993 and with 1990.

Although there is not a clear or direct correlation between decreased recruitment of medical students into psychiatry and the increased presence of managed care, one must wonder whether rapid changes in the field of psychiatry and problems associated with those changes have affected the teaching of medical students and their views about psychiatry. Dr. Alan Nelson, executive vice president of the American Society of Internal Medicine, attributed part of the increased recruitment into internal medicine to managed care. He stated, "U.S. medical students may be more interested in internal medicine partly because word is out that managed care companies are starting to pay internists higher beginning salaries" (Parker 1994, p. 1). Managed care emphasizes cost and efficiency and it affects the quality of care (Gabbard 1992; Tischler 1990). Managed care also intrudes on the physician-patient relationship (Sabin 1991). Educators have noted that financial realities impinge on the delivery of clinical care and that different types of care have actually been provided for similar patients, often as a function of financial considerations. Observations such as those cause much consternation for trainees (Lewis and Blotcky 1993) and may have a negative effect on medical students' feelings about psychiatry. Although vacant residency slots are currently being filled by international medical graduates, the nature of what we teach medical students, the types of clinical sites that serve as teaching experiences, and the future of residency programs vis à vis recruitment difficulties are all critically important (Weissman 1993).

Funding sources for psychiatry residency positions are also changing. Historically, postgraduate medical education has been subsidized through a variety of mechanisms involving cost distributions between public and private health insurance plans that financed the care of insured patients (Tasman and Riba 1993). This pattern of reimbursement has changed in the past decade (Department of Health and Human Services 1986; Relman 1984; Schwartz et al. 1985), and most residency programs are no longer able to completely cover direct and indirect costs of resident stipends through traditional reimbursement mechanisms. Because AMCs and their teaching hospitals continue to care for a high percentage of indigent and uninsured patients, and reductions in Medicare, Medicaid, and managed care reimbursements have contributed to decreasing revenues, paying residents' stipends has become an increasingly serious problem. To deal with such financial conundrums, the Association of American Medical Colleges (AAMC) has advocated a redraft of the section of the Health Security Act dealing with academic health centers. The AAMC advocates the creation of two all-payer funds; one fund would be allocated for medical schools, and the other fund would be earmarked for teaching hospitals. In this way, AMCs can compete more effectively in a managed care environment.

Apart from recruitment and reimbursement issues, changes in the generalist to specialist mix have been proposed in the 1994 Council on Graduate Medical Education (COGME) Fourth Report to Congress, ostensibly to improve access to health care (S. H. Weissman, memo to American Association of Directors of Psychiatric Residency Training, February 24, 1994). COGME has proposed changes in the generalist to specialist ratio so that 50% of all physicians will train and practice in the primary care fields of general internal medicine, pediatrics, and family practice. First-year residency positions would be limited to 110% of United States medical graduates. Medical school consortia would be established, including all teaching hospitals with graduate medical education programs. These consortia would be tasked so that 50% of their resident graduates would be in primary care. Finally, an all-payer pool would be established to fund graduate medical education using a surcharge on all health insurance as well as funding from Medicare direct payments. Other proposals suggest including obstetrics-gynecology in the group of primary care fields and varying the ratio of generalists to specialists. Those proposals, if enacted, could further decrease the total number of psychiatry residency positions and limit the number of international medical graduates eligible to train in psychiatry.

In view of the increased emphasis being placed on primary care, psychiatric educators are rethinking the future of psychiatry and psychiatric training (Meyer 1993). Gabbard (1992) expressed concern that the transition from residency to practice may be a "nightmare" because of inadequate education and residency training in managed care principles. Gabbard (1992) referred to this fate as "the big chill." He believed the dysphoria and demoralization that many residents experience upon graduating from residency can be traced to the anticipation of entering managed care systems. In reply, Sabin (1993) commented that residents are not being properly prepared for postresidency practice because academic psychiatrists are "morally myopic" when it comes to teaching residents managed care principles. Instead of focusing on the treatment of single patients, Sabin (1993) suggested that we think in terms of patient populations and patients who may need treatment but are not currently receiving it. Then we must determine how to most effectively use our limited resources.

Another problem related to education and training is that faculty educators are often rewarded for scholarship and research activities rather than for clinical and teaching abilities (Creditor 1993). Although most of the faculty are obligated to generate income either through research grants or clinical care, and most have teaching requirements as well, what is often valued by promotions committees and in tenure-track pathways are published peer-reviewed manuscripts, a national reputation in a specific area of expertise, and ownership of research grants. Furthermore, many faculty members were not trained or supervised in managed care systems and therefore may not be ideal candidates to teach the managed care process to medical students and residents. In Chapter 26, O'Connor asks, "Who will manage the managers?" We ask, "Who will supervise the supervisors?" (see Chapter 17).

A Faculty Development

To deal effectively with the evolving changes wrought by managed care, approaches must be multipronged and flexible. The following are general suggestions that faculty may find valuable in an attempt to keep pace with the demands of managed care.

Most faculty members probably already have some experience in managed care. However, they may be ill equipped by training or by personal value systems to convey some of the positive aspects and opportunities that exist in managed care systems. Even worse, they may convey negativism, demoralization, and disgust for managed care based on negative experiences in their own practice. At the very least, the faculty should be educated about the tenets of managed care and shown how to teach responsible managed care to residents and students (Sabin 1993). Managed care organizations may play a vital role in this process by serving as consultants to AMCs.

Faculty members need to receive personal counseling about their careers and to be told about the likelihood of promotion. It is extraordinarily difficult to feel positive about the field of psychiatry and about the care of patients if one's own position in the department is uncertain.

It is important for departments of psychiatry to respond to managed care proposals and win contracts that generate income. Departments must reward clinicians who provide excellent care and are willing to do managed care work. Being an excellent provider of managed care services cannot be an add-on to writing articles, lecturing, and trying to establish a national expertise. It has to stand on its own merit and be equal to or even more important than other missions and goals of the department. If such status is not achieved, the number of medical students choosing psychiatry will continue to decline, residents will continue to be unprepared on graduation, junior faculty members will continue to feel they will not survive the tenure-track promotion system, and the faculty will continue to feel demoralized (Lewis and Blotcky 1993).

The Psychiatrist of the Future

What will the psychiatrist of the future be doing? The answer to that question is critical given that academic psychiatrists will have primary responsibility for training future psychiatrists. Psychiatry has not been declared a primary care specialty. Nevertheless, will tomorrow's psychiatrists increasingly watch over their patients' medical ailments? The forces in favor of subspecialization in psychiatry appear to have quieted down. Might that imply that the value of specialization in psychiatry is being rethought so psychiatrists can position themselves closer to primary care physicians?

The didactic curriculum and clinical sites developed for medical students and residents must be reviewed and possibly revamped as the psychiatrist of the future is further defined. As treatment becomes short term, we must somehow build opportunities for trainees to have long-term relationships with patients and families. These opportunities will increasingly be found only in outpatient settings. For medical students, perhaps a 4- to 6-week clerkship is not optimal. Rather, a longitudinal clerkship over several months would enable students to observe treatment over a longer time, not just a snapshot in time.

If residents only treat patients for brief inpatient stays, then different ways to supervise them must be developed (Riba and Tasman 1993). Changes in the way supervision is done in an inpatient setting may help; however, it is becoming obvious that trainees must have long-term outpatient care as part of their clinical experience. In addition, teaching rounds, a mainstay of supervising residents on inpatient units, may need to be modified so that rounds take place perhaps twice a day, in the morning and afternoon. Weekend rounds, especially on Sundays, may also need to be instituted, an event that doesn't often take place in academic teaching hospitals. One has to be careful about adding clinical duties that do not contribute significantly to clinical care, because these additional duties can increase the cost of care.

Finally, as we place trainees in ambulatory sites off campus, what effect will this have on supervisors' time and income? Teaching medical students often imposes a substantial burden on private practitioners (Vinson and Paden 1994). Among primary care physicians in a HMO, adding teaching responsibilities decreased self-reported productivity and increased time at work (Kirz and Larsen 1986). Pawlson et al. (1989) determined that teaching a third-year medical student cost a private practice between $30 and $82 per student per day. In psychiatry, as the locus of treatment between inpatient and outpatient sites is redistributed, the impact of supervisory time and cost will have to be factored into the equation. New ways to pay for these expenses will have to be created.

Clinical Experiences in Managed Care Settings

There has been a definite ambivalence in sending medical students and residents to HMOs and other managed care settings for learning experiences. Educators have noted that managed care creates a "less predictable and secure environment for treatment," with reimbursement forcing clinicians to focus on symptoms and quick solutions rather than on complex and more interesting psychodynamic problems (Lewis and Blotcky 1993, p. 186). Why then would educators want to have trainees rotate in such environments?

There are many advantages for trainees; they may be initially uncomfortable but, with supervision, are able to learn and grow in managed care treatment settings. Because of the rapid turnover of patients in managed care settings, trainees have increased experience with initial evaluations and termination of treatment (Blackwell and Schmidt 1992). They are forced to define treatment goals and develop strong treatment plans to foster therapeutic success. HMOs often place a premium on providing continuity of care and integration of services (Blackwell and Schmidt 1992), both of which are difficult to teach in AMCs, where it is often impossible for house staff and students to follow patients from one setting to another. Because managed care emphasizes outpatient treatment, many medical schools are trying to shift clinical experiences to outpatient settings. Managed care settings offer many opportunities for teaching outpatient psychiatry. Finally, assigning residents to managed care clinical settings during training would obviate some of the problems described by Gabbard (1992), thus avoiding "the big chill" upon graduation.

Educators, especially medical student and residency training directors, need to establish alliances in the community where trainees are welcomed. Education of the staff at managed care settings is necessary to help map out the curriculum, provide supervision and oversight, and determine clinical responsibilities. Even mundane issues such as travel time for trainees, parking arrangements, and contractual agreements need to be operationalized. Establishing partnerships between departments of psychiatry and managed care entities may be difficult, but there is a growing literature indicating that it can be accomplished (Fox and Wasserman 1993; Kirz and Larsen 1986; Lewis and Blotcky 1993).

Making the Transition

A forgotten maxim is that trainees generally do best when there is minimal turmoil and chaos around them. Transitions and changes in the educational process must be thoughtful and well planned. Too often, educators are unaware of significant impending clinical and financial changes in a department that will directly affect training. With multiple missions in a department and multiple personnel, it is no wonder that a domino effect is created as a change in one problem area leads to a similar or worse problem down the line. Very often it is hard to anticipate the impact of institutional changes on trainees. If teaching faculty are not in the decision-making loop when important policies are made, they are likely to feel a loss of control and transmit feelings of demoralization to residents.

It becomes obvious, then, that changes that occur because of or related to managed care have to be carefully planned, and the potential impact of these changes on trainees must be constantly reassessed. The psychiatry department must be flexible and adopt plans to minimize the impact of managed care on trainees and have options or fall-back positions if the changes aren't beneficial.

Conclusion

Without a crystal ball or a psychic, it is certainly hard to predict the future. It is probably a safe bet, however, that academic psychiatry departments will survive managed care. It may be that only those departments housed within strong, visionary, and fiscally sound academic medical centers will be stable and secure. Greater integration and collaboration between departments of psychiatry and the medical community at large will be the primary mechanism of survival.

Improving the quality of care and access to treatment while contending with decreasing funding sources seems almost impossible. Yet patients need clinical care, medical students and residents require excellent supervision and sound clinical experiences, and multiple questions in the behavioral sciences require careful research. Sharpening the goals of treatment and evaluating treatment outcomes will help guide the utilization of resources and modify treatment based on reliable data. The training of medical students and residents must be clinically correlated with employment opportunities following graduation. Emphasis on ambulatory sites for students and residents makes sense if outpatient practice will be the focus of activity in the future.

Faculty members must be rewarded for their actual work as determined by the needs of the AMC in relation to its managed care book of business. Educating faculty members about new methods of service delivery and helping them adjust their research and clinical interests to managed care initiatives are also necessary for survival.

There is no simple road map for departments of psychiatry to follow in these changing times. A flexible and positive attitude toward managed care will no doubt be helpful. Strategies for success are multiple and varied. The challenge is to preserve the identity of academic departments of psychiatry, the education and training of medical students and residents, the research endeavors of investigators, and the clinical care of patients. Managed care will move psychiatry departments in the direction of rethinking and reshaping how these multiple and sometimes conflicting goals are achieved.

References

American Psychiatric Association Office of Research: Psychiatric Research Report, Vol. 8, No. 3. Washington, DC, American Psychiatric Association, September 1993

Blackwell B, Schmidt GL: The educational implications of managed health care. Hosp Community Psychiatry 43:962–964, 1992

Blumenthal D, Meyer G: The future of the academic medical center under health care reform. N Engl J Med 329:1812–1814, 1993

Borus JF: Economics and psychiatric education: the irresistible force meets the moveable object. Harvard Review of Psychiatry 2:15–21, 1994

Bulger RJ: Using academic health centers to help avoid health care's next crisis. JAMA 269:2548–2549, 1993

Cadman ED: The academic physician-investigator: a crisis not to be ignored. Ann Intern Med 120:401–410, 1994

Creditor MC: Medical education and health care reform. The Pharos 56(4):2–5, 1993

DeBakey M: Medical centers of excellence and health reform. Science 262:523–528, 1993

Department of Health and Human Services: Study of the Financing of Graduate Medical Education. Washington, DC, US Department of Health and Human Services, 1986

Ellwood P: Outcomes management: a technology of patient experience. N Engl J Med 318:1549–1556, 1988

Fox PD, Wasserman J: Academic medical centers and managed care: uneasy partners. Health Aff 12:85–93, 1993

Gabbard GO: The big chill: the transition from residency to managed care nightmare. Acad Psychiatry 16:119–126, 1992

Gonzales JJ: Outpatient consultation-liaison psychiatry: an unfilled promise? Gen Hosp Psychiatry 15:360–362, 1993

Hillman AL, Goldfarb N, Eisenberg JM, et al: An academic medical center's experience with mandatory managed care for Medicaid recipients. Acad Med 66:134–138, 1991

Huxtable R: Ne'er the twain shall meet. Nature 368:370–371, 1994

Iexxoni L, Schwartz M, Moskowitz M, et al: Illness severity and costs of admissions at teaching and nonteaching hospitals. JAMA 264:1426–1431, 1990

Iglehart T: The American health care system: teaching hospitals. N Engl J Med 329:1052–1056, 1993

Kirz HL, Larsen D: Costs and benefits of medical student training to a health maintenance organization. JAMA 256:734–739, 1986

Lewis JM, Blotcky MJ: Living and learning with managed care. Academic Psychiatry 17:186–193, 1993

Meyer RE: The economics of survival for academic psychiatry. Academic Psychiatry 17:149–159, 1993

Naisbitt, J: Global Paradox. New York, William Morrow & Co, 1993

Parker S: Match day '94: encouraging news for internal medicine. Internal Medicine News, April 1994, pp 1,8

Pawlson LG, Watkins R, Donaldson M: The cost of medical student instruction in the practice setting. J Fam Pract 10:847–852, 1989

Relman AS: Who will pay for medical education in our teaching hospitals? Science 226:20–23, 1984

Riba M, Tasman A: Residency training in psychotherapy on acute inpatient treatment services, in Less Time To Do More: Psychotherapy on the Short-Term Inpatient Unit. Edited by Leibenluft E, Tasman A, Green S, Washington, DC, American Psychiatric Press, 1993, pp 287–302

Sabin JE: The therapeutic alliance in managed care mental health practice. The Journal of Psychotherapy Practice and Research 1:29–36, 1991

Sabin JE: The moral myopia of academic psychiatry: a response to Glen O. Gabbard's "The big chill." Academic Psychiatry 17:175–179, 1993

Schwartz WB, Newhouse JP, Williams AP: Is the teaching hospital an endangered species? N Engl J Med 313:157–162, 1985

Tasman A, Riba M: Strategic issues for the successful merger of residency training programs. Hosp Community Psychiatry 44:981–985, 1993

Tischler GL: Utilization management and the quality of care. Hosp Community Psychiatry 41:1099–1102, 1990

Vinson DC, Paden C: The effect of teaching medical students on private practitioner's workloads. Acad Med 69:237–238, 1994

Weissman SH: Recommendations from the May 1992 conference to enhance recruitment of U.S. medical graduates into psychiatry. Academic Psychiatry 17:180–185, 1993

Weissman SH, Haynes RA, Killian C, et al: A model to determine the influence of medical school on students' career choices: psychiatry, a case study. Acad Med 69:58–59, 1994

Wyngaarden JB: The clinical investigator as an endangered species. N Engl J Med 301:1254–1259, 1979

Chapter 8

How Is Resistance to Managed Care Manifested?

Arthur Lazarus, M.D.

Managed care has been heavily promoted as a solution to the health care crisis in the United States. The impact of managed care on psychiatric treatment, in particular, has had significant implications. A survey of authorities cited managed care as one of the major forces shaping clinical practice in the field of mental health (Fazzi 1990). Several hundred organizations currently offer some form of managed mental health care, and about 50% of health maintenance organizations (HMOs) have contracted their mental health and substance abuse benefits to one of these organizations (Oss 1993). It has been estimated that managed care could soon account for half of all physicians' revenues (Solomon 1993) and be responsible for the closing of half of all U.S. hospitals by 2000.

Psychiatrists working in managed care systems have had to change their practice to accommodate increased information sharing, cultivate new relationships, and find new ways to cooperate. Rather than fight managed care, as many psychiatrists have done, former president of the American Psychiatric Association (APA) Paul J. Fink recommends, "Managed care is not the enemy—it is too late for that" (Wagner and Gartner 1993, p. 20).

However, early in the evolution of managed care, many psychiatrists appeared to resist practicing in a "managed" environment. Various managed care "abuses" were alleged, and in 1990 the APA began publishing a toll-free telephone hot line in *Psychiatric News* for the expressed purpose of "gather[ing] documented reports of patients harmed or put in jeopardy by managed care review decisions [and] countering some managed care organizations' arbitrary and capricious methods" (American Psychiatric Association 1990, p. 9).

An average of 200 calls per month were received by APA (1993b), and a summary of members' complaints was forwarded to President Clinton. Terms such as *managed chaos* and *minimized care*, singularly critical of managed care, appeared in trade newspapers. In 1994, the APA Assembly and Board of Trustees voted to expand its attack on managed care and to back litigation over managed care abuses. Advice to make the best of managed care has not been welcomed by the majority of the profession (Sherman 1991).

It is disconcerting that the managed care industry was criticized by APA while relatively little attention was given to well-recognized and documented transgressions in the public and private sectors. In fact, many abuses in the private domain preceded those in the managed care sector and ushered in an era of cost containment (Jellinek and Nurcombe 1993).

One psychiatrist commented: "It seems . . . that APA has pointed an unnecessarily unfriendly finger at managed care as a latter day 'evil empire'" (Moldawsky 1993, p. 16). Another psychiatrist (Prest 1992, p. 19), questioning the APA's continued publication of the toll-free telephone number, stated, "There is not, and I think never has been, a similar solicitation for information about providers. Does APA wish to have information about such practices as the Southern California hospitals (among others) that advertise in the Midwest and East for their weight-reduction programs, provide airfare for patients, and bill the insurance company for depression? Or about physicians who report suicidal ideation to reviewers, but do not make a chart note or order suicide precautions? If APA's concern were for the profession and the patient, I think such information would be solicited, compiled, and used as the basis for corrective action."

In 1992, the wording of the managed care "box" in *Psychiatric News* was changed to request information about successes as well as failures. Although some psychiatrists viewed this development as positive, others have remained skeptical of APA. Skeptics feel that the amended wording was a backhanded attempt to appease APA members who are heavily invested in managed care practice. Members practicing in managed care settings believe APA has failed to represent *their* interests in managed care. As a result, psychiatrists practicing in managed care firms and well-established HMOs have become increasingly alienated and disenfranchised from APA (Delmar 1991).

The majority of psychiatrists, however, have reacted negatively to managed care. Their complaints have centered on the intrusion of managed care into their professional roles. Psychiatrists are upset because they are frequently being second-guessed by faceless (and often nameless) insurance reviewers. Increased administrative burdens are being placed on them without any remuneration or obvious benefit. In essence, they claim that managed care has compromised their autonomy and their ability to advocate for patients.

Consequently, resistance to managed care has emerged in many areas throughout the United States. Examples of resistance include verbally abusing utilization reviewers, involving patients and families in insurance disputes, referring medically unstable patients into provider networks, failing to comply with managed care procedures, and targeting managed care firms for litigation. Rarely has this type of behavior been reported, however.

Verbally Abusing Utilization Reviewers

Psychiatrists who conduct utilization reviews may be verbally abused. Verbal abuse usually occurs during telephonic utilization review, typically after a denial of care is made by the reviewing psychiatrist, or merely because the attending psychiatrist was subjected to review, even when no denial occurs. In an effort to justify the need for continued care for his or her patient, the attending psychiatrist may raise his or her voice, shout, make insulting or rude remarks, or use offensive language. Some psychiatrists may become suspicious and tape record the review or threaten to report the reviewing psychiatrist to the state medical board, insurance commissioner, or professional society. In some instances, the attending psychiatrist will demand to know the name of the reviewing psychiatrist to give to the patient's family, presumably to exert further pressure to persuade the reviewing psychiatrist to certify treatment or reverse a denial.

Gabbard et al. (1991) described this form of alliance between the treatment team and the family against the insurance company as follows: "In many cases the insurance company has contractually agreed to a much higher level of benefits than they are actually willing to contribute to *an extended hospitalization* [emphasis added]. The family members involved may be forced to file a lawsuit against the insurance company to get the coverage that they have been guaranteed. (In describing this development, we do not mean to imply that the necessity of suing the insurance company for benefits is a pathological event. Families may be forced into this situation when they are denied benefits they have been promised.)" (pp. 321–322).

Reviewing psychiatrists, unlike most families, perceive an insurance benefit as an eligibility for treatment rather than an entitlement. They authorize benefits based on medical necessity, usually as defined in their company's utilization review criteria. Utilization review disputes can often be traced to differences in the way providers, patients, and utilization reviewers interpret these criteria and "protect" insurance benefits.

Case 1

A 63-year-old woman was psychiatrically hospitalized for an acute exacerbation of bipolar disorder. While she was hospitalized, the patient's progress was reviewed by a utilization review nurse in the hospital and a managed care nurse reviewer. After 2 weeks of hospitalization, the managed care nurse questioned certain aspects of the patient's treatment that could not be adequately answered by the hospital's nurse. Subsequently, a board-certified psychiatrist employed by the managed care firm was asked to discuss the case directly with the attending psychiatrist.

Several phone calls were made to the attending psychiatrist, but none were answered. When the attending psychiatrist was finally contacted, 2 weeks had elapsed and had not been certified for treatment. The attending psychiatrist, who had previously undergone reviews with the managed care firm, acted as if he were completely unaware of the rationale for the review. The managed care psychiatrist was put in a position of explaining a procedure with which the attending psychiatrist was already familiar.

As clinical information was exchanged, the attending psychiatrist became more irritated. He gave truncated responses to questions, precluding the reviewing psychiatrist from making independent assessments and judgments. For example, when the reviewing psychiatrist asked whether there were any vegetative disturbances of depression, the attending psychiatrist snapped, "I told you she was depressed and suicidal, what else do you need to know?"

On the basis of the scant information provided, the reviewing psychiatrist only certified the previous 2 weeks and informed the attending psychiatrist that another review would be necessary in 10 days. The attending psychiatrist objected and exclaimed, "Are you functioning like a clerk or a clinician?" The reviewing psychiatrist replied that his decision was based on clinical data as well as criteria established by the managed care company. The conversation was terminated after the attending psychiatrist begrudgingly consented to another review.

The course of utilization review described here is typical of the resistance that may be encountered by reviewing psychiatrists. The resistance is manifested in initial passivity and often gives way to open hostility. This type of exchange exemplifies what Olsson (1993) termed "our deepening crisis in collegiality" (p. 7). He observed, "One would think we favor consensual validation and cooperation, but far too often this is not the case. We seem to isolate ourselves into treasured theoretical camps and exude haughty omnipotence or muster defensiveness toward each other. We polarize ourselves by boycotting our own professional meetings, fostering divisive intragroup politics, and threatening suits against each other when ethical complaints are pursued, even in appropriate and open ways. These actions only serve to divide us further and make our profession more vulnerable."

The proliferation of managed care has created special challenges for physicians and patients. Schroeder et al. (1985) pointed out that both physicians and patients may feel trapped by managed care policies and must therefore rely on new or different strategies to reach sometimes divergent objectives. Managed care may change the physician-patient relationship in ways that neither likes. Under these circumstances, frustration on the part of the physician may easily turn into anger against the managed care psychiatrist. Gabbard et al. (1991) observed that the more adversarial and irrational the review process becomes, the more likely it is to interfere with treatment and, paradoxically, prolong hospitalization.

Involving Patients and Families in Insurance Disputes

Involving patients and families in insurance disputes is a form of protest that also represents resistance to managed care. Protesting appears to be a common strategy for dealing with disputed utilization review decisions instead of appealing adverse decisions by requesting a second opinion (Hall 1994).

One physician (Whittaker 1992) wrote, "I have recently started to refuse to speak with any representative of an insurance company unless the patient or a patient surrogate (family member, for example) is simultaneously on the line. This has served the . . . purpose of incorporating the patient into such decisions. I intend to continue this practice and urge my colleagues to consider it also" (p. 3434).

A psychiatrist (Drake 1992) wrote, "As an experiment, I have changed the way I operate with managed care companies . . . in an attempt to get the process of dialogue, conflict, and decision making back where it belongs—between the insured patient and his or her insurance company" (p. 18).

I believe that strategy may be self-serving, poorly thought out, and ultimately deleterious to patient care. It is cruel to lead patients and families into assaults against utilization reviewers, gatekeepers, or administrators of the managed care process. The attending psychiatrist must serve as an advocate for patients in these situations rather than passively watch them struggle with a process they may not understand. The patient's anxiety may be heightened as a result of the uncertainty of whether treatment will be reimbursed, leading to intensification of preexisting psychopathology and actual decompensation.

Case 2

A 52-year-old man was suffering from depression marked by anergia, excessive sleep, severe dysphoria, and auditory hallucinations directing him to kill himself. He rented a motel room with the intent of overdosing on medication. The patient also left a suicide note, but he never followed through with his plan. Instead, he telephoned his son, who arranged for psychiatric hospitalization.

After 1 week, the patient began to improve, and the auditory hallucinations had nearly remitted. Approval for additional hospitalization depended on the outcome of a chart review following the patient's discharge from the hospital. A social worker erroneously notified the patient that no further hospitalization could be certified. He became sad and withdrawn and was uncomfortable with the thought of leaving the hospital. Nevertheless, a therapeutic pass was issued. While home on pass, the patient overdosed on 350 mg of nortriptyline and 24 mg of lorazepam. He was distraught over the belief that his insurance coverage had been terminated. The voices had stated, "Now is your opportunity to do it (overdose)."

According to Appelbaum (1993), physicians are obliged to appeal an adverse decision affecting the care of their patients and continue treatment, irrespective of payment issues. In turn, I believe that managed care companies should offer at least two levels of appeal with physicians. Failing that, arbitration by an independent appeals panel should be offered (Lazarus 1994b). Although it may be tempting for the psychiatrist and other members of the treatment team to circumvent the appeals process and collude with the patient in the projection of all evil onto the insurance reviewer (Gabbard et al. 1991), shifting the responsibility for deciding about the necessity of care from the attending physician to the patient could be unethical (Pellegrino 1993).

Referring Medically Unstable Patients Into Provider Networks

I have observed another form of resistance to managed care wherein physicians refer medically unstable patients to managed mental health care companies for a psychiatric disposition (Lazarus 1994a). Psychiatrists and other physicians have become increasingly cognizant of carve-out managed care operations. They understand that many managed care companies, in addition to performing utilization review, are responsible for the assessment, triage, and treatment of patients through networks of select mental health providers. These providers typically consist of a variety of inpatient, outpatient, and partial hospitalization programs for mentally ill and chemically dependent persons. Because managed mental health care organizations have a contracted obligation to provide treatment, managed care networks may be accessed on demand and, regrettably, in lieu of more appropriate medical treatment.

The transfer of medically ill patients to contracted mental health providers usually represents a misunderstanding about the nature and limitation of psychiatric practice. In some instances, however, the pressure to admit or transfer medically ill patients stems from a fear that noncontracted providers will not be paid for treatment out of network. Occasionally, physicians from outside the network may insist that patients be treated in the network, simply to avoid dealing with difficult or undesirable patients, for example, those who are intoxicated or postoverdose.

The inappropriate transfer of patients into managed care networks is reminiscent of "dumping" more commonly seen in the public sector. Ansell and Schiff (1987) estimated that 250,000 critically ill patients are transferred annually for economic reasons. Dumping is illegal and is punishable by fines or sanctions against referring physicians and facilities under the Emergency Medical Treatment and Active Labor Act (Elliott 1993).

Case 3

A 27-year-old depressed man placed an electrically live wire in his mouth in a suicide attempt. He sustained numerous lesions in his oropharynx including third-degree burns of the mouth and tongue. In addition, he cut himself in the wrist and held the police at bay with a pair of scissors. He was eventually subdued and committed involuntarily for treatment.

The patient was hospitalized on the neurology service of a university hospital. He was seen in consultation by an otolaryngologist and a psychiatrist. The patient was unable to eat or drink as a result, in part, of the electrical burns in his mouth. He required hydration intravenously and skilled nursing support not available routinely on a psychiatric unit.

Several days after admission, the managed care company coordinating the patient's mental health benefits was contacted regarding transferring the patient to a psychiatric facility. The attending physician, a neurologist, reassured the managed care firm that the patient was medically stable and no longer required intravenous fluids. Accordingly, the transfer was approved.

However, when the patient arrived at the psychiatric facility, his condition was precarious. He was incontinent of urine and feces. He was still unable to take solids or liquids by mouth. Less than 24 hours remained on the patient's involuntary commitment, and there was insufficient time to prepare for mental health court. The patient had to be returned to the referring hospital for further treatment.

Psychiatric units in general hospitals are often pressured by other medical services to accept patients who may not be medically stable. Arguments often ensue over the placement of these patients even though it seems best for them to remain in an acute care medical setting until their condition has stabilized. A managed mental health care company has a gatekeeper role similar to a consultation-liaison service in a general hospital (Lazarus 1993). However, the managed care firm is at a greater disadvantage than the consultation-liaison service because it operates at arm's length from the actual treatment.

Triage coordinators for managed care firms must rely on the accuracy and credibility of information supplied by the caregivers to make a disposition. That reliance can be problematic if physicians try to "game" the system (manipulate information for personal or financial gain). For example, through a postpayment validation process, discrepancies may be found between information provided by the attending physician by telephone and data contained in the chart. Physicians should not distort information in their communications with managed care companies in the belief that companies will be more inclined to certify treatment.

Failing to Comply With Managed Care Procedures

Psychiatrists may be reluctant or unwilling to entrust patients to managed care personnel once patients have been psychiatrically treated or hospitalized out of the network. This situation occurs, for example, when managed care firms heavily penetrate an area, when patients are inadvertently admitted to noncontracted facilities, or when patients are forced to change their health plans and physicians as a result of job losses and changes in employment. The failure or refusal of physicians to conform to limitations inherent in HMO insurance policies, especially restrictions placed on the choice of provider, appears to be a common form of resistance to managed care.

Case 4

A 26-year-old woman drove to the emergency department of a community hospital after an argument with her husband. She had been depressed for several weeks. Her symptoms included vegetative disturbances of depression, alcohol abuse, and suicidal ideation without intent or plan. The results of her physical examination were normal.

In the emergency department, the patient commented, "I just want to talk to someone to make it all go away." She was tearful and despondent. She could not guarantee that she would not attempt suicide unless she was hospitalized. Therefore, the emergency department physician decided to hospitalize her in the psychiatric division of the hospital.

However, the hospital was not affiliated with the HMO's mental health provider network. The physician would not transfer the patient to a hospital that was under contract with the HMO. She was hospitalized even though the admission was not authorized.

By virtue of selective contracting, psychiatric patients are transferred from emergency departments of hospitals that have been excluded from provider networks to providers who have entered into exclusive arrangements with HMOs and managed care organizations. Psychiatrists and other physicians who do not participate in these networks may be reluctant to transfer patients into unfamiliar clinical surroundings simply at the request of an insurance company.

The Colorado Medical Society (1991), which has established guidelines relevant to patient transfers in managed care programs, has recommended that the transferring physician and the receiving physician jointly arrange for continuity of patient care between facilities. Out-of-network treatment should be authorized for critically ill patients until a transfer can be reasonably effected. The primary consideration in developing criteria for patient transfers should be the patient's clinical condition and needs; economic issues should be secondary (American Psychiatric Association 1994).

Targeting Managed Care Firms for Litigation

Claims of unfair managed care practices and concerns about the quality of care in HMOs have resulted in widespread litigation involving HMOs and managed care organizations (Sederer 1992). However, many managed care "horror stories" are anecdotal and sensational. In truth, most research comparing HMO care to that in indemnity plans has yielded mixed results or inconclusive results on health outcomes, suggesting that generalizations must be made with caution (Miller and Luft 1994; Relman 1994; Safran et al. 1994). Sederer and Summergrad (1993) reviewed studies bearing on criteria for hospital admission and concluded that preadmission certification and concurrent utilization review actually safeguarded quality rather than compromised it.

Nevertheless, lawsuits involving managed care organizations have been pursued without merit. In one instance, the chief executive of a managed mental health care company (a psychiatrist) was named as a defendant in a suit on the grounds that his employment by the company violated the Hippocratic oath. In another case, three attorneys were fined for filing lawsuits against a major HMO wrongly accusing the HMO of unfair business practices (Turner 1993).

Legal battles against managed care organizations have been waged in several states. There has also been corresponding litigation by managed care psychiatrists who have been unfairly criticized in public (cf. Psychiatric News, May 20, 1994, pp 1, 30).

An independent evaluation (Pierce 1991) of a troubled managed care operation in Connecticut revealed that psychiatrists who contracted with a managed care company were partly responsible for compromising care to patients in the network. Many of the psychiatrists in the network viewed the managed care company as an "enemy" from the beginning. They had no real interest in helping the firm succeed. Psychiatrists in the network appeared to be disinterested in managed care, failed to learn the company's procedures, did not advocate vigorously for their patients, and often unnecessarily involved patients in disputes with the managed care company.

Eist (1992) reviewed more than 90 APA district branch newsletters. He reported that "an overwhelming majority of the columns and commentaries described managed care as intrusive and destructive. They advocated different approaches in an attempt to deal with the problems managed care has created for patients and physicians. The approaches varied from trying to negotiate and even find areas where constructive cooperation could take place to all-out legal action against managed care firms and the development of legislation to curb destructive managed care practices" (p. 13). Eist (1992) observed that more than one-third of the states have enacted legislation to regulate the managed care industry, and other states were moving in the same direction. Certainly, constructive legislation, rather than vindictive litigation, is a healthier way to promote industry standards.

Case 5

A 22-year-old man was admitted to a partial hospitalization program of a private psychiatric facility for treatment of depression. The attending psychiatrist was contacted by two of the managed care company's reviewing psychiatrists during routine utilization review. He had previously participated in several reviews with the managed care company including the review described in Case 1.

The attending psychiatrist asked one of the reviewing psychiatrists whether the patient had given permission to conduct the review. The reviewing psychiatrist replied that he had never spoken to the patient, although he believed it was permissible to conduct the review based on the subscriber's agreement with the health plan as well as other documents. Additional time in the partial hospitalization program was approved based on the facts of the review.

Several weeks after the review, the attending psychiatrist wrote letters to both managed care psychiatrists asking them to radically alter their review activities with the managed care company. The attending psychiatrist believed that the reviewing psychiatrists had conducted themselves unethically because they did not have the contemporaneous informed consent of the patient to proceed with the review. The reviewing psychiatrists wrote the attending psychiatrist a letter inviting him to join them in a discussion and exploration of the issues in question. However, the attending psychiatrist refused to participate. He then filed a formal complaint with the state district branch of the APA alleging that the reviewing psychiatrists had violated medical ethics described in *The Principles of Medical Ethics With Annotations Especially Applicable to Psychiatry* (American Psychiatric Association 1993a).

The ethics committee of the district branch conducted a hearing into the matter. During the hearing, the attending psychiatrist reiterated his position that the reviewing psychiatrists did not have proper consent to conduct the review. He chose not to stay for the proceedings or to hear his accused colleagues' responses.

Evidence was introduced from state law as well as various contractual arrangements that, in fact, permitted the utilization review activities. In addition, the accused psychiatrists undertook a review of the literature related to informed consent and obtaining release of confidential information. A consensus of literature held that the attending physician had primary responsibility to verify consent and authorize communication with the insurance company and its review organization.

Furthermore, it was discovered that when the patient entered the partial hospitalization program he had, in fact, signed the hospital's release of information form that allowed telephonic utilization review. The attending psychiatrist was aware that his patient had signed this authorization, and the possibility of utilization review was discussed by the attending psychiatrist with the patient in anticipation of the review, but this information was never volunteered by the attending psychiatrist prior to the hearing.

The managed care psychiatrists were exonerated by the ethics committee. The legal costs incurred by the managed care company in defending the reviewing psychiatrists amounted to $17,000.

There is no question that managed care has entered the once sacred covenant between psychiatrist and patient; however, it hardly seems appropriate to decide the limits of confidentiality by a fiat. The reviewing psychiatrists in this case acted responsibly, ethically, and within the constraints of the law. On the other hand, the attending psychiatrist, by withholding relevant information and showing indifference to his colleagues' defense, acted in a questionable manner. When one probes beneath the surface in cases such as these, in which unwarranted or unsubstantiated claims hurled at managed care companies or individual psychiatrists employed by managed care companies are insincerely followed by litigation or professional arbitration, ulterior motives may be found.

Rapprochement

With managed care firmly rooted in the health care delivery system, psychiatrists are constantly being forced to reassess their identity and roles. They find themselves becoming increasingly responsive to a non–physician-controlled corporate system with values different from the medical profession's values. Managed care has been faulted for subscribing to the theory that less is more (i.e., when services are reimbursed through prepayment, clinicians may realize more profit by delivering less treatment) (Sharfstein and Beigel 1984).

Ethical dilemmas may arise as physicians attempt to balance their responsibilities to patients and to themselves as wage earners (Fink 1993). The inability to resolve that conflict may result in tension and fuel anger at the managed care industry. Nonetheless, rudeness should not be tolerated in any civilized dialogue. According to Oss (cited by Parker 1994), "more providers will get thrown out of networks for rudeness than [for] anything else" (p. 4).

Critics of managed care have pointed out that more than rudeness is at stake here. The development of managed care as an outgrowth of third-party reimbursement has encumbered the physician-patient relationship (Emanuel and Brett 1993; Schroeder et al. 1985). The third party has not been invited to participate in treatment, as a consultant would be. Moreover, some managed care companies have been slow to meet licensing and credentialing requirements that would demonstrate a concern for quality in the same way that any physician or hospital would be required.

Consequently, managed care organizations must be prepared to prove themselves and withstand skepticism. Sederer (1993) noted, "When proprietary managed care organizations make determinations on payment they explicitly disavow any responsibility for patient care and clinical outcome. Doctors and hospitals can never disavow these responsibilities. It is this difference which critically differentiates caregivers from cost containers" (p. 1434).

Managed care may affect psychiatric practice in many ways that psychiatrists could find disturbing. Psychotherapy, considered integral to private practice, will become increasingly restricted to nonmedical therapists and used primarily for symptom relief. Psychiatrists will be called on for brief medication-assisted therapy and for supervisory and administrative services, often in a multidisciplinary setting. They will be forced to reorganize their practice along medical lines. That is likely to cause a resurgence in the fields of emergency psychiatry and consultation-liaison psychiatry (Fink 1993). Not all psychiatrists will want to change their practice, however, and some may not be capable of doing so (Greco and Eisenberg 1993). Moreover, many psychiatrists do not endorse subspecialization.

To the extent that attacks on managed care have become a staple device of psychiatrists opposed to health reform in general, any plan that addresses reform must also take into account the behavior of physicians. Discontent within the medical profession appears to be an inevitable by-product of cost containment and other attempts to alter unnecessary utilization, so much so that Fuchs (1993) argued that "pain" is a prerequisite for changing health care policy. Unless physicians are willing to make sacrifices, they may be left out of crucial policy and decision-making committees.

Managed care and utilization review, in particular, have shocked the psychiatric community, but psychiatry is not the first specialty to be affected by managed care and it should not expect to receive special treatment (see Chapter 1). It is hoped that a peaceful era will follow this initial stage of uproar and protest. In the spirit of cooperation, Sabin (cited by Moran 1992) made several suggestions to help psychiatrists come to grips with this unavoidable alliance. I have modified Sabin's principles as follows:

- The attending psychiatrist should be open to suggestions from the managed care psychiatrist regarding changes in the treatment plan or level of care.
- When the attending psychiatrist and the managed care psychiatrist are in conflict, both should consult with peers.
- When two procedures or treatments are equally efficacious, the less expensive one is always preferable.
- When making reviewing decisions, the managed care psychiatrist must consider the feasibility of the recommendation in light of the patient's actual environment and resources.
- The attending psychiatrist must establish boundaries beyond which compromising quality of care will be considered unacceptable.
- It is reasonable for the attending psychiatrist to inquire about the criteria by which the managed care psychiatrist makes treatment recommendations and imposes limitations.

- Ultimately, both the attending psychiatrist and the managed care psychiatrist should act in accordance with individual conscience.

In addition, as recommended by the American Medical Association (McCormick 1994), utilization review organizations should apply for appropriate certification, base review criteria on scientific principles developed with providers, allow only physicians of the same specialty to deny coverage or payment, and respond promptly to prior authorization requests.

Conclusion

Managed care and the emphasis on utilization controls have been perceived by most providers as threatening and punitive. Resistance to managed mental health care has been shown in many ways. Examples include verbally abusing psychiatrists employed by managed care companies, involving patients and families in insurance disputes, referring medically unstable patients into integrated networks, refusing to cooperate with managed care procedures, and targeting managed care firms and psychiatrists for unwarranted litigation.

The factors that influence clinical decisions must balance the needs of the patient, providers, and society. The ability to achieve this balance will be a formidable task during the 1990s. As the managed care landscape changes, psychiatrists on both sides of the fence must unite and become proactive to ensure the integrity of the profession and the welfare of patients. Only in this way can the fence be transformed into a bridge.

References

American Psychiatric Association: APA seeks data on harmful effects of case management. Psychiatric News, July 20, 1990, p 9

American Psychiatric Association: The Principles of Medical Ethics With Annotations Especially Applicable to Psychiatry. Washington, DC, American Psychiatric Association, 1993a

American Psychiatric Association: APA's managed care phone complaints to go to Clinton. Psychiatric News, May 7, 1993b, pp 1, 16

American Psychiatric Association: Position statement on the continuity of care in the psychiatrist-patient relationship. Am J Psychiatry 151:632, 1994

Ansell D, Schiff R: Patient dumping: status, implications, and policy recommendations. JAMA 257:1500–1502, 1987

Appelbaum PS: Legal liability and managed care. Am Psychol 48:251–257, 1993

Colorado Medical Society: Guidelines for appropriate treatment of managed care plan subscribers requiring emergency medical care. Colorado Medicine 88:242–244, 1991

Delmar D: Some in managed care feeling alienated from APA. Clinical Psychiatry News, September 1991, pp 1, 13

Drake DE: A managed care experiment. Psychiatric News, December 4, 1992, p 18

Eist H: Managed care, ethics consume DB's attention. Psychiatric News, June 19, 1992, pp 13, 23

Elliott RL: Patient dumping, COBRA, and the public psychiatric hospital. Hosp Community Psychiatry 44:155–158, 1993

Emanuel EJ, Brett AS: Managed competition and the patient-physician relationship. N Engl J Med 329:879–882, 1993

Fazzi RA: Future/Perspectives in Mental Health. Holyoke, MA, Human Resource Association of the Northeast, 1990

Fink PJ: Earning a living in psychiatry: tomorrow's picture. Psychiatric News, January 1, 1993, p 14

Fuchs VR: No pain, no gain: perspectives on cost containment. JAMA 269:631–633, 1993

Gabbard GO, Takahashi T, Davidson J, et al: A psychodynamic perspective on the clinical impact of insurance review. Am J Psychiatry 148:318–323, 1991

Greco PJ, Eisenberg JM: Changing physicians' practices. N Engl J Med 329:1271–1274, 1993

Hall RCW: Legal precedents affecting managed care: the physician's responsibilities to patients. Psychosomatics 35:105–117, 1994

Jellinek MS, Nurcombe B: Two wrongs don't make a right: managed care, mental health, and the marketplace. JAMA 270:1737–1739, 1993

Lazarus A: Disputes over payment for hospitalization under mental health "carve-out" programs. Hosp Community Psychiatry 44:1134–1136, 1993

Lazarus A: Dumping psychiatric patients in the managed care sector. Hosp Community Psychiatry 45:529–530, 1994a

Lazarus A: Using an appeals panel to mediate mental health care UR disputes. Medical Interface 7(8): 56–58, 76, 1994b

McCormick B: Managed care and medicine in "fairness" fight. American Medical News, May 9, 1994, pp 1, 34

Miller RH, Luft HS: Managed care plan performance since 1980: a literature analysis. JAMA 271:1512–1519, 1994

Moldawsky RJ: Managed care (letter). Psychiatric News, June 18, 1993, p 16

Moran M: APA needs positive vision of what good managed care will look like, expert advises. Psychiatric News, January 17, 1992, p 6

Olsson PA: Our deepening crisis in collegiality. Psychiatric Times, January 1993, p 7

Oss ME: Considerations in structuring behavioral health service delivery in managed competition models. Open Minds 7(5):4–6, 1993

Parker S: The risky business of joining managed care. Clinical Psychiatry News, June 1994, pp 3, 14

Pellegrino ED: Can the doctor's burden be shifted to the patient? The Pharos 56:34, 1993

Pierce C: Psychiatrists who worked with MCC are held partly to blame. Clinical Psychiatry News, July 1991, p 20

Prest JR: Managed care box. Psychiatric News, November 20, 1992, p 19

Relman AS: Medical insurance and health: what about managed care? N Engl J Med 331:471–472, 1994

Safran DG, Tarlov AR, Rogers WH: Primary care performance in fee-for-service and prepaid health care systems: results from the medical outcomes study. JAMA 271:1579–1586, 1994

Schroeder JL, Clarke JR, Webster JR Jr: Prepaid entitlements: a new challenge for physician-patient relationships. JAMA 254:3080–3082, 1985

Sederer LI: Judicial and legislative responses to cost containment. Am J Psychiatry 149:1157–1161, 1992

Sederer LI: Cost containment and the profit motive (Dr. Sederer replies). Am J Psychiatry 150:1434, 1993

Sederer LI, Summergrad P: Criteria for hospital admission. Hosp Community Psychiatry 44:116–118, 1993

Sharfstein SS, Beigel A: Less is more? today's economics and its challenge to psychiatry. Am J Psychiatry 141:1403–1408, 1984

Sherman C: Advice to make the best of managed care draws fire. Clinical Psychiatry News, July 1991, p 26

Solomon RJ: Preparation could help you survive in a changing market. American Medical News, January 4, 1993, p 32

Turner DI: Three lawyers must pay U.S. Healthcare $27,553. The Philadelphia Inquirer, July 8, 1993, pp E1, E9

Wagner J, Gartner C: Highlights of the 44th Institute on Hospital and Community Psychiatry. Hosp Community Psychiatry 44:18–22, 1993

Whittaker CK: If called by the insurance company, call in the patient on the call. JAMA 268:3434, 1992

Chapter 9

Is Managed Care Ethical Care?

James E. Sabin, M.D.

During a discussion of the issue of trust, I asked a patient at the health maintenance organization (HMO) in which I've practiced for 20 years what he thought I should say in this chapter. My patient, with whom the therapeutic alliance is strong but who is highly skeptical about the goodwill of organizations and bureaucracies replied, "You can tell them I don't doubt that managed care provides a service of some kind, but to claim that this is any form of the traditional profession is a fraud and a travesty on the profession." Clinicians in workshops on the ethics of managed care regularly challenge the workshop topic in a similar vein, "Let's face it. Managed care has nothing to do with ethics. It's simply a matter of the bottom line!"

In this chapter I want to argue the opposite perspective—that managed care has a coherent, defendable ethical foundation and that for ethical reasons it should become the prevailing pattern of practice. I will further contend that managed care takes seriously, and seeks to apply elements of, traditional medical ethics that have largely been ignored by educators (Sabin 1993) and the mental health professions (Sabin 1994a).

Managed care advocates must acknowledge, however, that managed care techniques have sometimes been used to achieve rapid savings through what insiders call "slash and burn" programs. These are the programs that Sharfstein (1990) appropriately called "mangled care." Genuine managed care (Goldstein 1989), by contrast, seeks to produce the maximum value (outcome) for a population from the resources available, not simply to contain costs. In this chapter I attempt to specify the ethical premises of genuine managed care. Although poorly managed care is mangled care, unmanaged care is mangled ethics.

The Ethical Premises of Managed Care

The rapid evolution of health care into a managed system is—and should be—unstoppable, but it is far from certain that this evolution will yield an improved product. The broadsides against managed care seen so frequently in professional journals and the press are too global to have any useful influence. For real quality improvement we need rigorous critical evaluation of the emerging system by the standards of genuine managed care. Unfortunately, because the ethical basis of managed care is not widely understood, this crucial form of rigorous clinical and ethical evaluation is all too rare.

I have suggested elsewhere (Sabin 1994b) that ethical clinicians practicing in managed care settings espouse four principles to supplement the codes of ethics already established by the mental health professions. These principles (adapted slightly), which I present as assertions but which need to be debated, modified as needed, and—I believe—adopted, lay out clear implications for what clinicians, organized systems, and the public should demand of managed care:

> Principle 1: Ethical clinicians should dedicate themselves to caring for their patients in a relationship of fidelity and at the same time act as stewards of society's resources.

When health care was largely a one-to-one transaction between the patient and the clinician, paid for by the patient with no involvement of collective (third-party) funds, the clinician could closely approximate a position of pure advocacy for the patient, although even in that setting clinicians also "advocated" for themselves by setting office hours, fees, and similar conditions that were not solely for the benefit or at the request of the patient. The prevalent model of the clinician's fiduciary responsibility[1] to patients—which posits that clinicians who consider societal interests in their clinical roles are unethical double agents (Simon 1987)—comes from this long-gone world in which the health care system consisted of multiple one-to-one contracts between individual patients and individual clinicians.

---

[1]Although *fiduciary* is the more commonly used term, I prefer to follow Morreim (1991) in using the term *fidelity*, which better conveys that the clinical encounter has a more moral than a legal quality.

The use of collective resources creates a different social compact that imposes new obligations on all participants—clinicians, patients, and health care organizations. The Preamble to the *American Medical Association's Principles of Medical Ethics*—which form the basis of the American Psychiatric Association's ethical code (American Psychiatric Association 1993b, p. 1)—promises a moral vision that will include some type of balance between patient-centered (fidelity) and communitarian (stewardship) ethics:

> As a member of this profession, a physician must recognize responsibility not only to *patients, but also to society*, to other health professionals, and to self [emphasis added].

Unfortunately, the promise is not fulfilled. Neither the annotated *Principles of Medical Ethics* (American Psychiatric Association 1993b) nor the separately published *Opinions of the Ethics Committee* (American Psychiatric Association 1993a) offers any explication of the responsibility that the physician—qua physician—bears toward society.

This is an extremely serious omission. Because the American Psychiatric Association *Principles* and *Opinions* do not reinforce the communitarian ethic of the *Principles* Preamble or clarify the ways in which ethical clinicians (or programs that are targeted to populations) should pursue positive ideals of social justice, many clinicians are conflicted, confused, and even anguished when asked to consider the welfare of society (stewardship) as well as individual patient welfare (fidelity). Community mental health systems have long expected clinicians to consider populations as well as individuals (Shore 1992), but this moral outlook is new in the managed insurance programs under which the middle class receives its health care. At least part of the assertion that "managed care has nothing to do with ethics" arises from the relatively recent extension of communitarian values from the public sector to a private sector that had not considered collective as well as individual welfare.

In all areas of health care there are many clinical situations in which individual clinicians have strong opinions about the "right" way to practice but for which panels of experienced clinicians and health service researchers would see a range of legitimate alternative paths toward the desired clinical outcome. The ethics of managed care gives very clear guidance for how to proceed in these circumstances:

> Principle 2: Ethical clinicians should recommend the least costly treatment alternative unless they have substantial evidence that a more costly intervention is likely to yield a superior outcome.

In the highly fragmented United States health care system—with 1,500 different insurers and a comparable number of public federal, state, county, and city systems—it is extremely difficult for clinicians to see the ethical rationale for this approach to practice (Daniels 1986). Not surprisingly, a participant at a American Psychiatric Association (1991) conference on ethics in managed care stated—without contradiction from other participants—that "when [two or more treatments] were equally effective, even though one might be less expensive, it was not appropriate or ethical for the reviewer to say ['use the less expensive treatment']" (p. 81). This moral outlook, which is still widely prevalent among American clinicians, is a second source of the claim that "managed care has nothing to do with ethics."

By contrast, in the United Kingdom and Canada, where citizens levy taxes on themselves to support health care for the entire population, the relationship between societal resources, parsimonious practice patterns, and individual welfare is much clearer. Thus, the British Medical Association (1988) tells physicians they have a positive *ethical duty* to use the most economic option that achieves the clinical objectives. It explains this duty as follows:

> Finite resources can never match potentially infinite demands or expectations. The inevitable consequence is that a decision to allocate a particular sum to a particular service will produce underfunding of another service. This will result in a number of possible outcomes (e.g., ward closure/staff reductions/increased waiting lists) all of which may increase morbidity . . . [consequently] *it is the doctor's ethical duty to use the most economic and efficacious treatment available*" [emphasis added]. (p. 72)

When systems use managed care techniques to achieve wider access and more overall benefit for a population, clinicians can manage costs aggressively and allocate their own time stringently in good conscience. In the United Kingdom and Canada, clinicians can be confident that parsimonious forms of practice promote the greatest good for the greatest number, because savings in the care of one patient will be used to meet the health needs of another. They can also be confident that their patients have given the equivalent of informed consent for this practice style (neither country uses the term *managed care*) through the legislative process.

In the complex and chaotic United States nonsystem, however, clinicians are uncertain as to whether managed care should be seen as a potential aid to achieving improved access and outcomes for patients and populations or as "a takeover of mental health practice by business interests, with devastating effects on patients, practitioners and the professions" (Edward and Shore 1993, p. A14). In all likelihood both have been true in the past and are possible paths in the future. The third principle reflects the particular need for clinicians to influence the ethical quality of managed care programs by acting as advocates for *health system ethics* as well as *individual patient ethics.*

> Principle 3: In their stewardship role, ethical clinicians need to advocate for justice in the health care system, just as in their clinical role they need to advocate for the welfare of their patients.

A full consideration of what *justice* means for health care requires extended discussion (see, for example, Daniels 1985 and Morreim 1991). In practical terms, however, there are three major dimensions quality improvement–minded critics of managed care should examine as a prelude to advocating for justice in the health care system.

First, clinicians and the public should insist that managed systems truly enhance the effectiveness of the health care (effectiveness = outcome/dollars spent) delivered to the affected population. There is nothing in the concept of justice that precludes for-profit health care enterprises, as long as the for-profit structure produces better outcomes per dollar spent than the alternatives. Many public mental health systems contract with private vendors—including for-profit entities—on the basis of their belief that doing so will provide greater value to the public. Clinicians, however, will bitterly resist managed care and portray it as having "nothing to do with ethics" unless they perceive it as striving to produce the best results the available resources can produce for the affected population.

Second, clinicians and the public should demand that a process of genuine informed consent has taken place. This process entails much more than small print in an insurance contract. Insofar as different insurance programs rest on different philosophies of care, these philosophies should be articulated clearly enough to allow participants in a system supposedly governed by competitive principles to choose in accord with their preferences and at the same time to bear the consequences (including costs) of their choice. In single-payer systems like Canada's, the question of how much of the available resources are to be devoted to health care is part of the political process. The public can legitimately ask for more health care, but it must then struggle with the question of what trade-offs to make. In the United States, the structure of the system appears to be designed to allow political leaders and the public to indulge in "the wishful thinking that we can have it all as long as we get the flowcharts and systems theory right" (Gaylin 1994, p. A41). Ultimately, true informed consent about managed care will require a more honest political dialogue than has occurred to date.

Finally, clinicians and the public must demand that all Americans have access to an adequate standard of health care. The American Psychiatric Association states that "a psychiatrist should not be a party to any type of policy that excludes, segregates, or demeans the dignity of any patient because of ethnic origin, race, sex, creed, age, *socioeconomic status* [emphasis added], or sexual orientation" (American Psychiatric Association 1993b, p. 3). If a company provides full insurance to full-time salaried employees, but offers no coverage to part-time hourly employees, an ethical clinician would have to advocate for change in what appears to be discrimination according to socioeconomic status. Although the American Psychiatric Association's annotation does not include reference to discrimination on the basis of health status, if a managed program sought to exclude patients with preexisting conditions, the ethical clinician would be obligated to participate in lobbying for a change in that policy.

> Principle 4: Ethical clinicians insist that potentially beneficial interventions should only be withheld on the basis of explicit standards that have been established with participation of the affected populations and that are acknowledged with the individual patient.

Principle 4 addresses the politically explosive issue of rationing. Most thoughtful observers of health care, unless they are running for public office, acknowledge that rationing is inevitable, and the truly honest among them admit that it already occurs.

Rationing policy can be done in at least four very different ways:

1. The most common form of rationing in the current American health care system is "accomplished" by leaving people out of the system of care, as through uninsurance and underinsurance. If we regard health care as a basic good that should be available to all members of a first-world economy, we must condemn this form of rationing as unethical.
2. The form of rationing most familiar to mental health clinicians occurs by way of arbitrary benefit limits. Most of the value provided by psychotherapy and hospital care can be achieved within the constraints of 20 outpatient visits or 30, 45, or 60 hospital days per year—but not all. Those individuals who would benefit from resources beyond what an insurance cap allows, and who could not receive that benefit within the cap by more effectively managed care, are being rationed.
3. Rationing can be accomplished by a system like that used in Oregon, under which priorities among treatment condition pairs were set with wide public participation. It is the legislature that then decides how far down the prioritized list to go by deciding how much money it is prepared to allocate to health care. Interestingly, psychiatric and substance abuse conditions fared very well in this kind of priority-setting process.

4. Rationing can occur in the course of establishing criteria for determination of medical necessity. Most forms of insurance use the concept of *medical necessity* to specify the range of interventions the insurance will cover. With regard to managed care, an Institute of Medicine study concluded that "UR [utilization review] decision(s) invariably turn on whether a treatment or service is 'medically necessary'" (Helvestine 1989, p. 172).

However, despite its ostensibly straightforward, scientific connotation and the implication that medical facts might themselves determine what was necessary to do, medical necessity is a highly value-laden concept that presupposes a prior process of moral reasoning (Sabin et al. 1991). No treatment is *necessary* in itself—only as a *means* to an agreed-on *end*—and deciding on the ends or goals of treatment is a moral process.

To be useful, a model for defining medical necessity must make distinctions between necessary forms of treatment and not-necessary treatments that the public and clinicians regard as fair, will be administrable in the real world, and will lead to results that society is prepared to pay for (Sabin and Daniels 1994). Managed care systems have emerged because the payers for health care—business and the various levels of government—have demanded a reduction in their expenditures. Administrative systems, such as capitation and utilization review, have been developed to achieve the desired savings. However, the kind of public dialogue needed to develop understanding of the choices and trade-offs involved in achieving the cost savings and to create a widespread sense that the system is fair has not yet taken place.

That dialogue will have to address two basic issues. First, what conditions should insurance cover? Should coverage be limited to schizophrenia, bipolar illness, and what some advocates call the other "diseases of the brain"? Or, should counseling for conditions like marital distress or job dissatisfaction—which may not be illnesses in the DSM-IV (American Psychiatric Association 1994) sense but which can cause substantial suffering—be covered as well? Second, within whatever scope of coverage is agreed to, what types of treatment goals should be covered? Should insurance be limited to stabilization and acute problem resolution, or should work with character adjustment also be covered?

It is easy to agree that appendectomy for acute appendicitis is medically necessary because there is widespread agreement that 1) a ruptured appendix can be fatal, 2) saving the life of an otherwise healthy person is desirable, 3) appendectomy can cure the condition, and 4) there is currently no alternative form of treatment. It is not so easy, however, to agree on whether continued hospitalization is "needed" for the limited but real risk associated with ambiguous suicidal impulses or whether insurance should regard long-term treatment focused on a destructive relationship pattern as medically necessary for a patient with a severe personality disorder who has just been treated for acute suicidality resulting from a failed relationship. Managed care programs craft answers to those questions, but without a much wider discussion that political leaders have not yet been willing to foster, it is difficult for those programs to elicit support and understanding. Those who prefer different definitions of medical necessity often conclude that "managed care has nothing to do with ethics."

The following case (elements of which are presented in Sabin 1992 and Sabin and Daniels 1994) illustrates how many of the ethical issues discussed above actually emerge in managed care practice.

Case Example: The Lost Administrator (L.A.)

Part A. L.A.'s first contacts with mental health treatment at her HMO led to a complaint. "I am very discouraged with what I have experienced in your mental health area. Approximately 3 months ago I had an appointment with X. I was uncomfortable with the emphasis placed on a limited number of sessions. While I understand that your program offers short-term therapy up to 20 sessions, I got the impression that availing oneself of 15 to 20 sessions was discouraged. I would hope that my treatment would not take this long but needed to know that should it, I would not feel pressure to complete it early. Today I saw Y, who also strongly emphasized your policy, and we never even discussed what my issues might be. I am hoping you can recommend someone to me who would be sympathetic, encouraging, and at least as concerned with my counseling as he or she is with your policies. Thank you!"

Discussion—Part A. In terms of Principle 1, L.A. experienced the initial contacts as driven by stewardship ("policies") without the necessary fidelity ("my issues"). Her experience exemplifies the fundamental clinical and ethical concern about managed care.

Part B. On meeting L.A,, her new clinician said: "I know you have felt put off by my colleagues and my organization. But can we put that aside to focus on you, what the problems are, and what you really need?" L.A. was visibly relieved and fully cooperative.

Discussion—Part B. The new clinician simply followed L.A.'s clear request—that her concerns be attended to with fidelity. In her complaint L.A. made clear that she recognized the fact that resources were limited and had to be managed. She was prepared to comanage her care, but she wanted to be listened to.

Part C. L.A. reported that she was the third child and only daughter in a family of five. By the time of her birth her father already had severe diabetes. Throughout her childhood he experienced progressive complications including amputation, heart disease, kidney failure, and loss of vision. He died when she was 16. He was severely critical of her, and L.A. felt that her mother had been overwhelmed by his illness and the financial burdens and was emotionally unavailable to her. L.A.'s mother confirmed that L.A. had been a precociously responsible, undemanding child and that she herself had indeed felt overwhelmed and unavailable when L.A. was growing up.

Now, at 35, L.A. was moderately successful in her work as an administrator and had many friends. However, she felt intensely "empty" and "lost," especially in love life, and perceived herself as defensively detached in all areas of life. She had been involved with a series of men who had been attached to others or unwilling to make a commitment and not drawn to men who might have been more reliable. In outpatient psychotherapy 7 years earlier she had become increasingly frightened until she interrupted treatment precipitously after 18 months.

Her therapist believed that a time-limited therapy with a preplanned termination as described by Mann (1973) might allow intense work with her maladaptive defenses and fear of loss. As the focus for the therapy he proposed the following: "Ever since you were a young girl you have acted independent and appeared self-sufficient, but you have always felt desperate and needy inside yet scared to get really close to someone and to let go in love." He recommended 10 further sessions with a specified termination but was explicit that although he expected the approach to work, L.A. could return if it did not. L.A. described the plan as follows: "We've planned an 'abandonment' to work with my fear . . . we're going to believe that the final appointment will be the last . . . but I know you wouldn't ultimately abandon me if I need help."

Discussion—Part C. Here we see the clinician and patient applying Principle 2 in a responsible manner. Mann's form of therapy is especially effective at mobilizing conflicts involving separation and loss. The clinician recommended the least costly treatment alternative but built in a plan to assess the results.

Part D. L.A. returned 3 months after the termination. She was pleased that she had been able to end a destructive relationship about which she had previously felt "paralyzed," but she continued to feel depressed. Although not acutely suicidal, she could not imagine continuing life were her mother to die. She was not willing to try antidepressant medication. She and her therapist agreed to meet approximately every 3 weeks to work in a format that combined elements of cognitive-behavioral and interpersonal therapy. She committed herself to try new behaviors to challenge the defensive pattern. After 10 months, however, she recognized that she was not able to do this and agreed to join a weekly psychotherapy group on a fee-for-service basis outside the HMO.

Discussion—Part D. Although many clinicians might argue that L.A. required intensive individual psychotherapy to change, the evidence from her own earlier experience of therapy suggested otherwise. Her clinician believed that ongoing therapy would be needed, but he recommended what he believed was the least costly treatment alternative that might achieve the outcome objectives. When the limits of this approach became clear, he recommended group psychotherapy as a potentially beneficial intervention. The HMO benefit (up to 20 prepaid visits) would not pay for this potentially beneficial treatment. L.A. and her therapist acknowledged that she was encountering rationing.

Part E. The individual and group psychotherapy continued for 2½ years with significant but partial benefit. Despite an earlier intense reluctance to use a medication, L.A. was now willing to try an antidepressant, which led to further improvement.

Discussion—Part E. L.A. and her clinician had developed a strong alliance in the course of comanaging her care. This alliance allowed her to try an intervention that she had previously been reluctant to accept. Well-managed care is done collaboratively by clinician and patient—not by a clinician to or on the patient.

Conclusion

Managed care has emerged in a characteristically American way. It has evolved more as an effort to fix the problem of health care costs by technical (managerial) means than through open political and ethical debate about choices and trade-offs. As a result of this absent process, many clinicians and members of the public simply do not understand what is happening in the health care system. Until political leaders are ready to educate the public about the real issues and choices, clinicians, managers, and other health care activists will have to undertake this effort themselves.

Managed care is based on a distinctive moral perspective familiar to clinicians and patients in the public sector but new to the sectors serving well-employed and wealthy persons.

Ethical (or genuine) managed care is a form of population-based practice that seeks to allocate substantial but nevertheless limited resources to achieve maximum utility, not simply cost containment. This ethic puts into practice the "responsibility . . . to society" (p. 1) referred to in the Preamble to the American Psychiatric Association's Principles of Medical Ethics but not developed in the American Psychiatric Association annotations or opinions. Clinicians who embrace the communitarian ethic of managed care will have to adopt a practice style in which they preferentially recommend trying the least costly plausible intervention first. It is entirely appropriate to debate whether our society should embrace this kind of communitarian ethic with regard to health care. If, however, the answer to the question "Is managed care ethical care?" is that "managed care has nothing to do with ethics," it is at best a misunderstanding and at worst a form of moral arrogance or deliberate disinformation.

References

American Psychiatric Association: Transcript Summary: Ethics in Managed Care Conference (October 25–26, 1991). Washington, DC, American Psychiatric Press, 1991

American Psychiatric Association: Opinions of the Ethics Committee on the Principles of Medical Ethics: With Annotations Especially Applicable to Psychiatry. Washington, DC, American Psychiatric Association, 1993a

American Psychiatric Association: The Principles of Medical Ethics: With Annotations Especially Applicable to Psychiatry. Washington, DC, American Psychiatric Association, 1993b

American Psychiatric Association: Diagnostic and Statistical Manual of Mental Disorders, 4th Edition. Washington, DC, American Psychiatric Association, 1994

British Medical Association: Philosophy and Practice of Medical Ethics. London, British Medical Association, 1988, p 72

Daniels N: Just Health Care. Cambridge, England, Cambridge University Press, 1985

Daniels N: Why saying no to patients in the United States is so hard: cost-containment, justice, and provider autonomy. N Engl J Med 314:1381–1383, 1986

Edward J, Shore K: The trauma of managed mental health care. New York Times, February 15, 1993, p A14

Gaylin W: Faulty diagnosis. New York Times, June 12, 1994, p A41

Goldstein LS: Genuine managed care in psychiatry: a proposed practice model. Gen Hosp Psychiatry 11:271–277, 1989

Helvestine WA: Legal implications of utilization review, in Controlling Costs and Changing Patient Care? The Role of Utilization Review. Edited by Gray BH, Field MJ. Washington, DC, National Academy Press, pp 169–204, 1989

Mann J: Time-Limited Psychotherapy. Cambridge, MA, Harvard University Press, 1973

Morreim EH: Balancing Act: The New Medical Ethics of Medicine's New Economics. Dordrect, Netherlands, Kluwer Academic Publishers, 1991

Sabin JE: The therapeutic alliance in managed care mental health practice. Journal of Psychotherapy Practice and Research 1:29–36, 1992

Sabin JE: The moral myopia of academic psychiatry: a response to Glen O. Gabbard's "The big chill." Academic Psychiatry 17:175–179, 1993

Sabin JE: Caring about patients and caring about money: the American Psychiatric Association code of ethics meets managed care. Behavioral Science and the Law 12:317–330, 1994a

Sabin JE: An ethics credo for managed mental health care practice. Hosp Community Psychiatry 45:859–860, 869, 1994b

Sabin JE, Daniels N: Determining "medical necessity" in mental health practice. Hastings Cent Rep 24(6): 5–13, 1994

Sabin JE, Forrow L, Daniels N: Clarifying the concept of medical necessity, in Proceedings of the Group Health Institute. Washington, DC, Group Health Association of America, 1991, pp 693–707

Sharfstein SS: Utilization management: managed or mangled psychiatric care? Am J Psychiatry 147:965–966, 1990

Shore M: Managed care: reinventing the wheel. Hosp Community Psychiatry 43:205, 1992

Simon RI: The psychiatrist as a fiduciary: avoiding the double agent role. Psychiatric Annals 17:622–626, 1987

Section III

Utilization Review

Chapter 10

When Is Psychiatric Hospitalization Required?

Martin G. Allen, M.D.

When I entered psychiatric residency 30 years ago, the daily charge for psychiatric inpatient care (including professional care, given primarily by residents) was $40. Now, the charge for inpatient psychiatric treatment often exceeds $1,000 per day.

Escalating medical costs, in all fields of medicine, have led to efforts by the government, insurance companies, and businesses to control costs—first by reviewing care for medical necessity and more recently by "managing" psychiatric care by referring patients to "providers" (therapists, institutions) who have special expertise in treating the problem described by the patient and have negotiated reduced-fee contracts. Therapists have joined panels of providers who have pledged to provide symptom-focused, problem-oriented mental health care. Managed care organizations refer patients to these professionals in the "least restrictive environment" appropriate for the treatment of that patient.

The Origins of Utilization Review

The motivation and impetus for developing utilization review and managed care are based on the fact that health care costs have become an increasing percentage of the gross national product and corporate expenses (Office of National Cost Estimates 1990), and there is increasing competition for limited health care dollars. Private insurance, the government, and corporations are consequently demanding increased control over health care expenses.

Mental health expenditures increased because of the existence of indemnity insurance, which led to the proliferation of psychiatric hospitals in the 1980s. Private psychiatric hospitals actively advertised and recruited patients for hospital treatment (Jellinek and Nurcombe 1993). Inpatient care became the initial focus of utilization review. Policymakers and reviewers looked first at costs, standards, and criteria for inpatient psychiatric care, because it is the most "restrictive," most expensive form of treatment.

The expansion and development of alternatives to inpatient care became the focus of increased study. Since the late 1960s, studies have shown that partial hospitalization (day hospitalization) is effective for many patients who would have been hospitalized for psychiatric or substance abuse problems (Allen and Phillips 1993; Fink et al. 1978; Greene and De La Cruz 1981; Herz 1982; Kiesler 1982; Mason et al. 1982; Mosher 1983; Washburn et al. 1976). Residential treatment, a less intensive form of psychiatric care, was developed, and new maintenance medications—including injectable long-term (depot) medications and lithium—made the outpatient management of both long-term and short-term patients more realistic. Consequently, managed care did not arrive out of nowhere; it evolved over many years from a multiplicity of historical factors.

The history of psychiatric peer review, utilization review, and managed care also has its origins in the development of the community mental health centers in the 1960s. These centers, which had limited budgets, were charged with providing basic care to a population. As a result, choices had to be made to provide the most cost-effective, economical care to the greatest number of people. Medicare physician review organizations and insurance companies began to review cases and consider ways to limit the yearly increases that were becoming commonplace (Allen 1994). In 1979, the American Psychiatric Association became interested in quality assurance and utilization review (Kuzmicki and Penner 1987) and began a program of reviewing psychiatric care for cost-effectiveness and quality. Subsequently, in the 1980s, insurance companies and independent organizations developed utilization review programs. From these came managed care. These organizations negotiated reduced-fee contracts with providers (hospitals, psychiatrists, partial hospitals, and substance abuse programs) and focused on cost control and efficient delivery of mental health care by referring patients to the least restrictive, most appropriate level of care.

What has been the effect of all these changes? Anderson (1989) presented a summary by the National Medical Audit. The study showed that specialized utilization review, coupled with a specialized preferred provider organization (PPO), can greatly reduce expenses and prevent "unnecessary" inpatient utilization for mental health. In 201 cases reviewed between July 1, 1987, and June 30, 1988, the mean number of inpatient days per case was 18.2 for nonspecialized review and 9 days for the combination of specialized utilization review with a PPO.

Arispe (1991) reviewed Group Health Association data for 1989. The study reported that although 3% of all medical admissions were for mental health, mental health discharges represented 10% of hospital days. The median number of hospital days per 1,000 for the independent practice group was 36, whereas network model plans had a median stay of 17 days. Comparing average length of stays, independent practice groups had a mental health average length of stay of 10.9 days, compared with 5.2 days for network plans. These figures show that within the health maintenance organization (HMO) model—in which cost and utilization were already controlled—additional reviews and network control resulted in an average length of stay half that of independent provider groups. Length of hospital stay averaged 20–40 days in 1986, compared with 10 days in 1990 (Jellinek and Nurcombe 1993).

Another study of the effects of managed psychiatric care was reported by Callahan et al. (1994). The authors reported the effects of managed care on the mental health and substance abuse treatment costs for the 375,000 participants in the Massachusetts Medicaid program in fiscal year 1993. Overall, the managed care program saved $47 million, a 22% reduction from expected expenditures.

In summary, utilization review, especially when combined with PPOs, has resulted in a substantial reduction in hospital days. However, some have questioned whether the quality of care is maintained under such circumstances (Sharfstein 1990). This is a controversy that is certainly not settled (see Chapter 13). In 1990, *Psychiatric News* published the results of a study reporting that length of stay was not related to long-term outcome (Pogge et al. 1990). Many studies have reported similar outcomes comparing full hospitalization to partial hospitalization for both psychiatric care and substance abuse treatment.

Concepts and Definitions

The concepts and definitions of managed care are especially relevant to inpatient treatment and have been summarized in detail elsewhere (Allen 1994; Mattson 1992). The first concept is that of "medical necessity" discussed in detail in Chapter 12. Medicine has defined illness for centuries in terms of signs and symptoms. Therefore, medically necessary treatment is defined as services that are appropriate and necessary to treat the symptoms of a medical condition. For psychiatry, determining medical necessity first requires a medical diagnosis, defined in DSM-IV (American Psychiatric Association 1994) by signs and symptoms that require treatment. Medically necessary treatment is defined as the practices and procedures that are generally acceptable in medical practice to cure, improve, stabilize, or control an illness. The services are not primarily for the convenience of the patient, the family, or the physician.

Next is the question of *appropriate* treatment for a particular condition. Frequently, there may be several treatments that are considered appropriate and helpful for a psychiatric condition. When treatments are equally effective, managed care then asks, "Is treatment provided in the least costly manner?" That question involves the concept of cost-effectiveness.

In summary, when determining allocation of resources, managed care asks, "Is there an illness that needs to be treated?," "Is the treatment appropriate for that illness," and "Is it cost-effective?" Effectiveness refers to treatment likely to result in improvement or at least stabilization of the patient. The concept of cost-effectiveness includes the belief that patients can and should be treated in the "least restrictive environment," also known as a "lower level of care." The inability of a patient to utilize a lower level of care (such as partial hospitalization or outpatient treatment) is demonstrated by a failure to keep appointments; runaway behavior; debilitating anxiety, psychosis, or depression; failure to take prescribed medications; suicidal, homicidal, or violent behavior; significant medical complications that specifically require hospital treatment; failure to care for oneself; or a significantly complex clinical presentation that requires continuous observation to make a definitive treatment plan. In such cases, inpatient psychiatric hospitalization is appropriate and necessary.

Consequently, the concepts of least costly alternative and least restrictive environment are oriented toward the most efficient allocation of resources and treatment in a setting that maintains the greatest contact with the external world in order to maintain functioning. This strategy diverts patients from inpatient hospitalization, thereby reducing the likelihood of regression and dependency and facilitating reentry into the world as a functioning member of society.

Criteria for Hospitalization

Utilization review criteria for inpatient treatment can be characterized in several ways. Underlying the criteria for both preadmission review and concurrent review is that hospitalization is used for stabilization and safety (Sabin 1994) rather than for definitive, complete treatment. With this concept, inpatient hospitalization is viewed in most cases as a relatively short-term episode in a continuum of care with partial hospitalization or outpatient treatment or both. Many studies of partial hospitalization and day treatment programs have shown that partial hospitalization is often as effective as and less restrictive than inpatient hospitalization. As a result, many insurance programs now include partial hospitalization treatment and often cover more days of partial hospitalization as a trade-off for inpatient hospital days.

An additional factor in hospitalization admission criteria is the type of treatment being considered for a particular patient. Certain hospital programs specialize in brief treatment but are less able to handle longer stays or provide specialty programs such as for eating disorders, electroconvulsive therapy (ECT), children, or long-term intensive treatment. Therefore, managed care currently addresses both the presenting clinical condition of the patient and the specific institutional program that is being considered for admission. Inpatient hospitalization may be viewed as short term (currently up to 2 weeks), intermediate (2–4 weeks), and long term. Residential treatment criteria are often considered separately, as are criteria for partial hospitalization or custodial care. In the following section, I discuss criteria for each of these types of care. The American Psychiatric Association, in the *Manual of Psychiatric Quality Assurance* (Wilson 1992), specifies the following criteria for acute inpatient treatment:

- Danger to self
- Danger to others
- Court-ordered admission
- Failure of outpatient treatment
- Concurrent medical and psychiatric illnesses

Any of the criteria can justify inpatient admission but only after a threshold of severity is reached. Consequently, for patients to be considered dangerous to themselves, more than passive suicidal ideation is required. Even chronic suicidal ideation is usually insufficient to justify a hospital admission. Rather, only when there is persistent suicidal ideation with a specific plan, a recent serious suicide attempt, command hallucinations, or persistent, serious self-mutilating acts (such as cutting or burning oneself) has the "threshold" been reached to necessitate hospital admission. Factors that increase suicidal risk are considered, for example, a history of suicide in the family, dead relatives or loved ones with whom one wishes to join, anniversary reactions, and previous suicide attempts.

Consequently, danger to oneself is based on a clinical assessment of the seriousness of the risk. Occasional suicidal or homicidal ideation, or even persistent suicidal ideation without life-threatening gestures, attempts, or plan is currently considered by managed care standards as appropriate for treatment in an outpatient or partial hospital setting, whereas serious life-threatening suicidal or homicidal attempts or persistent serious ideation with a feasible plan and history of previous attempts justifies inpatient admission. In the same way, danger to others needs to be assessed carefully and clinically to determine the degree of risk and seriousness of the threat. Consequently, current utilization review and managed care procedures require that a patient be clinically assessed, carefully and thoroughly, prior to admission. Previously, patients would often walk into a hospital—or be recruited by a hospital marketing program or radio or TV advertisements—and be admitted to a hospital without a careful clinical assessment and preadmission review.

The other admission criteria listed in the American Psychiatric Association *Manual of Psychiatric Quality Assurance* (Wilson 1992) also are more actively reviewed and questioned by managed care companies. For example, court-ordered admissions are not automatically certified by managed care. The thinking is that a court order of hospitalization for evaluation or treatment does not mean that inpatient treatment is medically necessary.

Similarly, failure of outpatient treatment as a reason for hospitalization would be more actively questioned in current utilization review. For example, an evaluation would be made before admission to determine whether some other treatment (another form of therapy, a different therapist, different medications) has been tried or might be useful. More intensive outpatient treatment, partial hospitalization, or specialty treatment (e.g., specialized group therapy, eating disorders programs, couples or family therapy) might also be considered before certifying inpatient treatment. For example, in the *Manual of Psychiatric Quality Assurance,* one reason given for hospital admission is that of "frequent binging and purging, over 4 times daily, in a bulimic patient for a period of over two weeks" (Wilson 1992, p. 117). That kind of problem might be an indication for a more specialized outpatient eating disorders program or partial hospital program, unless the patient has severe electrolyte imbalance, cardiac arrhythmia, other major medical complications, or severe weight loss (e.g., below 75% of lean body weight). Other examples given in the manual—a marked deterioration in personal hygiene, persistent refusal by the patient to comply with medication, or failure to show symptomatic or functional improvement in an affective or psychotic illness—would not necessarily be certified as medically necessary for an inpatient admission by many managed care organizations.

Case Examples

Case 1. An obsessional man who was unable to function had been judged to have "decreased mental capacity." He was not taking his medications nor coming to therapy sessions with any regularity. Inpatient hospitalization was requested to provide control and structure for the patient. However he was not psychotic, homicidal, or suicidal. Managed care did not certify inpatient care but rather certified partial hospitalization to provide the necessary structure, medication management, and therapy.

Case 2. An elderly paranoid woman with organic mental syndrome had turned off the heat in her house in January. The patient had been delusional for more than 40 years, but never treated. She had been started on haloperidol by an internist, but the dose was not increased because of side effects. After 4 weeks, there was no change in her mental status, so hospitalization was recommended. However, with managed care involvement, a suggestion was made to switch to another neuroleptic medication so the dose could be increased. A change in her living arrangements was also recommended. The patient improved, and a move to a supervised group home was arranged.

Case 3. A patient was judged acutely suicidal by an employee assistance counselor. Nevertheless, he traveled unaccompanied hundreds of miles to the hospital. The hospital staff also said he was acutely suicidal. Yet the medical records revealed that the day after admission he was given an unaccompanied pass off the hospital grounds. These facts raised questions about the seriousness of his suicidality, resulting in a denial of certification for the hospitalization.

Case 4. A 65-year-old man had problems in his second marriage. His wife wanted to leave him. His only previous history was that in his 40s he had been treated as an outpatient for depression after a divorce. He had never had vegetative symptoms of depression, and he was never suicidal, homicidal, or psychotic. His wife took him to a hospital, and the hospital recommended lengthy inpatient treatment. The utilization reviewer questioned the necessity of inpatient treatment but did certify outpatient therapy (including couples therapy).

In summary, admission criteria for inpatient hospitalization are currently based on the severity of the illness, the intensity of the treatment, and a history of failure of less intensive forms of treatment. Admission is usually not certified for a chronic condition by itself (e.g., where there is no acute exacerbation), in lieu of incarceration for illegal activities, the convenience of the patient or his or her family, fear of relapse, behavioral or characterological changes when the behavior itself is not life threatening, or an alternative living environment (e.g., residential treatment for adolescents). At the same time, if an adolescent is a runaway, has not cooperated with treatment, or is acting out to such an extent that he or she cannot engage in treatment without some form of "holding," then residential treatment or inpatient treatment is considered medically necessary and appropriate. Currently, even treatments such as ECT or detoxification for substance abuse can be accomplished on an outpatient basis.

Criteria for inpatient hospitalization take into account the specific needs of the patient, the specific inpatient program to address those needs, and the severity of clinical symptoms that have been carefully and completely evaluated by a trained mental health clinician. Inpatient psychiatric treatment is certified when there is serious, life-threatening suicidal or homicidal behavior or plan; serious threat to basic adaptive skills necessary for survival; a floridly psychotic decompensation; ineffective outpatient treatment; serious concomitant medical illness that can only be managed in a hospital; or a dysfunctional family system that is so destructive (e.g., recurrent violence, rape, or incest) that the patient needs to be removed from the home for stabilization and transition to another environment.

Long-Term Hospitalization

Certification for long-term hospitalization, like all other forms of hospitalization, is based on a careful clinical assessment of the patient as well as an evaluation of the previous treatment history, especially the hospitalization history. In addition, as with regular hospital care, long-term hospitalization takes place in a variety of settings (Wilson and Phillips 1992a, 1992b), including residential treatment centers, state hospitals and other public facilities, hospitals that specialize in long-term intensive psychodynamic treatment, and some partial hospitalization programs. Often, long-term hospital care is used when a patient has failed to improve after several shorter inpatient hospital stays.

In the past, residential treatment care was often used in cases where adolescents (or others) needed a semistructured setting separate from a dysfunctional (or nonpresent) family. Currently, residential treatment—although still most often recommended for adolescents—is viewed as a transition from inpatient care or as a temporary supportive environment but measured more in weeks to months rather than years.

The following are examples of utilization review criteria for admission to residential care treatment:

- Inability to recover or stabilize from an acute illness or to maintain improvement after several acute inpatient or partial hospitalization treatments followed by outpatient care.

- History of failed attempts at reintegration into the family and community life following several acute or partial hospitalizations.
- Presence of severely dysfunctional (e.g., incest, violence) factors in the family or other support systems with severe social, school, or work disruptions.
- Recurrent truancy or runaway behavior (adolescents).
- Recurrent loss of impulse control (e.g., hypersexual, suicidal, or violent behavior of a chronic nature) that needs more structure and supervision than the family, foster home, or school can provide.
- Chronic substance abuse, not responsive to previous inpatient or outpatient treatment.
- Chronic, severe school phobia, not responsive to outpatient or partial hospital treatment (including medication trials).

Long-term inpatient psychiatric hospitalization is usually considered when briefer hospitalizations have led to readmissions. This pattern is sometimes referred to as the "revolving door." In such cases, some patients—especially those who are verbal and can benefit from an intensive, long-term working-through process—may be certified by managed care for longer stays. These include patients with severe character pathology who are repeatedly mutilating themselves or are prone to frequent decompensation. Extended hospital treatment is also certified for patients who need specialized treatment, such as ECT, after failure of antidepressant medication trials. Also included are patients with eating disorders of a life-threatening nature and patients who have a severe dissociative disorder or multiple personality disorder.

The current treatment of multiple personality disorder and dissociative disorder is controversial (Chu 1992; Frankel 1993; Putnam and Loewenstein 1993). Many therapists believe that an intensive, long-term working through and integration of alters are essential to the successful treatment of such patients. Others see such treatments as time consuming, expensive, regressive, destabilizing, and often not resulting in lasting improvement. Inpatient programs that concentrate on treating patients with multiple personality disorder often use specialized techniques such as hypnosis, amytal interviews, group therapy, psychodrama, and other abreactive techniques such as primal scream therapy. In an era of insurance limitations, such as 30 inpatient days per year or a lifetime limited dollar amount of treatment, financial constraints become additional factors in the consideration of the type of psychiatric care realistically available to these patients.

At present, many managed care companies are reluctant to certify long-term, regressive, abreactive treatment, not only because of contractual lifetime insurance limits, but also because managed care views such treatment as counterproductive, destabilizing and inappropriate.

Long-term treatment may also be certified for patients in partial hospitalization programs, although partial hospitalization is usually certified for shorter stays. Although partial hospitalization (day hospital, day treatment) is used as an alternative to inpatient care (when a patient is not seriously suicidal, violent, or unmanageable) or to facilitate reentry into the community from an inpatient hospital stay, partial hospitalization may be used on a longer term basis as a rehabilitative setting for chronically ill patients or for certain patients (e.g., adolescents, geriatric patients, those with substance abuse problems) when a more intensive, structured treatment program is indicated than can be given in two or three outpatient sessions a week. Acting-out patients with severe borderline disorder often respond to a structured day hospitalization program. For partial hospitalization to be effective, adequate resources are needed to monitor and support evening and weekend activities.

It should be noted that although many partial hospitalization programs are 5 or 6 days (or evenings) a week, many patients can benefit from day treatment programs that are reduced in frequency to 2 or 3 days a week.

Like inpatient treatment, many partial hospital programs provide a combination of treatments including individual therapy, medication management, group therapy, family therapy, and other activities—including occupational therapy, music therapy, art therapy, stress management, and overall institutional support that maintains an emergency response system. In such programs, fragile chronic patients can maintain productive work and school activities and contact with their family (when not destructive) and can often improve.

Clinical criteria for admission and continued stay in partial hospitalization programs are not unlike those for full inpatient programs, except the mental disorder is less severe. Candidates for partial hospitalization must have a major diagnosable disorder, specific symptoms and behaviors that can be identified; their treatment must be focused on the amelioration of symptoms, with medication and behavioral management.

The last major category of long-term hospitalization is for patients needing custodial care. Custodial patients are those who have reached their optimal levels of functioning and thereby have achieved maximum benefit from acute and intermediate treatment services. These patients often have tried a variety of treatments and therapies in a variety of inpatient, partial hospital, and outpatient settings. The use of the term *custodial* implies chronicity with limited hope for improvement.

Custodial care—usually given in state or Veterans Affairs hospitals in the United States—constitutes supportive and maintenance services provided to minimize the deterioration of patients whose psychiatric problems have resulted in serious, continuous impairment in life functioning. In the current managed care environment, custodial care is rarely certified by managed care programs because in the United States, such patients historically have been supported and maintained in state hospitals or state clinic programs. Nonetheless, utilization review may have a significant impact on the treatment of patients in long-term care facilities. The following is an example.

Case 5. A woman in her mid-30s had many hospitalizations, including several long-term, intensive inpatient treatment programs. Her diagnosis varied from major depression with borderline personality disorder, to schizoaffective disorder, to bipolar affective disorder. Many medications—separately and in combination—were tried. Then a course of ECT was utilized. No treatment was helpful. Custodial care in a state hospital was planned. In the managed care review, the reviewing psychiatrist discussed the case at length with the treating psychiatrist and ended the conversation by saying, "Well, doctor, the only medication you haven't tried is Tegretol." Ten days later, when another call was made to review the case, the doctor reported that Tegretol was started, the patient was much better, had a successful pass with her mother, and the mother said, "I have my daughter back again." The patient was discharged to outpatient care rather than to the state hospital.

Conclusion

As utilization review and managed care have become more prevalent, changes in both medical and psychiatric care have occurred. Inpatient stays have become shorter and limited to severe psychiatric problems. Patients and their families are expected to go home from inpatient treatment sooner or to a lower level of care. As a result, there has been an increase in partial hospital and structured outpatient programs.

The transition to partial hospitalization, structured outpatient, or regular outpatient care is facilitated by a continuum of care, in which there is a smooth transition from inpatient to outpatient care and a quicker transition and reintegration into community and family life. The degree to which continuity of care can be achieved through managed care networks or hospital-affiliated networks expedites the likelihood of an effective, smooth transition and reintegration into family and occupational life. Residential care is also viewed as transitional in most instances, in contrast to the previous view.

It is likely that certification for hospitalization by managed care will occur less often and be of shorter duration. There is an increased likelihood of partial hospitalization as an alternative to inpatient care, and other options are likely to expand.

One option is the use of an observation bed (also called a *23-hour bed*). This is a procedure in which a patient is admitted to an emergency department for evaluation, acute stabilization, and acute detoxification (in the case of substance abuse). Every effort is made to use medication and crisis-oriented therapy to stabilize and transfer the patient in less than 24 hours. This effort requires active use of medications; arrangements for careful evaluation from family, co-workers, or others; and making arrangements with family for support and transition to partial hospitalization or outpatient treatment.

Another modality is the use of crisis intervention teams (crisis stabilization units, in-home treatment, mobile evaluation teams) to quickly and actively go to the patient at home or work. Professional personnel, trained in crisis management and acute stabilization, function to stabilize an acute situation and divert treatment toward nonhospital settings if possible. Organizations such as Positive Alternatives to Hospitalization and Acute Community Crisis Evaluation Service System are already functioning.

Whatever the future brings, it is most likely to include increased government controls, capitated care, large multispecialty groups—some of which will include mental health care and others that will not—and even shorter hospital stays in both inpatient and partial hospital programs.

References

Allen MG: Understanding and coping with utilization review and managed care. Psychoanalysis and Psychotherapy 11:113–118, 1994

Allen MG, Phillips KL: Utilization review of treatment for chemical dependence. Hosp Community Psychiatry 44: 752–756,1993

American Psychiatric Association: Diagnostic and Statistical Manual of Mental Disorders, 4th Edition. Washington, DC, American Psychiatric Association, 1994

Anderson DF: How effective is managed mental health care? Business and Health 34–35, 1989

Arispe IE: 1991 Sourcebook on HMO Utilization Data. Washington, DC, Group Health Association of America, 1991

Callahan JJ, Shepard DS, Beinecke RH, et al: Evaluation of the Massachusetts Medicaid Mental Health/Substance Abuse Program. Waltham, MA, Brandeis University, 1994

Chu JA: The critical issues task force report: the role of hypnosis and amytal interviews in the recovery of traumatic memories. International Society for the Study of Multiple Personality and Dissociation News 10(3):6–9, 1992

Fink EB, Longabaugh R, Stout R: The paradoxical underutilization of partial hospitalization. Am J Psychiatry 135:713–716, 1978

Frankel FH: Adult reconstruction of childhood events in the multiple personality literature. Am J Psychiatry 150:954–958, 1993

Greene LR, De La Cruz A: Psychiatric day treatment as alternative to and transition from full-time hospitalization. Community Ment Health J 17:191–202, 1981

Herz MI: Research overview in day treatment. Int J Partial Hosp 1:33–44, 1982

Jellinek MS, Nurcombe B: Two wrongs don't make a right: managed care, mental health, and the marketplace. JAMA 270:1737–1739, 1993

Kiesler CA: Mental hospitals and alternative care. Am Psychol 37:349–360, 1982

Kuzmicki KV, Penner NR: Cost containment: the American Psychiatric Association's psychiatric case management program. QRB Qual Rev Bull 13:21–25, 1987

Mason JC, Louks JL, Burmer GC, et al: The efficacy of partial hospitalization: a review of recent literature. Int J Partial Hosp 1:251–269, 1982

Mattson MR (ed): Manual of Psychiatric Quality Assurance. Washington, DC, American Psychiatric Press, 1992

Mosher LR: Alternatives to psychiatric hospitalization. N Engl J Med 309:1579–1580, 1983

Office of National Cost Estimates: national health expenditures, 1988. Health Care Financ Rev 11(4):20–33, 1990

Pogge DL, Miller R, Stavridis G, et al: Length of stay not related to long-term outcome. Psychiatric News 25:11, 1990

Putnam FW, Loewenstein RJ: Treatment of multiple personality disorder: a survey of clinical practices. Am J Psychiatry 150:1048–1052, 1993

Sabin JE: The impact of managed care on psychiatric practice. Directions in Psychiatry 14:1–7, 1994

Sharfstein SS: Utilization management: managed or mangled psychiatric care? Am J Psychiatry 147:965–966, 1990

Washburn S, Vannicelli M, Longabaugh R, et al: A controlled comparison of psychiatric day care and inpatient hospitalization. J Consult Clin Psychol 44:665–675, 1976

Wilson GF: Utilization review for adult short-term hospitalization, in Manual of Psychiatric Quality Assurance. Edited by Mattson MR. Washington, DC, American Psychiatric Press, 1992, pp 115–120

Wilson GF, Phillips KL: Utilization review criteria for adult extended hospitalization, in Manual of Psychiatric Quality Assurance. Edited by Mattson MR. Washington, DC, American Psychiatric Press, 1992a, pp 121–126

Wilson GF, Phillips KL: Residential treatment centers: quality assurance and utilization review guidelines, in Manual of Psychiatric Quality Assurance. Edited by Mattson MR. Washington, DC, American Psychiatric Press, 1992b, pp 173–180

Chapter 11

Should the ASAM Criteria Be Adopted as a National Standard?

Jonathan D. Book, M.D.
Henry T. Harbin, M.D.
Clarissa C. Marques, Ph.D.
Chip Silverman, Ph.D., M.P.H.
Suzanne Lizanich-Aro, R.N., M.P.H.
Arthur Lazarus, M.D.

With control of health care costs high on the nation's agenda, the substance abuse treatment field sorely needs a universally accepted set of criteria for maintaining utilization of substance abuse services. Published in 1991, the American Society of Addiction Medicine (ASAM) criteria were based on the Cleveland criteria and the criteria of the National Association of Addiction Treatment Providers, which were both developed in 1987 (Hoffman et al. 1991). Although the ASAM criteria and

Adapted from Book J, Harbin H, Marques C, et al: "The ASAM and Green Spring Alcohol and Drug Detoxification and Rehabilitation Criteria for Utilization Review." *American Journal on Addictions* 4:187–197, 1995. Used with permission.

their predecessors have received only limited critical or empirical evaluation to date (McKay et al. 1992; Mee-Lee 1993), they obviously constitute a major effort and have rapidly become widely known as a fully articulated set of criteria sponsored by a prestigious medical group. Filling a vacuum in the field, the ASAM criteria have already begun to influence the thinking of some policymakers and regulators. A few states have even begun to consider adopting the ASAM criteria as the cornerstone of their legislative efforts to control the costs of substance abuse treatment.

The research on substance abuse treatment has been significantly advanced since the ASAM criteria development began. In this chapter, we show how the new knowledge gained from these advances in research can be used to support the need for expanded work on the ASAM criteria, particularly in the area of outpatient levels of care and treatment. In addition, we show how the effectiveness of the ASAM criteria can be maximized when combined with other medical necessity criteria such as those developed by managed care organizations. In doing so, we draw heavily from our experience at Green Spring Health Services (GSHS), a national behavioral health care company with a network of more than 25,000 individual providers serving more than 10 million subscribers.

Development of Green Spring's Medical Necessity Criteria

GSHS (1992) has developed clinical criteria and procedures based on many years conducting utilization review. Our criteria are determined by the severity of illness and intensity of service across a continuum of treatment levels. The criteria have been derived from extensive practice in the peer review field, provider input, experience in performing utilization management, and outcomes research literature. The criteria were reviewed and critiqued by a national advisory board with expertise in the field of addiction research and treatment. The GSHS criteria guide insurers in making certain that reimbursed treatments are specific to patient conditions and that the treatments have been provided at the least restrictive level believed to be effective for the individual patient.

GSHS has provided its clinical criteria as well as detailed procedures for conducting utilization review free of charge to all institutional providers in a proactive fashion and, on request, to any individual mental health or substance abuse practitioner. This policy has allowed providers to become knowledgeable about these criteria and to make sound decisions about the criteria before the review takes place. GSHS's commitment to an open and clear clinical decision-making process has minimized confusion regarding utilization review decisions and has facilitated a positive relationship between GSHS and the provider community.

GSHS's criteria are constantly being evaluated against patient outcome measures as well as by extensive input from professional providers. GSHS's current medical necessity criteria were last revised in 1993. Additional criteria for some levels of care have been developed since 1993 and are currently being revised. The most recent revisions were based on the following data sources:

- Written and verbal input from a multitude of professionals who have been reviewed by GSHS.
- The latest outcome studies in the field of psychiatry and substance abuse.
- The most recent drafts of related publications by national professional associations including ASAM and the American Psychiatric Association.
- GSHS's National Mental Health Advisory Committee and its National Substance Abuse Advisory Committee. These advisory committees have nationally recognized authorities in the fields of substance abuse and mental health who represent well-known academic institutions and national professional associations.
- Input from the senior clinical and medical leadership of GSHS and from criteria previously developed by Blue Cross and Blue Shield Plans.

Each revision has led to a decrease in ambiguity in the interpretation of the criteria and continues to incorporate the technological advances in the field of mental health and substance abuse. Because GSHS has made its criteria public to all providers, most reviews are accomplished with professionals who have a copy of the criteria. As a result, GSHS has access to feedback on the criteria from a variety of professional providers and regularly reviews these valuable contributions so that improvements resulting from this information are incorporated into each revision.

The GSHS criteria share many of the basic assumptions that are credited to the development of the ASAM criteria and their predecessors according to Hoffman et al. (1991, pp. 4–6). These assumptions include the following:

- Substance abuse treatment should be "individualized, quality clinical care based on patient assessment and treatment planning" (p. 4);
- Providers must "demonstrate both fiscal accountability . . . and a rational clinical decision-making process" (p. 4);
- "Escalating health care and insurance costs were viewed as factors in the treatment of substance abuse disorders in the same way as with other medical problems" (p. 4);
- "The preferred level of care was the least intensive level that could accomplish the treatment objectives while providing safety and security for the patients" (p. 6).

GSHS Versus ASAM Criteria

GSHS is both a provider and manager of substance abuse treatment; its clinicians use many clinical tools while providing treatment and evaluating the effectiveness of services including, but not limited to, the GSHS Medical Necessity Criteria for Detoxification and Rehabilitation Treatment. In some cases, GSHS staff also employ the ASAM criteria as a treatment planning guide. It is GSHS's position that the criteria sets are complementary and that benefits may be gained through their combined use. For example, the ASAM criteria are useful to clinicians precisely because the criteria draw their attention to a wide range of treatment issues that may require some form of intervention. However, because of perceived limitations of the ASAM criteria, when GSHS is acting primarily as a utilization review agent, it uses the GSHS criteria to determine level of care. In general, we believe that choosing between different sets of criteria should be based on their respective merits for that purpose, as revealed in a critical analysis of their differences and implications.

The ASAM criteria appear to have a broader treatment rationale and purpose, which may limit their usefulness for utilization review. The ASAM criteria were designed as a patient placement criteria tool to help guide treatment decisions within levels of care by assessing six dimensions of patient functioning: 1) acute intoxification or withdrawal potential, 2) biomedical conditions and complications, 3) emotional or behavioral conditions or complications, 4) treatment acceptance or resistance, 5) relapse potential, and 6) recovery environment. GSHS, in fact, has found the ASAM criteria useful for elucidating components of treatment and uses them to assist in planning clinical treatment. However, GSHS has also found wide variability and inconsistency in the application of ASAM criteria in the determination of medical necessity for substance abuse treatment across facilities, programs, and providers nationwide.

Our analysis reveals that the ASAM criteria have shortcomings when employed as a tool for utilization management and that legislative adoption of the ASAM criteria in their current state of development could have an effect opposite to the one that legislators intend. Public officials are seeking objective means of reducing the cost of substance abuse treatment while protecting the quality of care. Their chief method is to reduce unnecessary hospital and residential care and replace it with outpatient treatment wherever therapeutically defensible. Although the ASAM criteria may appear to move the field in that direction, without the refinement the recent literature suggests they may actually restrict the use of outpatient treatment and tend to recommend use of the most expensive and restrictive forms of treatment for patients who do not need them. In the words of one of the authors of the ASAM criteria (Mee-Lee 1992), "The ASAM criteria bring to the field guidelines that can help clinicians, payers and policy makers broaden the treatment options. The criteria place a greater emphasis on the continuum of care which must include outpatient levels of care and encourage flexible movement up or down the continuum. At the same time, the criteria uphold the legitimacy of inpatient levels of care and protect and guard clinical integrity and patient care" (p. 21).

Although GSHS also believes that inpatient or residential care is legitimate, GSHS maintains that outpatient care is the treatment of choice in most cases. Residential care is necessary and, therefore, legitimate for substance abuse treatment only under a limited set of circumstances where patient needs indicate that inpatient care is the appropriate treatment modality. Indeed, the Brandeis University Institute for Health Policy Study on Substance Abuse (1993), funded by the Robert Wood Johnson Foundation, found that 82% of all substance abuse treatment was conducted on an outpatient basis in 1991.

The disparity between the ASAM criteria and the GSHS criteria stems from several key structural differences between the two criteria sets. Compared with the ASAM criteria, the GSHS criteria employ more levels of care (six to four), specifically including an additional level for supervised residential treatment, such as halfway houses, and having a level of care for intensive outpatient treatment that is separate from partial hospitalization (Table 11–1). For many patients, these intermediate forms of outpatient care are lower-cost, functional equivalents of residential treatment. We would like to see ASAM expand its criteria to include the complete continuum of treatment alternatives while allocating limited residential treatment resources to patients more precisely on the basis of need for that level of treatment.

In GSHS's extensive experience in conducting utilization review and determining medical necessity in substance abuse treatment facilities and programs nationwide, we have consistently experienced providers using and, in some cases, distorting the ASAM criteria to support residential treatment as the primary solution to a very wide range of patient problems (assessment dimensions). The range of problems include whether the patient

- is heavily intoxicated or has potential for a withdrawal process;
- has biomedical conditions or complications;
- has emotional or psychological conditions or complications;
- is in denial or is resistant to treatment;
- is in imminent danger of relapsing;
- has an unsupportive home or work situation;

Table 11–1. Levels of care in the ASAM and GSHS criteria systems

Level of care	ASAM criteria	GSHS criteria
Hospital	Medically managed	Acute care
Residential	Medically monitored	Subacute care
Halfway house	NA	Supervised/residential
Partial hospitalization/ day treatment	Partial hospitalization/ day treatment[a]	Partial hospitalization/ day treatment
Intensive outpatient	Intensive outpatient[a]	Intensive outpatient
Outpatient	Outpatient	Traditional outpatient

Note. ASAM = American Society of Addiction Medicine. GSHS = Green Spring Health Services. NA = not applicable.
[a]ASAM criteria do not distinguish between partial hospitalization/day treatment and outpatient intensive levels of care.

- lacks transportation to treatment;
- is in danger of physical, emotional, or sexual attack or victimization; or
- has a job where continued substance use might put him or her or others at risk.

Because there is little empirical evidence linking many of these factors to patient outcomes or services that can only be delivered in a residential setting, the GSHS criteria assume that these problems can often be addressed effectively and efficiently by less restrictive and less expensive levels of care.

Although it may not have been the initial intent, the ASAM criteria appear to be structured and used in a manner that favors residential treatment over outpatient treatment as the treatment of choice for persons with significant substance abuse problems. Among today's substance abusers, few can satisfy the ASAM outpatient criteria. For example, although a patient who has failed to complete an outpatient detoxification in the past or is in danger of relapsing while attending only a self-help group may need only an intensification of outpatient services, ASAM recommends that this patient has to satisfy just one of five other assessment dimensions (e.g., is in denial or has unsupportive family members) to be placed in residential treatment. Furthermore, to be eligible for admission to outpatient treatment in the ASAM system, a patient can have only minimal risk of severe withdrawal (i.e., not being physiologically dependent on opiates nor having used cocaine or amphetamines on consecutive days or even as often as the frequency of the program contact [once a week in most cases]). The patient must also have successfully completed an outpatient detoxification program in the past or have support services that ensure commitment to completion and continued care. The patient can have only a mild coexisting emotional condition and can have little or no risk of harming self or others. He or she must be willing to attend all scheduled activities and must not need a structured milieu program. Finally, the patient must have a supportive family and work environment and be able to get to treatment, or the patient must have demonstrated motivation and willingness to make the changes necessary to obtain these things.

Experienced clinicians would hardly be surprised if few substance abusers, including many who have successfully completed outpatient treatment, could satisfy all of these requirements. Indeed, *The Report of the 1991 ASAM Invitational Roundtable Conference on Patient Placement Criteria for Psychoactive Substance Abuse Disorders* (American Society of Addiction Medicine 1991) describes the overemphasis on inpatient modalities as a drawback of the ASAM criteria and criticizes the criteria by noting that "patients may be placed in a higher level of care than needed" (p. 8). Thus, in our view there is insufficient empirical evidence at this time for state legislatures to take the unusual step of adopting the ASAM criteria in an unamended form above all other available criteria sets.

Standards

There are additional areas and issues that might also shed some light on redefining the ASAM criteria to support more cost-effective treatment. Comparison of the GSHS and ASAM criteria regarding inpatient care clearly indicates that GSHS criteria require patients to meet higher standards even when the content of the criteria are effectively the same. For example, the GSHS residential criteria require that a patient lives in a "severely dysfunctional living environment" (Green Spring Health Services 1992, p. RTC-2), whereas the ASAM counterpart requires only that "the patient lives in an environment (social and interpersonal network) in which treatment is unlikely to succeed" (Hoffman et al. 1991, p. 42). Although both criteria are open to variation in measuring the key concepts, we believe that there is far more latitude in deciding the characteristics of environments in which treatment is unlikely to succeed. Similarly, the GSHS criteria insist that "there must be actual evidence for, or clear and reasonable inference of serious, imminent physical harm to self or others, directly attributable to the continued abuse of substances which would prohibit treatment in an outpatient setting" (Green Spring Health Services 1992, p. RTC-2), whereas the ASAM criterion requires only that "there is danger of physical, sexual, and/or severe emotional attack or victimization in the patient's current environment which will make recovery unlikely without removing the individual from this environment" (Hoffman et al. 1991, p. 43). The standards of evidence in the GSHS criterion are clearly greater, and the danger must be caused by continued substance abuse rather than by general social or psychological conditions in which patients find themselves. This factor also weighs heavily toward supporting a broader continuum of treatment choices. Clearly though, the field would benefit from a more objective assessment of the dysfunctional environment and also whether such an environment makes a differential impact on treatment outcome.

Treatment Failure and Residential Treatment

Despite the lack of convincing scientific proof that residential treatment is more effective than outpatient treatment, the ASAM criteria appear to assume that the more severe a patient's status is on its six dimensions, the higher the level of care that he or she should receive. That is, there appears to be a linear relationship between the assessment dimensions and the level of care.

In GSHS's experience, various problems using the ASAM criteria follow from this assumption of linearity. Patients may have biomedical complications (e.g., cognitive deficits) that limit their ability to benefit from standard residential or hospital treatment. They may instead need long-term institutionalization or supervised living arrangements. Similarly, psychiatric problems may become so severe that the person cannot effectively participate in or benefit from residential substance abuse care or treatment in an acute care hospital's substance abuse unit. Psychiatric hospitalization, perhaps on a dual-diagnosis unit, would be a more appropriate treatment regimen. Some patients are so deeply in denial and so resistant to obtaining treatment that they lack sufficient motivation to cooperate with treatment or to achieve a positive long-term outcome. Similarly, some patients may so wish to return to drinking or using drugs that they attempt to leave the facility or smuggle drugs into it. Although it appears to be reasonable to respond to relapse by intensifying recovery efforts incrementally, intensification can take many forms both within and across levels of care. Residential treatment is clearly no panacea; many patients relapse repeatedly following residential treatment and eventually exhaust their insurance benefits. In some cases, they then succeed as outpatients in a publicly funded program or on their own. Finally, some patients live in situations so dangerous to recovery (e.g., married to a major drug dealer) that little can be gained if the situation is not changed or there must, at least, be commitment to change before entering treatment, be it inpatient or outpatient.

GSHS's criteria require mental competence and restorative potential and assume that responsible use of limited health care resources dictates against providing highly expensive residential treatment to persons who are clearly not yet ready for it or are no longer able to realize its benefits and could be placed in another type of appropriate setting (e.g., halfway house). Assuming there is not a need related to patient dangerousness, this principle of mental competence and restorative potential could be incorporated in the ASAM criteria.

Is There a Treatment of Choice for Substance Abusers?

We have recently witnessed a major shift in the treatment field's view about what constitutes the optimum course of treatment for substance abusers. In the past several decades clinical professionals and treatment facilities have adopted a particular model of treatment for substance abuse, often referred to as the *Minnesota Model* or the *chemical dependency model* (Geller 1992). Originally developed for alcoholic patients in three Minnesota treatment facilities, this model has responded to the recent epidemic of substance abuse among middle- and working-class populations (McAuliffe 1990). In contrast to the poor, inner-city heroin addict traditionally found in methadone clinics and therapeutic communities, these new substance abusers were employed, possessed health insurance, and were treated in hospitals or freestanding residential chemical dependency facilities (often far from home). The treatment regimen routinely consisted of detoxification and rehabilitation for a period of 28 days. Despite the professional context, the psychosocial clinical model employed in chemical dependency facilities followed the Twelve-Step Fellowship principles of Alcoholics Anonymous (AA). Upon discharge, patients were typically referred for aftercare to local self-help groups (e.g., AA or Narcotics Anonymous) or to local professionals for individual or group aftercare counseling (Geller 1992). In the event of relapse, another stay at the residential facility was commonly prescribed.

Eventually, the chemical dependency model of treatment came under attack (e.g., see Chiauzzi and Liljegren 1993). Analysis indicates that the detoxification component of the Minnesota Model implies a biomedical theory for substance abuse that emphasizes the central role of physiological dependence, to which medical management and monitoring are logical responses. However, basic research beginning in the 1950s (Nichols et al. 1956) demonstrated that animals would self-administer a withdrawal-inducing drug such as morphine even if the animals were not physiologically dependent. Subsequent studies demonstrated that self-administration of drugs such as amphetamines did not always produce physiological dependence. In some studies, animals became powerfully attached to the effects of cocaine even though there is no powerful physiological dependence evident in animals. Many theorists have interpreted this body of research as demonstrating that physiological dependence is not an essential condition of addiction (Edwards et al. 1982; McAuliffe and Gordon 1974). Although physiological dependence is a symptom of addiction, people may be physically dependent without any drug–seeking behavior, and some people are addicted to drugs such as stimulants without marked physical dependence. According to this view, the essence of addiction is behavioral drug reinforcement, including but not limited to reinforcement stemming from avoidance of unpleasant withdrawal symptoms when they are present.

The American Psychiatric Association (1994) and the World Health Organization (Edwards et al. 1982) revised their diagnostic criteria for substance dependence to reflect this change in the scientific understanding of the etiology of substance abuse. For example, DSM-IV (American Psychiatric Association 1994) includes tolerance and withdrawal as two of seven criteria of psychoactive substance dependence, but they are no longer required to be present to make the diagnosis of psychoactive substance dependence. The other five DSM-IV criteria are behavioral in nature. Any three of the seven are sufficient for making a diagnosis.

Epidemiological and clinical developments supported this new understanding of substance abuse and suggested that inpatient or residential detoxification and rehabilitation may be clinically unnecessary in many cases and that residential treatment was no more than the beginning of treatment. Field studies showed that many severe substance abusers, such as those with addiction to alcohol, heroin, or cocaine, were able to stop drug use on their own and to remain drug free (Biernacki 1986; Shaffer and Jones 1989; also see Chiauzzi and Liljegren 1993). Many patients tended to enter treatment at an earlier stage in their disease (Hoffman et al. 1991); consequently, advanced stages of physiological dependence and medical complications were no longer as prominent as in earlier times. Many alcoholic patients and patients with drug addictions presenting for treatment do not therefore require around-the-clock medical attention. Clinical studies showed that substance abusers could be detoxified safely and effectively as outpatients (Galloway and Hayner 1993; McDuff et al. 1993). In a leading reference work on substance abuse, the head of a New York drug detoxification unit stated unequivocally, "Anyone can be withdrawn successfully from a narcotic or a sedative-hypnotic-anxiolytic substance in an outpatient setting" (Alling 1992, p. 402). Even among those substance abusers who might require residential treatment on medical grounds, there is wide variation in the amount of medical attention required, indicating that there was little justification for the industry's longstanding habit of assigning all patients to the same length of stay.

Furthermore, as patient populations have increasingly shifted their drugs of abuse from alcohol, sedatives, and heroin to marijuana, hallucinogens, and cocaine (i.e., from drugs for which withdrawal is an important clinical feature to drugs for which it is not), the medical monitoring or intensive medical management of physiological withdrawal has become a less prominent feature of chemical dependency treatment. Although a cocaine withdrawal syndrome has recently been described in the literature, it consists mainly of psychological symptoms such as depression (Gawin 1991). Subjective craving is also said to be a cocaine withdrawal symptom, but most observers who have no stake in demonstrating that there is a cocaine withdrawal syndrome requiring residential treatment view craving as a symptom of addiction rather than as a symptom of physiological withdrawal. In any case, none of the symptoms of the cocaine withdrawal syndrome routinely require the intensive, 24-hour-per-day medical or psychiatric monitoring or management found in residential or inpatient treatment facilities. There is thus no clear rationale for requiring medical management or even medical monitoring in an inpatient setting for detoxification for uncomplicated cases of cocaine addiction, currently the major diagnostic group admitted to chemical dependency facilities.

Clinical research, primarily on alcoholic patients (Hayashida et al. 1989) but including some studies of other substance abusers (Amini et al. 1989), has failed to confirm the widely held assumption that residential treatment would produce better patient outcomes than would outpatient treatment in the broad cross-section of patients (Annis 1985–1986; Miller and Hester 1986). Scientific investigations covering several decades and several countries consistently have found no significant differences in the outcomes of patients randomly assigned to inpatient versus outpatient care. Although a study by Walsh et al. (1991) found that hospitalization followed by self-help participation was superior to referral for self-help participation alone, the study did not include an experimental condition for *professional* outpatient treatment or professional treatment of any kind, which would have made the study's results more clearly relevant to the issue at hand.

There is also experimental evidence that leads one to question whether the duration of residential treatment within the normal range has any measurable effect on patient outcomes (Annis 1985–1986). The recent Institute of Medicine report on drug abuse treatment (Gerstein and Harwood 1990) points out that controlled studies have not found that longer programs have yielded a better outcome than shorter treatment intervention (Bien et al. 1993; Ericksen 1986; Miller and Baca 1983; Powell et al. 1985; Walker et al. 1983).

A common response to the experimental research that failed to find a difference between residential and outpatient treatment was that the effects of residential treatment were masked by the inclusion of clients who did not need residential treatment. Presumably, if patients had been matched to treatment according to need, the results would have been more positive. This patient-matching hypothesis has received little experimental support thus far; other explanations of the research results are possible and should be explored. It is entirely possible, however, that more sensitive research will show the superior value for inpatient treatment for some subgroups of patients.

In one of the few relevant studies reported thus far, McKay et al. (1992) attempted to assess the validity of the Cleveland criteria (the original basis for the development of the ASAM criteria) for inpatient rehabilitation by comparing placement criteria at admission and treatment outcomes for 70 cocaine-addicted patients and 73 alcoholic patients who were assigned to day treatment. Thirty-five of the patients did not meet the Cleveland criteria for inpatient treatment, whereas 108 patients did. The latter group were therefore mismatched to day treatment and could be expected to have poorer outcomes than the former group if the Cleveland criteria were valid. When the authors compared the outcomes, there were no significant differences between the groups.

A major shortcoming of the chemical dependency model was the relative neglect of outpatient treatment that should have followed discharge from residential treatment. Of special importance are intermediate levels of outpatient care, as either primary care or aftercare. Even for those persons who achieved abstinence through residential or inpatient care, the bulk of the recovery process occurs only after the person has returned home to remain drug free. For many patients, the usual referral to self-help groups or to counseling for once or twice a week during a period of a few months did not provide the requisite amount of support to sustain long-term recovery. Many clinicians in the substance abuse field have now widely embraced the notion of a continuum of care that is most intensive at first and *gradually* declines in intensity as the patient recovers. However, until recently, the treatment system, especially with respect to treatment for illicit drugs, lacked a range of intermediate levels of care (e.g., halfway or recovery houses, day treatment, evening care) that could provide patients with the different levels of support they required as they progressed in recovery. Moreover, when clients became overwhelmed and relapsed, even briefly, there was no slightly more intensive level of care to refer them to, and as a result, the relapse typically worsened until a return to residential care was apparently warranted.

Finally, the great inflation in health care costs and the increasing trend toward including substance abuse treatment in health insurance benefit packages led to concerns about the high cost of substance abuse services. A month-long residential stay typically exceeded $10,000, sometimes substantially more, and frequently patients returned to residential treatment repeatedly.

The cost of a year of outpatient treatment was often only one-half to one-third, or even less, of the cost of a month of residential care and several months of aftercare. Studies also suggested that patients treated in residential settings have an increased propensity to use inpatient treatment settings again in the future without any offsetting improvement in outcome (Miller and Hester 1986). Not only does this point to higher costs at the time of treatment, but also to higher costs over time as the patient has a tendency subsequently to seek treatment in a more expensive treatment setting. To be equally cost-effective, residential treatment would have to produce long-term outcomes (e.g., abstinence rates) several times higher than those obtained through outpatient treatment. In light of the results of experimental studies reported to date, it appears unlikely that residential treatment can be easily justified on the grounds of cost-effectiveness for the typical substance-abusing patient. Thus, residential treatment may be a reasonable expense for only those special cases in which the complications of addiction are more severe, the patient's life is in danger, or other forms of treatment have failed. Although this may have been the intent in the design of the ASAM criteria, the definition of severity by substance abuse providers has led to a default recommendation of residential treatment.

Conclusion

Armed with the latest clinical research and theory, managed care companies such as GSHS have challenged the widely held assumption in the industry and among the lay public that residential treatment is the essence of routine substance abuse treatment. To the extent that the treatment of choice depends on patient characteristics, we have established criteria that assume most clients could be treated effectively on an outpatient basis (with a continuum of outpatient care including partial hospitalization, halfway houses, intensive outpatient, less intensive outpatient, aftercare, and long-term follow-up) and that residential treatment is required only when specifically indicated by particular conditions. Our view has gained increasing acceptance despite the organized efforts of persons who either have interests in maintaining the status quo or who sincerely believe that, despite scientific evidence to the contrary, they can best serve their patients—at least some of them—by providing them with the most intensive and expensive care available.

We believe that the ASAM criteria are helpful in treatment planning, but we have concluded that they are not adequate in medical necessity review for utilization management in their current form and should not be prematurely legislated as required criteria for level-of-care determinations. We have recommended several areas for revision in light of recent literature and changes in patterns of practice corresponding to this literature and the availability of a broader array of outpatient treatment services. We believe that such changes would yield improved cost-effective treatment because treatment would be more accurately matched to the needed level of care. In addition, with better matching of patients to level of care, better research on patient outcomes will be possible.

References

Alling F: Detoxification and treatment of substance abuse, in Substance Abuse: A Comprehensive Textbook. Edited by Lowinson JH, Ruiz P, Millman RB, et al. Baltimore, MD, Williams & Wilkins, 1992

American Psychiatric Association: Diagnostic and Statistical Manual of Mental Disorders, 4th Edition. Washington, DC, American Psychiatric Association, 1994

American Society of Addiction Medicine: Report of the 1991 Invitational Roundtable Conference on Patient Placement Criteria for Psychoactive Substance Use Disorders. Washington, DC, American Society of Addiction Medicine, 1991

Amini F, Zingberg NJ, Burke EL, et al: A controlled study of inpatient vs. outpatient treatment of delinquent drug abusing adolescents: one year results. Compr Psychiatry 23:436–444, 1989

Annis HM: Is inpatient rehabilitation of the alcoholic cost effective? Con position. Adv Alcohol Subst Abuse 5(1–2):175–190, 1985–1986

Bien TH, Miller WR, Tonigan JS: Brief interventions for alcohol problems: a review. Addiction 88:315–336, 1993

Biernacki P: Pathways from Heroin Addiction: Recovery Without Treatment. Philadelphia, PA, Temple University Press, 1986

Brandeis University Institute for Health Policy Study on Substance Abuse: Substance Abuse: The Nation's Number One Health Problem, Key Indicators for Policy. Princeton, NJ, Institute for Health Policy, Brandeis University for the Robert Wood Johnson Foundation, 1993

Chiauzzi EJ, Liljegren S: Taboo topics in addiction treatment: an empirical review of clinician folklore. Journal of Substance Abuse Treatment 10:303–316, 1993

Edwards G, Arif A, Hodgson R: Nomenclature and classification of drug and alcohol-related problems: a shortened version of a WHO memorandum. Br J Addict 77(1):3–20, 1982

Ericksen L: The effect of waiting for inpatient treatment after detoxification: an experimental comparison between inpatient treatment and advice only. Addict Behav 10:225–248, 1986

Galloway G, Hayner G: Haight-Ashbury free clinics' drug detoxification protocols: part 1: opioids. J Psychoactive Drugs 25:157–158, 1993

Gawin F: Cocaine addiction: psychology and neurophysiology. Science 251:1580–1586, 1991

Geller A: Rehabilitation programs and halfway houses, in Substance Abuse: A Comprehensive Textbook. Edited by Lowinson JH, Ruiz P, Millman RB, et al. Baltimore, MD, Williams & Wilkins, 1992

Gerstein D, Harwood H: Treating Drug Problems, Vol 1. Washington, DC, National Academy Press, 1990

Green Spring Health Services, Inc: Utilization Review Criteria 1992. Columbia, MD, Green Spring Health Services, Inc., 1992

Hayashida M, Alterman AI, McLellan AT, et al: Comparative effectiveness and cost of inpatient and outpatient detoxification of patients with mild-to-moderate alcohol withdrawal syndrome. N Engl J Med 320:358–365, 1989

Hoffman NG, Halikas JA, Mee-Lee D, et al: Patient Placement Criteria for the Treatment of Psychoactive Substance Use Disorders. Washington, DC, American Society of Addiction Medicine, 1991

McAuliffe WE: Health care policy issues in the drug abuser treatment field. J Health Polit Policy Law 15(2):357–385, 1990

McAuliffe WE, Gordon RA: Testing Lindesmith's theory of addiction: the frequency of euphoria among long-term addicts. Am J Sociology 79(4):795–840, 1974

McDuff DR, Schwaartz RP, Tommasello A, et al: Outpatient benzodiazepine detoxification procedure for methadone patients. J Subst Abuse Treat 1993, 10: 297–302, 1993

McKay JR, McLellan AT, Alterman AI: An evaluation of the Cleveland criteria for inpatient treatment of substance abuse. Am J Psychiatry 149:1212–1218, 1992

Mee-Lee D: The ASAM patient placement criteria for adolescent addictions treatment. Addiction & Recovery January/February, 1992, pp 20–22

Mee-Lee D: Patient placement criteria for chemical dependency: progress toward validation. Behavioral Healthcare Tomorrow 2(2):28–31, 1993

Miller WR, Baca LM: Two year follow-up of bibliotherapy and therapist directed controlled drinking for problem drinkers. Behavior Therapy 14:441–448, 1983

Miller WR, Hester RK: Inpatient alcoholism treatment: who benefits? Am Psychol 41:794–805, 1986

Nichols JR, Headlee CP, Coppock HW: Drug addiction I. Addiction by escape training. Journal of the American Pharmaceutical Association Scientific Edition 45:788–791, 1956

Powell BJ, Penick EC, Read R, et al: Comparison of three outpatient treatment interventions: a twelve-month follow-up of men alcoholics. J Stud Alcohol 46:309–312, 1985

Shaffer HJ, Jones SB: Quitting Cocaine: The Struggle Against Impulse. Lexington, MA, Lexington Books, 1989

Walker RD, Donovan DM, Kirlahan DR, et al: Length of stay, neurophysiological performance and aftercare: influences on alcohol treatment outcome. J Consult Clin Psychol 51:900–911, 1983

Walsh DC, Hingson RW, Merrigan DM, et al: "A randomized trial of treatment options for alcohol-abusing workers. N Engl J Med 325:775–782, 1991

Chapter 12

Who Decides What Is Medically Necessary?

Armin U. Kuder, LL.B.
Marcia B. F. Kuntz, J.D.

Determining what is medically necessary is fundamental to decisions about providing and paying for medical services. Apart from broad policy questions as to what should and should not be deemed medically necessary, once the concept is used to determine payment, managed care systems must establish a mechanism for determining what is medically necessary and who makes that decision in specific cases. Historically, physicians made the determination, insurers usually deferred to those decisions by covering the costs of the services provided, and if there was a dispute, it was resolved by a court.

The medical world has changed, and a number of other entities have joined in the process of defining medical necessity: insurers writing policies, federal and state governments, utilization reviewers, and health care managers. In this chapter we explore the question of who has the final word when conflicts arise.

Defining Medical Necessity

The need to determine what treatment is *medically necessary* is at the heart of any health care insurance or payment system. The concept, then, must be the cornerstone of any attempt to *manage care*, yet there is no simple or generally accepted definition of the concept among insurers, reviewers, and managed care organizations.

Medical necessity is used to mean something less than "life-or-death necessity," with the intent "to exclude coverage for care that is harmful, of no benefit, or nonstandard."[1] It is often considered interchangeable with the equally elusive concept of *medical appropriateness*.[2]

However, the elusiveness of these terms does not prevent utilization reviewers at all levels, whether in the governmental or private sector, from assessing whether a procedure or course of treatment is or was medically necessary in determining whether it should be paid for by someone other than the physician or patient. Some private insurance policies use the term without defining it.[3] Others use equivalent terms to connote a meaning of medical necessity: for example, *necessary medical services*, *medically required*, *necessary for medical care of illness*, *required in connection with illness*, and *medical expenses incurred for reasonable and necessary treatment of bodily injury*.[4]

Many policies use a checklist of criteria for a determination of medical necessity. One plan offered by an insurer in the District of Columbia, for example, defines the term as follows:

> Medically Necessary. Those services or supplies provided by a Hospital, physician or other Provider of health care services to diagnose or treat an illness, injury or medical condition in [sic] which the Health Plan Medical Director shall determine are:
> (1) appropriate and necessary for the symptoms, diagnosis or treatment of the medical condition;
> (2) provided for the diagnosis or direct care and treatment of the condition;
> (3) not provided primarily for cosmetic purposes;
> (4) not primarily Custodial Care (including domiciliary and institutional care);
> (5) not provided primarily for the convenience of the Member, the Member's attending or consulting physician or another health care provider;
> (6) are consistent with those benefits which are covered by the Health Plan; and
> (7) performed in the least costly setting or manner appropriate to treat the member's condition.[5]

The provision for mental health care in many insurance policies reflects prior decisions about what care is medically necessary, even if the term is not used. In the foregoing example, the last paragraph would exclude therapy designed to maintain a certain, less than ideal, level of function. Other insurance policies specifically limit coverage of mental illness to treatment of conditions the physician can assert are temporary and likely to be improved by treatment, as opposed to treatment for chronic illness. Many states now require that insurers provide a certain minimum level of mental health care for their policyholders, and insurers have responded by capping their coverage of mental health care at those minimum levels. Even these limited levels of treatment are reduced further. For example, in the group benefits contract of George Washington University Health Plan, Inc., at p. 42, cited above, in addition to the specified limits on mental health coverage, the plan provides that benefits for the treatment of mental and nervous disorders "will not be provided to Members who, in the opinion of a Plan Mental Health Provider or Medical Director, would not be responsive to treatment or therapy."

The attempts to limit and define treatment have not changed the fact that most payment plans and systems still rely on the broader terms. Coverage under Medicare and Medicaid is governed by general medical necessity principles. The Medicare statute, since its enactment in 1965, has disallowed payment for expenses that "are not reasonable and necessary for the diagnosis or treatment of illness or injury or to improve the functioning of a malformed body member. . . ."[6] The Supreme Court has suggested that the Medicaid statute should be interpreted to require states to cover all "medically necessary services."[7]

Even today, health care reform initiatives use the broad concept of *medical necessity.* For example, coverage under the Health Security Act, proposed by the Clinton administration, was to be controlled by medical necessity determinations. Coverage was not to be provided for "an item or service that is not medically necessary or appropriate."[8] Medical services were limited throughout the plan to those that are "medically necessary" or, in some sections, "medically indicated."[9] Regulations were to be promulgated to carry out the general limitation to treatment that was medically necessary.[10] Still, there was no attempt in the act itself to define the term or to guide the drafters of the regulations.

Asserting that medical necessity governs payment decisions under most private and public medical coverage systems is only to begin the inquiry on how reimbursement decisions are made. When contracts or statutes go beyond the general terms themselves and define or limit what will be called necessary, the process has begun to take form, and be limited, but even those attempts at definition are less than definitive.

Increasing Importance and Complexity of Medical Necessity Determination

As the curtailment of health care costs becomes a major priority in the health care industry, the payers of health care costs have taken a more active role in determining which medical services will be paid. In what commentators have labeled a "transition from the provider-based utilization review of the 1960s and 1970s to utilization management by third parties in the 1980s,"[11] payers have appropriated, to the extent they have been capable, the task of giving substance to the term *medical necessity.*

Several factors have affected this transition. First, government and private purchasers of insurance have "intensified involvement . . . in efforts to contain health care costs."[12] For example, in 1982, Congress established peer review organizations "to monitor the appropriateness and quality of medical care provided to Medicare beneficiaries."[13] It imposed a prospective payment system on Medicare for inpatient services, whereby hospitals are paid a fixed amount per case, with rates predetermined for each type of case, or diagnosis-related group.[14] Larger private employers have begun self-insuring; the proportion of companies surveyed in 1986 who have moved to self-insurance has increased from 19% in 1980 to 59%.[15]

Studies that raise questions about the exactness of medicine as a science provide a second stimulus in this transition to third-party review.[16] Studies have suggested that as many as one-fourth to one-third of all medical services performed are "of little or no benefit to patients."[17] There is great variability in the consumption of medical services across geographical areas.[18] Utilization of services varies widely based on cost.[19]

Other factors have contributed to the transition to third-party review: 1) an increasing abundance of resources that makes case-by-case evaluation possible and 2) an increasing concern on the part of purchasers of medical coverage (in the case of the government and large private employers that self-insure, the purchasers are also the insurers) with coordinating cost containment, both from the point of view of eliminating excessive medical services and of ensuring that quality is maintained.[20]

The more aggressive involvement in utilization review on the part of third-party reviewers, including insurers, has manifested itself in several ways. Policies requiring evidence of medical necessity have increased greatly in number over the past 15–20 years. More recently, insurers have begun writing policies to restrict coverage to only those medical services that *in the insurer's determination* are medically necessary.[21] Also, many policies now exclude experimental procedures or those performed primarily for investigative or educational purposes.

Of perhaps equal or greater significance, purchasers and insurers have recently instituted another dramatic change in utilization review. They have begun to require both prospective and concurrent review of treatment decisions in the belief that this approach will prevent the incurring of unnecessary medical costs. The review methods for nonemergency cases include evaluation of the location or level of care, precertification, ongoing review of hospitalization decisions, second-opinion requirements for surgical decisions, and intensified management of high-cost cases.[22]

Prior and concurrent reviews present a new set of factors for patients, physicians, insurers, and courts to consider in making decisions about the medical necessity of particular medical services. Patients must decide whether to undergo treatment despite a denial of coverage. Physicians must determine whether sound medicine requires that they nonetheless provide the medical service.[23] Insurers have to weigh whether to risk incurring additional liability when the services they have refused to cover are not provided to the patient.[24] Even courts are faced with decisions about whether to order perhaps extremely high cost procedures prospectively, without full records, knowing that a failure to do so could result in denial of treatment to the patient.[25]

The court in *Wickline v. State*[26] summarized the concern of everyone involved in medical necessity determinations thus:

> A mistaken conclusion about medical necessity following retrospective review will result in the wrongful withholding of payment. An erroneous decision in a prospective review process, on the other hand, in practical consequences, results in the withholding of necessary care, potentially leading to a patient's permanent disability or death."

Wickline is a groundbreaking case in that it begins to set standards for liability on the part of managed care reviewers for denials of coverage prospectively or concurrently. Ms. Wickline claimed that the discontinuance of eligibility under California's medical assistance program (Medi-Cal) caused her premature discharge from the hospital, which resulted in complications in her recovery from surgery and, ultimately, amputation of her right leg. Medi-Cal had approved 10 days of hospitalization for treatment of Leriche's Syndrome. The patient's treating physician concluded that it was *medically necessary* that the patient remain in the hospital for another 8 days. Her physician submitted the necessary forms to Medi-Cal, whose consulting physician authorized only 4 of the 8 additional days requested. The consulting physician testified that based on the information provided he determined that a longer stay was not medically necessary. The patient was discharged by two physicians after 4 additional days, pursuant to Medi-Cal's limited authorization. At home, the patient's leg became infected and had to be amputated. Her treating physician testified that had she remained in the hospital for the additional days requested, her progress could have been observed, and she would not have suffered the loss of her leg.

Although the court reversed a verdict against Medi-Cal, holding that the treating physicians, and not Medic-Cal, were the principal cause of the patient's early discharge, it went on to articulate a standard for third-payer liability in prospective review situations:

> Third party payers of health care services can be held legally accountable when medically inappropriate decisions result from defects in the design or implementation of cost containment mechanisms as, for example, when appeals made on a patient's behalf for medical or hospital care are arbitrarily ignored or unreasonably disregarded or overridden.[27]

After *Wickline*, the same appellate court decided the case of *Wilson v. Blue Cross of Southern California,*[28] standing more forcefully for the proposition that third-party insurers and reviewers can be held liable for injuries to patients resulting from a prospective denial of a claim. In that case, the insured was hospitalized for major depression, drug dependency, and anorexia on the determination of his treating physician that he needed 3 to 4 weeks of care. After 10 days, the insurer announced that it would not pay for further inpatient care. The decedent was discharged and committed suicide 3 weeks later. The court held that the concurrent reviewer, which had made the decision not to pay for further hospitalization, could be found liable for the decedent's death. Although so far, courts in other jurisdictions have found that plaintiffs asserting claims against third-party reviewers failed to show that the reviewer's decision was a legally cognizable cause of the plaintiff's injuries, the *Wilson* court said, "There is substantial evidence that Western Medical's decision not to approve further hospitalization was a substantial factor in bringing about the decedent's demise."[29] *Wilson* explicitly rejects the *Wickline* panel's suggestion that the physician is principally liable for treatment decisions. These cases could have far-reaching effects on prior and concurrent review cases. The cases highlight the increasing complexity of deciding what is medically necessary.

However, an important limitation to *Wilson*'s holding regarding the potential liability of utilization reviewers quite likely exists for plans governed by the Employee Retirement Income Security Act (ERISA).[30] In general, ERISA plans are those funded and administered by employers for the benefit of their employees, although the issue of which plans are or are not covered by ERISA is complicated and largely unresolved. In the case of *Corcoran v. United Healthcare, Inc.,*[31] the court held that a utilization reviewer of an ERISA plan is not subject to a malpractice action for the reviewer's decision to deny coverage. Under *Corcoran*, the reasoning in *Wilson* concerning the potential liability of utilization reviewers does not apply to the review of ERISA plans. Although the *Corcoran* court recognized that prospective denial of coverage might directly influence medical treatment decisions, the court said that the reviewer's decision constituted a "benefit determination" as well as a medical determination, placing the decision under the rubric of ERISA and its restrictions on the types of lawsuits that plaintiffs can bring.[32]

How Are Medical Necessity Determinations Made?

In the real world of medical treatment and payment, most patient-physician-insurer relationships do not start with a legal opinion or decision. Patients decide whether to receive a particular medical service or course of treatment for a problem, based on options explained by the health care provider and, in nonemergency situations, on whether the insurer is likely to pay. If the patient opts for treatment, the patient or treatment provider applies to a third-party coverer for payment or reimbursement, and the third party pays after limited review.

It is the extraordinary situation in which the third party refuses to pay. Insurers issue absolute denials of payment in fewer than 2% of all cases, although in many more cases, insurers negotiate with physicians to modify the proposed treatment program during some stage of the review process.[33] The low 2% figure should not be interpreted as an indication that payment decisions are made rigorously, consistently, or nonarbitrarily.[34] Nevertheless, the small percentage of contested cases do set standards that govern the conduct of the parties in the vast body of daily treatment and payment decisions. So we must turn to how those conflicts arise and then how they are resolved.

What the Physician and Insured or Patient Decide

The first party making a decision regarding treatment coverage is the patient, or the insured, if the two are different. In searching for a health insurance policy or deciding whether to join a health care plan, the insured in theory carefully reads policy provisions and performs a cost-benefit analysis and assessment of risk in determining the breadth of coverage he or she wants to pay for. It is a separate, albeit important, policy decision whether the insured should be held strictly accountable for this initial decision in later determinations of whether insurers should be forced to provide coverage in particular cases.

Once the patient chooses a plan and it appears that the third-party payer will refuse to pay, the patient and physician have several options. Only if coverage is denied prospectively can the patient refuse the treatment. Whether prospective or retrospective, patient and physician can look to each other to absorb treatment costs. They can hire a lawyer and file suit or attempt settlement.[35] Failing that, they can ask a court for a decision.

What the Insurer Decides

There are a number of ways in which insurers attempt to control decisions about medical necessity and, therefore, about coverage. The principal way is through the drafting of their insurance policies.

In drafting policies, insurers can simply exclude certain medical services. When these exclusions are clear, they probably prevent some disputes. It is likely that patients do not bother in most cases to seek payment for services that are clearly excluded, such as fertility services, sex reassignment surgery, hearing and visual aids, and orthodontia. Again, however, health insurance providers cannot anticipate all types of treatment and, therefore, must resort to more generally worded exclusions, such as exclusions for procedures that are not medically necessary. This word choice, or a phrase like it, gives rise to disputes about what services are covered and what services are not.

A number of insurers have attempted to take control of the review process by stipulating in their contracts that they will have the power to determine medical necessity. Most courts have upheld these provisions, while requiring that the insurer undertake in good faith an independent determination of the medical necessity of the services for which coverage is requested.

For example, an insurance policy at issue in *Franks v. Louisiana Health Services & Indemnity Company.*[36] excluded payment for hospitalizations that were not medically necessary (i.e., in the insurer's judgment hospitalizations that were ordered for medical services that could have been provided in an outpatient arrangement without harming the patient). The court did not take issue with the exclusion itself, finding that the insurer had an obligation to conduct its own good faith analysis of medical necessity. Here, the court held that the insurer had properly done so, and its refusal to pay for the hospitalization of the insured's children for flu symptoms was supported by the evidence.

Because of a requirement imposed on insurers that they act in good faith, despite policies giving them free reign over medical necessity determinations, courts have ordered coverage in some instances. In the case of *Lopez v. Blue Cross of Louisiana,*[37]the court ordered coverage for the hospitalization of the insured for depression, despite the insurer's right in the policy to make medical necessity determinations. The court said that in this case, the insurer did not adequately meet its obligation to investigate the claim. The court said that it should have examined the patient rather than relying merely on the records and should have provided a good reason for its decision.

Congress has provided another means by which insurers can remove control of medical necessity determinations from physicians. ERISA restricts review by courts of insurers' decisions in certain circumstances.[38] Under the statute, if an ERISA plan gives the plan administrator or fiduciary discretionary authority to determine eligibility for benefits or to construe the plan's terms, then the administrator's or fiduciary's decisions with respect to claims are subject to considerable deference by a court assessing the claim.[39] Under these circumstances, courts can review a decision regarding coverage for treatment only for whether it was "arbitrary and capricious" or, put another way, whether it constituted an "abuse of discretion."[40] As insurers seek to take more authority away from treating physicians, courts have become more active in resolving disputes, applying a standard of good faith in one form or another.

How the Courts Decide

Whether as interpreters of contracts or statutes, courts ultimately decide whether an insurer must pay for a particular medical service if medical necessity is disputed. There are at least three ways that courts resolve the issue of whether a procedure for which coverage is sought is medically necessary. They sometimes defer to the responsible physician's determination that a procedure is medically necessary. They sometimes defer to the insurer. Finally, courts sometimes impose an objective standard and make the determination themselves based on evidence offered by the parties.

When courts defer to the treating physician, they do so usually because the insurer has not attempted to provide otherwise in the policy. When the policy itself or an applicable statute does not provide who decides medical necessity, judges generally start their analysis by deciding whether there is an ambiguity in the contract or statute. If a court finds that there is no ambiguity, it "is bound to adhere to the insurance contract as the authentic expression of the intention of the parties, and [the contract] must be enforced as made where its language is plain and certain."[41] Without a finding of ambiguity, the contract must be interpreted on its face without any reference to the parties' intent.

The law provides generally that if the insurance contract as a whole or the exclusion from coverage is ambiguous, the ambiguity should be interpreted against the insurer.[42] If there is an ambiguity, the insurance contract "will be construed most strongly against the insurer and liberally in favor of the insured."[43]

It is within this legal framework that courts in several jurisdictions have analyzed who makes the decision about medical necessity and, finding that the term or its equivalent is ambiguous, will defer to the physician and against the insurer. For example, the insurance policy at issue in *Shumake v. Travelers Insurance Company.*[44] provided payment for "covered medical expenses" which were "necessarily incurred," where *covered medical expenses* were defined as costs incurred upon the recommendation and approval of the patient's treating physician and "required in connection with" the patient's treatment. Summarizing a body of cases, the *Shumake* court said that *necessary* can have any of three possible meanings: "appropriate," "wise in light of facts known at the time rendered," and "reasonably calculated to shorten and relieve an ordeal of agonizing pain and thereby effectuate the most rapid recovery possible. . . ."[45] Because of its multiple meanings, the court said the term was ambiguous, and such ambiguity should be interpreted against the insurer. Furthermore, the court said that in the absence of a provision giving the insurer the discretion to determine medical necessity, the physician's determination is entitled to deference. The court, accordingly, ordered the insurer to reimburse the insured for the cost of laetrile treatments received by the insured for cancer.[46]

Where the contract or statute gives the insurer more specific authority, the courts have deferred to the insurer. ERISA requires that courts review insurer decisions only for whether they were arbitrary and capricious. The statute requires that insurers establish and adhere to an internal appeal process, and a failure to do so may result in a finding against the insurer for the procedural error. Similarly, courts sometimes defer to insurers' decisions about medical necessity when the policy provides that such determinations shall be made by the insurer, as previously discussed. These insurers must follow their own rules, and the courts impose a requirement that they act in good faith in determining medical necessity (i.e., they cannot act arbitrarily).

In the absence of specific requirements of ERISA or similar contracts, some courts impose an objective standard in medical necessity determinations. They do so by finding that *medically necessary*, or its equivalent, is not an ambiguous term. Rather, they say, the term has a clear, objective meaning and should be interpreted without consideration of the parties' intent and "according to the ordinary meaning of the words used."[47] In defining what is medically necessary, the *Free v. Travelers Insurance Company* court recognized the same definitions as those later cited by the *Shumake* court, but found that the coexistence of several possible definitions did not give rise to ambiguity.[48]

Leading California medical necessity cases have adopted a somewhat different analytical framework for giving objective content to the term *medically necessary.* Rather than deliberating over whether the term is clear or ambiguous, in *Sarchett v. Blue Shield of California*[49] and *Hughes v. Blue Cross of Northern California*,[50] the courts suggest that the appropriate analysis is to look at whether the physician's recommended treatment is reasonable and consistent with prevailing community standards. In *Sarchett,* the insured attempted to argue that the insurance contract was "ambiguous as to who decides whether hospitalization is medically necessary." The insured argued that the ambiguity should be resolved by making the treating physician's decision unreviewable. The court's analysis of the ambiguity of the contract was confined to a determination that the contract was not ambiguous as to who decides medical necessity, the policy clearly providing that in the event of a dispute over coverage, the decision is to be made by an impartial review committee and subject to further review by arbitration. In response to the insured's assertion that a subscriber under a Blue Shield policy enters into the agreement with the expectation that he or she will be covered for hospitalization recommended by the treating physician, the court said, rather:

> the subscriber expects coverage because he trusts that his physician has recommended a *reasonable treatment consistent with good medical practice* [emphasis added]. Consequently we believe the subscriber's expectations can be best fulfilled not by giving his physician an unreviewable power to determine coverage, but by construing the policy language liberally, so that uncertainties about the reasonableness of treatment will be resolved in favor of coverage.

While speaking clearly in favor of the ability of insurers to question physician decisions, the court in this case found for the insured, holding that the insurer had violated its duty of good faith to inform the insured of the contractual right to impartial review and arbitration of the insurer's denial of the claim.

The *Hughes* court expanded on the *Sarchett* principle regarding the insured's expectations, stating that in assessing a claim, the insurer must act in good faith, which "demands a construction of medical necessity consistent with community medical standards that will minimize the patient's uncertainty of coverage in accepting his physician's recommended treatment."[51] Without this standard, the court said, the patient bears the risk of "accept[ing] the advice of his treating physician . . . [[and] incurring liability not likely foreseen at the time of entering the insurance contract."[52]

Hughes involved Blue Cross's denial of coverage for the hospitalization of the insured's son, who had severe psychiatric problems that rendered him suicidal and incapable of functioning as an outpatient. The court found that the Blue Cross medical review department lacked a complete file necessary to assess the insured's claim. The file did not include a discharge summary or a statement by the attending physician of the patient's history, treatment, or diagnosis. The court said that Blue Cross's psychiatric consultant charged with reviewing the case was not aware of significant information contained in the patient's records. Testimony indicated that he spent on average only 12 minutes per claim and rejected 30% of claims he reviewed. His denial was contrary to the recommendations of three treating physicians and an independent psychiatric consultant. Most important, he disclaimed any responsibility to obtain missing information before making his recommendation. The court said that a jury could reasonably infer that the consulting psychiatrist "employed a standard of medical necessity sufficiently at variance with community standards to constitute bad faith."[53]

The policy at issue in *Jacob v. Blue Cross & Blue Shield*[54] excluded coverage for medical services that were not medically necessary, which it defined as services that, in accordance with acceptable medical standards of practice, could not be denied without harming the patient. The court found that the language in the policy was clear and said that the insurer had adequately established that it had an objective basis for denying coverage for immunoaugmentative therapy undergone by the insured's son for cancer.

The *Sarchett* and *Hughes* decisions (as well as the insurance policy at issue in *Jacob*) seem to reflect an effort to implement a standard for medical necessity that incorporates a broader view of the issues confronting our health care system. Defining medical necessity as dictated by community standards goes beyond such concerns as the unfair bargaining position of the insurer, awarding insureds more coverage than they believed they were paying for, and whether specific procedures had been followed. This approach is not without precedent. Judges and juries traditionally have been arbiters of community standards of not just medicine, but due care generally.

Exclusions for Experimental or Investigative Procedures

The combined forces of rapidly emerging medical technology and a heightened awareness of the need to control costs have given rise to a number of cases involving experimental procedures. Most insurance policies contain explicit provisions excluding coverage for *experimental* procedures or those done for the purpose of investigation. In addition, insurers have argued successfully in particular cases that a requirement of medical necessity in a policy provides a justification for refusing coverage for experimental procedures.[55] "The 'experimental' exclusion common in health insurance policies responds to a growing concern that most current medical procedures were adopted without ever having been tested rigorously and that at least some of the procedures commonly used today have limited or no medical value."[56] Many of the cases discussed above in the context of the determination of medical necessity generally involved claims for coverage of the cost of procedures denied by the insurer because they were experimental and, therefore, unnecessary.

It is largely in the context of the experimental exclusion that Hall and Anderson assert that "the inclination of judges to adopt every conceivable argument in favor of coverage has essentially precluded insurers from exercising any meaningful oversight of medical appropriateness."[57] They suggest that there is a direct correlation between the degree to which a particular procedure is experimental and the severity of the illness; desperate situations call for desperate measures, and judges, they suggest, are particularly reluctant to deny coverage where the insured faces a life-threatening illness. The result of this way of thinking has been a few phenomenally high awards in non-ERISA cases.[58]

This questioning view of experimental exclusion cases is supported by Ferguson et al.[59] reviewing six cases involving claims for technologies that had been previously determined to be unsafe, ineffective, or inadequately assessed. The authors found that in some cases contract law dictated a result for the insured. They also found a great reluctance on the part of judges to consider highly technical information about the efficacy and safety of certain technologies and a tendency to rely excessively on expert witnesses with vested interests in a finding that the particular technology at issue should be covered by the insurer.

This view of experimental exclusion cases may be for the most part accurate, but studies suggest that problems with coverage decisions may lie with insurers as well. Another study found that the frequency of approval of clinical trials for autologous bone marrow transplantation for breast cancer bore little relation to medical or scientific information and "often seemed arbitrary and capricious."[60] The authors found further: "Of two requests to the same insurer by similar patients in the same protocol, one request might well be approved and the other denied."[61] It appears that the difficulty faced by the health care industry in developing an operative concept of *experimental* parallels that faced by the industry generally with respect to the concept of *medical necessity.*

Special Problems in Mental Health Care

Establishing a workable system of utilization review in the mental health care area may be particularly difficult because of a lack of consensus among psychiatrists over approaches to treatment.[62] "There are many treatment techniques but relatively few rigorous experiments documenting their differential efficacy."[63] A decision about the medical necessity of mental health services among treating therapists and utilization reviewers will therefore depend on the values placed by the professionals involved on particular procedures.

Although such lack of consensus may exist in other medical specialties, it is perhaps particularly evident in mental health care because of the disparity in insurance coverage for mental disorders compared with disorders deemed to be physical in nature. This disparity continues in the face of rapidly increasing costs for mental health care benefits.[64] Several states have mandated minimum benefits to be provided by insurers, but predictably these "minimum benefits have become the standard instead of simply the allowable mimimum."[65]

In addition to limiting coverage to the statutorily mandated levels, insurers have other ways of precluding coverage of mental health care costs. They can dispute the medical necessity of particular procedures. They can draw distinctions in policies between acute and chronic care and exclude treatment for care that they determine falls in the latter category. According to one commentator, third-party insurers, in confirming the necessity for outpatient treatment, require documentation that a psychiatric condition is associated with a diminished capacity to meet role requirements or carry out activities of daily living. Consideration is given to the potential for exacerbation of an illness that previously resulted in inpatient care or partial hospitalization. The need for physician monitoring of a patient's treatment regimen is also taken into account.[66]

For inpatients, Tischler writes, the standards are stricter:

> The criterion for admission typically is the presence of significant psychiatric symptoms, such as thought disorder, severe depression or anxiety, uncontrolled substance abuse, marked disorganization, or organicity. The extent to which patients are dangerous to themselves or others, their ability to care for themselves, and the availability of social supports are weighed. Coexisting medical conditions, impaired impulse control, pathological interactions with the family or social environment, the need for special services or skilled observation, and court mandates are also considered.[67]

In states that have not mandated minimum levels of health care coverage, insurers can simply refuse to cover treatment of mental disorders. In cases involving such policies, plaintiffs have gone to great lengths to prove to the court that the relevant treatment is for a physical as opposed to a mental condition. Specifically, in one case, an insured argued successfully that his daughter's bipolar disorder was physical in origin.[68] Another court ruled that a policy's limitation of coverage for "mental illness or nervous disorders" to $10,000 per year should not be read to include autism and ordered the insurer to pay the full costs of hospitalization for the insured's child.[69] These cases are arguably pyrrhic victories for advocates of increased coverage for mental health care, as insurance companies can, and have, simply broadened the exclusions in their policies in an effort to encompass cases such as these.[70] Thus, cases involving mental health coverage bear a double burden. They have received much more restrictive treatment in insurers' drafting of policies, and courts struggle with a lack of clear objective data or community standards.

Conclusion

Ultimately, courts decide what is medically necessary. Nevertheless, under evolving review procedures, some courts defer to the treating physician; some defer to the decision of the reviewer or health care manager; and some courts make independent determinations; but in all cases, what the payment contract provides will limit the court's area of discretion.

"Who decides what is medically necessary?" is certainly not an eternal question. It would be more accurate to ask who decides the issue today. Courts will continue to be the final arbiters, but their decisions will be influenced by the changing terms of health insurance policies, by the increasingly frequent utilization of review agreements, by evolving community standards, and by the quality of the medical evidence presented when a particular issue finally reaches court. Physicians and others seeking to influence the contours of medical necessity cannot wait until courts speak. They first must make themselves heard by payers, review organizations, and public bodies establishing the policies that the courts will construe.

Notes

1. Hall M, Anderson G: Health insurers' assessment of medical necessity, U Pa L Rev 140:1637–1712, 1646 n.27, 1992 [Hereinafter "Hall and Anderson"]
2. Id.
3. Helvestine W: Legal implications of utilization review, in Controlling Costs and Changing Patient Care? The Role of Utilization Management. Edited by Gray BH, Field MJ. Washington, DC, National Academy Press, 1989, p 197, n.6
4. Annotation, What Services, Equipment, or Supplies Are "Medically Necessary" for Purposes of Coverage under Medical Insurance, 75 ALR4th 763-874, 768, 1990
5. Group Health Benefits contract issued by The George Washington University Health Plan, Inc., at p. 6 (1995)
6. 42 U.S.C. §1395y(a)(1)(A) (Suppl. 1994)
7. This point was made by Hall and Anderson, in reading Beal v Doe, 432 U.S. 438, 444 (1977), in which the Supreme Court made the relatively noncommittal statement that "serious statutory questions might be pre-

sented if a state Medicaid plan excluded necessary medical treatment from its coverage."

Indeed, abortion cases illustrate the extent to which the meaning of *medically necessary* can be politicized. See, e.g., Doe v Bolton, 410 U.S. 179, 191 (1973) (upholding as not unconstitutionally vague language in Georgia statute prohibiting a physician from performing an abortion except when it is "based upon his best clinical judgment that an abortion is necessary," and noting that definition of *necessary* brings to bear psychological as well as physical well-being); Beal v Doe, 432 U.S. 438, 449–451 (1977) (Brennan, J., dissenting) (pregnancy being "unquestionably a condition requiring medical services," once it is established that treatment of some sort is necessary, Medicaid statute does not dictate type of treatment).

8. H.R. 3600, 103rd Cong., 1st Sess. §1141 (1993)
9. E.g., Id. at §§1114(e)(2)(A) and 1120(b)(1)
10. Id., at §1154
11. Controlling Costs and Changing Patient Care? The Role of Utilization Management. Edited by Gray BH, Field MJ. Washington, DC, National Academy Press, 1989, p 43 [Hereinafter "Gray and Field"]
12. Id.
13. Hall and Anderson, at 1653
14. Bovbjerg R, Griffin C, Carroll C: U.S. health care coverage and costs: historical development and choices for the 1990s. Journal of Law, Medicine & Ethics 21:141–160, 1993
15. Gray and Field, at 41
16. Id., at 43–44
17. Id., at 45
18. Id., at 44–45
19. Id., at 44; see, e.g., Ellis R: Reimbursement systems and the behavior of mental health providers. International Journal of Law and Psychology 14:347, 1991
20. Gray and Field, at 41
21. Hall and Anderson, at 1647
22. Hall and Anderson, at 1653; Utilization Management: A Handbook for Psychiatrists, Washington, DC, American Psychiatric Association, 1992. Initial studies suggest that prior review does result in lower hospital use and expenditures, and provide no conclusions one way or the other regarding the effect on the quality of patient care. Gray and Field, at 110
23. See Sarchett v Blue Shield of California, 729 P.2d 267 (Ca. 1987) (en banc); Hughes v Blue Cross of Northern California, 263 Cal.Rptr. 850 (Cal.App. 1989)

24. Hughes v Blue Cross of Northern California, 263 Cal.Rptr. 850 (Cal.App. 1989)
25. See, e.g., Wickline v State, 239 Cal.Rptr. 810, 812 (Cal.App. 1986)
26. Id.
27. Id.
28. 271 Cal. Rptr. 876 (Cal. App. 1990)
29. Id., at 883
30. 29 U.S.C. §1001 et seq.
31. 965 F.2d 1321 (5th Cir. 1992)
32. Id., at 1332
33. Gray and Field, at 77
34. See, e.g., Peters WP, Rogers MC: Variation in approval by insurance companies of coverage for autologous bone marrow transplantation for breast cancer. N Engl J Med 330:473–477, 1994 [Hereinafter "Peters and Rogers"]
35. Id., at 474–75 (suggesting efficacy of hiring attorney when faced with denial of coverage by an insurer)
36. 382 So.2d 1064 (La.App. 1980)
37. 386 So. 2d 697 (La. App. 1980), rev'd in part on other grounds, 397 So. 2d 1343 (1981)
38. See Firestone Tire and Rubber Co. v Bruch, 109 S.Ct. 948 (1989)
39. Id.
40. Id. Further, under ERISA, courts can award to plaintiffs medical costs and attorneys' fees, but not "extracontractual damages" for traditional common law claims, such as damages for pain and suffering. Corcoran v United Healthcare, Inc., 965 F.2d 1321 (5th Cir. 1992). It is unclear at this point whether courts can award punitive damages under ERISA. See Hall and Anderson, at 1662 n.90
41. 43 Am Jur2d, Insurance §271, at 343 (2d Ed. 1982)
42. See, e.g., Free v Travelers Ins. Co., 551 F.Supp. 554 (D.C. Md. 1982); Dallis v Aetna Life Insurance Co., 574 F.Supp. 547, 552 (N.D. Ga. 1983) 768 F.2d 1304; Van Vactor v Blue Cross Association, 365 N.E.2d 638, 643 (Ill. App. 1977)
43. Van Vactor v Blue Cross Association, 365 N.E.2d at 643
44. 383 N.W.2d 259 (Mich. App. 1985)
45. Shumake v Travelers Insurance Co., 383 N.W.2d at 262–63 [citations omitted]; see also Dallis v Aetna Life Ins. Co., 574 F. Supp. at 547
46. See also Dallis v Aetna Life Insurance Co., 574 F. Supp. at 551–52 (finding that *necessary*, under policy precluding payment for treatment that is not necessary, is ambiguous and should be construed against the insurer, court denies insurer's motion for summary judgment on issue of

the medical necessity of immunoaugmentative therapy for cancer treatment); Tudor v Metropolitan Life Insurance Co., 539 N.Y.S.2d 690 (1989) (holding burden is on the insurer to establish that procedures for which plaintiff sought coverage were not *medically necessary* under the applicable policy); Abernathy v Prudential Insurance Co., 264 S.E.2d 836 (S.C. 1980) (ordering coverage for depilatory treatment, where court found ambiguity in policy that excluded coverage for treatment that was not medically necessary, and physician recommended treatment)

47. Free v Travelers Insurance Co., 551 F.Supp. 554, 558 (D.Md. 1982)
48. One might postulate that these cases are largely result-driven, that is, that a judge or appellate panel of judges will decide, consciously or not, whether a particular treatment seemed reasonable, and fit that result into the legal framework for analyzing the ambiguity of the terms employed
49. 729 P.2d 267 (Ca. 1987) (en banc)
50. 263 Cal.Rptr. 850 (Cal.App. 1989)
51. Hughes v Blue Cross of Northern California, 263 Cal.Rptr. at 857
52. Id.
53. Hughes, 263 Cal.Rptr. at 857
54. 758 P.2d 382 (Or.App. 1988)
55. See, e.g., Jacob v Blue Cross & Blue Shield, 758 P.2d at 382
56. Hall and Anderson, at 1638
57. Hall and Anderson, at 1644
58. In the recent case of Fox v Health Net (Reported in "Looking Beyond Fox v. Health Net," *Managed Health Care* 4(3):1, March 1994), the jury awarded the plaintiff $77 million in punitive damages, $12.1 million in compensatory damages, and $212,000 for medical expenses for the insurer's refusal to cover a procedure it deemed experimental in the treatment of the plaintiff's cancer. (This case has since settled for an undisclosed lower amount. Bergthold LA, Sage WM: Medical Necessity, Experimental Treatment and Coverage Determination: Lessons from National Health Care Reform. Washington, DC, National Institue for Health Care Management, October 1994)
59. Ferguson J, Dubinsky M, Kirsch P: Court-ordered reimbursement for unproven medical technology. JAMA 269:2116–2120, 1993
60. Peters and Rogers, at 476
61. Id.
62. Tischler GL: Utilization management of mental health services by private third parties. Am J Psychiatry 147:967–973, 1990; Zusman J: Utilization review: theory, practice, and issues. Hosp Community Psychiatry 41:531–536, 1990

63. Tischler GL, at 969. Dr. Tischler notes that the problem of a lack of consensus among professionals regarding treatment techniques is not unique to psychiatry, but he analyzes the ramifications of this uncertainty on mental health coverage decisions. Id.
64. See Hastings DA: Legal and regulatory issues in managed mental health care, in The Insider's Guide to Managed Care: A Legal and Operational Roadmap. Washington, DC, The National Health Care Lawyers Association, 1990
65. Seltzer DA: Limitations on HMO services and the emerging redefinition of chronic mental illness. Hosp Community Psychiatry 39:137–139, 1988
66. Tischler GL, at 967
67. Id.
68. Arkansas Blue Cross and Blue Shield, Inc. v Jane Doe, 733 S.W.2d 429 (Ark.App. 1987) (en banc)
69. Kunin v Benefit Trust Life Insurance Co., 696 F. Supp. 1342 (C.D.Ca. 1988), 910 F.2d 534 (1990)
70. Appelbaum PS: Litigating insurance coverage for mental disorders. Hosp Community Psychiatry 40:993–994, 1989

Chapter 13

How Effective Is Utilization Review?

William M. Glazer, M.D.
Geoffrey V. Gray, Ph.D.

Most payers believe that there are three main strategies to control health care costs (Tischler 1990). These approaches include shifting the economic risk from the payer to the provider, using organized service delivery systems, and employing utilization review. Since the 1970s, these three tactics have intensified as efforts to contain costs have failed.

To *shift risk* to providers, payers have attempted to change benefit design and pricing methodologies through the use of prospective payment, discounts, and so forth. The fact that capitation has emerged as the leading financial strategy of managed care testifies to the failure of utilization review alone to effectively control costs. With capitation, costs can be prospectively controlled with a certitude that payers need. The Clinton administration's health care plan proposed to formalize and regulate purchasing coalitions that would influence providers to accept financial risk for the care that they deliver.

As payers began to recognize the value of multiple levels of care for psychiatric patients, more flexible benefit designs allowing *organized service delivery systems* have evolved. Programming for psychiatric patients is expanding beyond the traditional inpatient or outpatient dichotomy that promoted the use of the most expensive inpatient services (Glazer and Bell 1993). Currently, the health care system is responding vigorously to the expectations that health care will be delivered in a more efficient manner. Newer forms of integrated delivery systems such as physician-hospital organizations, foundations, practices without walls, and managed services organizations are beginning to compete with the more traditional health maintenance organization (HMO) and preferred provider organization (PPO) structures.

The History of Attempts to Control Health Care Costs

Utilization review (UR), the focus of this chapter, has been defined by the Institute of Medicine (1989) as "techniques used by or on behalf of purchasers of health care benefits to manage health care costs by influencing patient care decision-making through case-by-case assessment of care prior to its provision." UR has emerged in various forms. It can be conducted on a prospective, concurrent, retrospective review, or second-opinion basis. It can occur *internally*, where it is implemented within a service delivery system, as is dictated by the standards of the Joint Commission on the Accreditation of Healthcare Organizations (JCAHO). It also occurs *externally*, when a third- or fourth-party administrator—that is, a managed care organization—is given the contractual authority by the payer to assess and authorize payment for clinical care via telephone, chart review, second opinion, or on-site review. In this form, UR is a meta-assessment—that is, an assessment by a reviewer of an assessment that has been made by a provider. The fundamental concern of UR is to ascertain whether there is a congruence between the severity of illness and intensity of service. Thus, the focus of UR is on the decision concerning treatment allocation, not on the technical characteristics of that treatment. Implicit in the activity of UR is the notion that there are practice guidelines for treatment intensity that correlate with severity of illness.

Historically, UR has been related to the quality improvement process in general. Thus, UR is interrelated with peer review, practice guidelines, and provider profiling. Wilson (1992) traced the beginning of UR to the peer review function that emerged in the 1970s when the professional standards review organizations monitored the medical necessity of hospital care for Medicare patients. In the 1980s, the professional standards review organization system was replaced by peer review organizations (PROs), organized on a statewide basis to review the medical necessity of admission and continued stay for Medicare psychiatric inpatients. A recent study of the peer review process concluded that its reliability was poor and recommended higher standards to improve the approach (Goldman 1992). A description of a California-based company's experience with the PRO format supported the widely held assumption that clinicians learn little from the peer review process (Feldman and Rundall 1993).

More recently, clinical guidelines have become an important component of UR (see Chapter 4). Although JCAHO published standards for acute care psychiatric facilities years ago, the behavioral health field has only a few guidelines and no broadly accepted formal national standards. Efforts to implement practice guidelines—such as those of the American Psychiatric Association and the Agency for Health Care Policy and Research—provide broad brush strokes identifying the boundaries of acceptable practice, but compared with like efforts in other areas of medicine such as cardiology or anesthesiology, they are in their infancy. In part because biological validators for psychiatric illnesses are as yet unavailable (Glazer 1992), psychiatry is a long way from developing practice guidelines or standards. In other areas of medicine, studies evaluating the effect of published guidelines on medical practices indicate slow response from providers. Thus, special efforts will be required to introduce guidelines into practice (Wilson et al. 1991).

Whereas UR assesses the appropriateness of specific decisions, *provider profiling* evaluates the appropriateness of the broad pattern of decisions made over time. With provider profiling, rates of performance are measured and compared with other providers on an individual or group basis. Eventually, these data will also be compared with national standards. The focus of provider profiling usually includes price, patient satisfaction, access, and the quality improvement process. In psychiatry, activity in this area is limited to a single facility or to individual providers. Rarely does it cover all services associated with an episode of care. Because managed psychiatric treatments involve multiple services, managed behavioral health care organizations will eventually have to place their focus more on network profiles than individual providers or institutions.

Studies of the Effectiveness of Psychiatric Utilization Review

Little is known about the impact of psychiatric UR on the cost or quality of care, and there are many questions. Few studies are available to prove the common assumption that psychiatric UR is cost-effective. Of the existing studies, none provide the requisite information on outcomes to answer that question. In this section we review existing data as well as identify some of the crucial methodological and conceptual questions that need to be considered by researchers.

In one of the earliest studies of the psychiatric precertification process, investigators working in an HMO described their experience handling 421 patients treated under capitated versus fee-for-service arrangements (Blackwell et al. 1988). The HMO was mandated by the state of Wisconsin to treat 28,000 Medicaid enrollees under a prepaid mental health insurance arrangement. In response to this mandate, the HMO set up a quality monitoring committee that approved all treatment for the prepaid group in advance. The fee-for-service patients were treated in the HMO's usual open-ended manner. One-year follow-up data were obtained on a retrospective basis for the entire cohort. The results indicated no statistically significant difference between the amount of outpatient services provided to the two groups. Although the authors concluded that this study indicated that case review had little effect on quantity of care, several important weaknesses limit such an inference. Putting aside the uncontrolled nature of the study, it failed to report utilization data for the rest of the program (i.e., no inpatient utilization figures were presented at all). Additionally, in the absence of outcome measures such as recidivism rates, work productivity, consumer satisfaction, quality of life, and so forth, it is impossible to know what the impact of precertification UR was on the Medicaid population.

It would be important to compare the impact of internal and external UR on the financial and clinical outcomes of care. Managed care companies argue that internal UR serves the purposes of the provider, whereas providers make the same argument in reverse. One study conducted by Mercer Meidinger Hansen, Inc. (Anderson 1989) randomly reviewed 201 mental health and chemical dependency hospitalizations that occurred between July 1, 1987, and June 30, 1988. These cases had undergone UR via three different service configurations: a specialized PPO with UR (70 cases), specialized UR only (67 cases), and nonspecialized UR (64 cases). The study found that the mean number of approved inpatient days per case was greatest for the nonspecialized UR organization (18.2 days) compared with 16 days in the specialized UR only and 9 days in the specialized UR-PPO structure. Although the cost of less intensive substitute services was not measured, the author assumed that the overall savings achieved by the specialty UR-PPO organization compared with the other two formats were substantial. Outcomes reflecting the quality of the services delivered by the three types of organizations were not measured, but independent psychiatric reviewers found little difference in quality of care as indicated by the medical records. The implication of this study is that UR works best when it is conducted as a part of the delivery system. However, without total cost and clinical outcome measures, one can only speculate about these data.

Using inpatient claims from the Aetna database for 1988 and 1989, Gotowka and Smith (1991) compared the outcomes of confinements exposed and unexposed to concurrent inpatient UR. They found that the UR process reduced utilization and cost measures without increasing readmissions or recidivism rates. Of course the chief concern about such research is that it does not attend to the employee to patient level of analysis; rather, it focuses on claims. Additionally, this study failed to control for benefit design and geographical effects. Nevertheless, studies such as these delineate important trends and support the assumption that UR reduces costs without impairing the quality of care.

Neuwirth and Noone (1992) presented a 5-year case study of the impact of a managed care strategy consisting of a service network and UR on the utilization pattern for substance abuse treatment within a company of 17,000 employees and their dependents living in a single metropolitan area. Their outcome was impressive—less utilization of the benefit following the implementation of a managed care approach. This study does not help to determine the effectiveness of UR alone because the UR function is inextricably combined with a service network strategy. It does lend support to the conclusions of the Anderson study (1989), however.

These studies demonstrate numerous methodological issues that need to be considered in testing the effectiveness of UR. When conducting observational studies such as these, it is crucial that comparison groups have similar characteristics, such as disease severity, physical and psychological stress, and so forth. In addition other characteristics need to be comparable: demographic, geographic—that is, local practice patterns and mental health care market area considerations (Wickizer et al. 1989)—and benefit design influences.

The Evolution of Utilization Review

Psychiatry, like other medical specialties, is undergoing a major shift in its clinical decision-making paradigm. Figure 13–1 presents the economic context within which this paradigm shift exists. In the fee-for-service model, mental health care is reimbursed on a *cost-plus* basis. In such a scenario, where the dominant value is effectiveness for the patient, the major risk is that of overtreatment. The antithetical position involves capitation. Capitation solves the problem of cost overruns but brings with it its own unique problems. Mechanic and Aiken (1989) concluded that "doctors on capitation do not behave in the benevolent fashion theory but instead allow other goals, values, and orientations to affect how they practice. They appear less tolerant of their patients' demands" (p. 16). The ideal solution combines the best aspects of fee for service and capitation and results in a synthesis that balances cost with quality of care. As vertically integrated systems and financial risk sharing dominate health care delivery systems, the challenge is to maintain the emphasis on effectiveness that drove the fee-for-service, solo practitioner model.

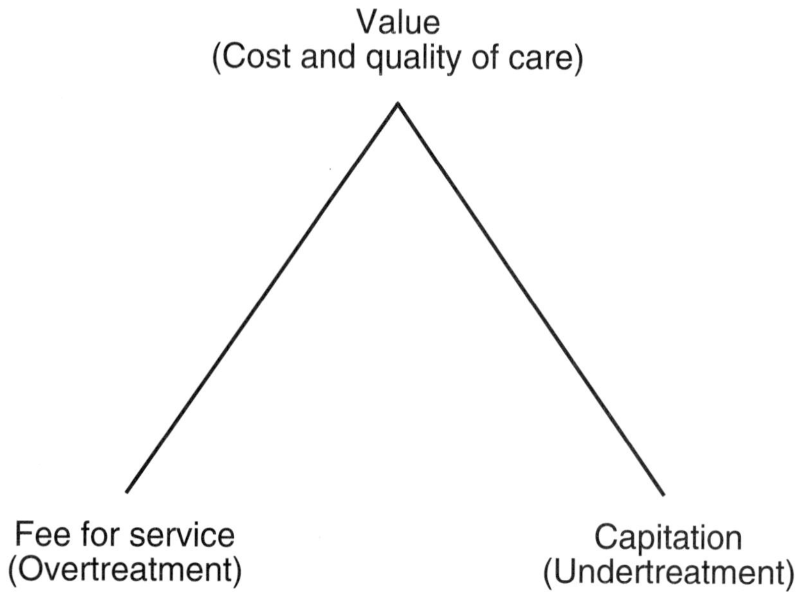

Figure 13–1. Paradigm shift in health care economics.

A recent study by the Rand Corporation (Rogers et al. 1993) found that in capitated systems psychiatrists are far less likely to diagnose and treat clinical depression than their fee-for-service colleagues. If overtreatment is the Achilles' heel of fee-for-service medicine, then the problem for capitation is its mirror opposite: undertreatment. With no incentive to practice "in the benevolent fashion theory," providers may seek to avoid cases, minimally treat, risk patient welfare, and even deny necessary care.

In the United States, UR has played a central role in the early stages of this paradigm shift. Interestingly, this has not been the case for our European counterparts. For example, the British system's socialized form of health care delivery first emphasized organized service delivery systems while relying on cooperation, goodwill, and responsible decision making by providers. However, with their inability to curb rising health care costs, they are now bringing in prospective reimbursement methodologies *and* UR. In the United States, of the three cost-saving mechanisms previously mentioned—shifting the economic risk from the payer to the provider, the use of organized service delivery systems, and UR—it is UR that has taken center stage in the behavioral health care arena. UR has flourished while most psychiatrists, even psychiatric managed care companies, have not yet generated sound and generalizable risk-sharing mechanisms. UR has become the focus of attention while the psychiatric profession has only begun to develop treatment models in HMOs, PPOs, and other forms of integrated practice. The private sector is quickly learning about integrated mental health systems from the public sector, and it is already predictable that the two will compete, blend, and eventually merge. As mentioned in the introduction of this chapter, professional guidelines and provider profiling are in embryonic or at best infantile stages of development. Given this state of the profession, it is no wonder that many psychiatrists still believe that managed care equals UR!

Such a view could not be further from the truth. UR is an evolving tool, a transitional object if you will, that will transform along with psychiatric delivery systems where accountability, outcomes, and value are the dominant considerations. As the first two mechanisms to reduce health care costs take hold, the role and function of UR will change.

Utilization Review as a Sentinel Effect

UR is evolving in a manner depicted in Figure 13–2. The initial level of UR simply involved the use of a sentinel effect. Until the late 1980s, managed care or PROs attempted with greater or lesser success to alter treatment decisions simply by placing a reviewer over the shoulder of the practitioner. The limitations and potential bias inherent in this type of approach explain why most managed care companies have already extended their UR methodology to the next level.

Utilization Review as a Set of Relevant Clinical Dimensions

As practitioners have revolted against what they experienced as intrusive and sometimes inappropriate forms of management, managed mental health care organizations have evolved to the second level shown in Figure 13–2: the identification of relevant clinical dimensions for review. There have been a few efforts to define relevant clinical dimensions for purposes of UR. The earliest example was the development of checklists (Warner et al. 1961; Whittington 1966) of experimental criteria for hospitalization designed to help mental health professionals perform evaluations in the newly created community mental health centers. Researchers at Yale (Flynn and Henisz 1975; Henisz et al. 1981) modified, then studied, the validity of the Whittington Scale (reliability data were never reported); and other groups expanded and replicated this work (Costello et al. 1991; Newmark et al. 1977). The Whittington Scale (Whittington 1966) consisted of 12 questions about the patient's behavior, mental status, and physical condition as well as the mental health professional's consideration of the patient's clinical status.

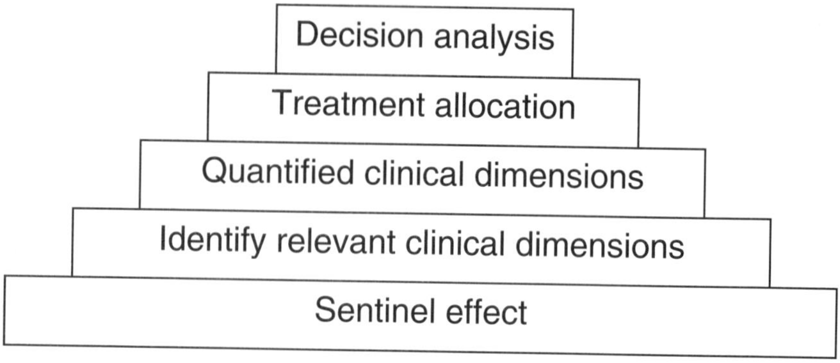

Figure 13–2. The evolution of the utilization review function.

Strumwasser et al. (1991) reviewed 539 records of hospitalized patients for appropriateness of hospitalization using an instrument developed by InterQual (1987) and modified by Blue Cross and Blue Shield of Michigan. Thirty-eight percent of the inpatient days of care were deemed unnecessary. It is important to point out that the reliability of the InterQual tool was never established, yet this group applied a modified version to assess medical necessity of psychiatric treatment.

It should be apparent that more effort in the development of UR tools in psychiatric practice is needed. Some authors published model scales (Grossman 1987). Guidelines for UR are emerging (Allen et al. 1988; Goodman et al. 1992; InterQual 1987; Sederer and Summergrad 1992), but the reliability and validity of these efforts remain to be demonstrated. Currently, proprietary companies have begun to identify broad areas of concentration (Goodman et al. 1992): illness severity, treatment intensity, treatment effectiveness, and others. By doing so, they have at least provided a map of the terrain, but the identification of relevant clinical dimensions for review leaves a great deal to the imagination. Unless these relevant clinical dimensions are defined precisely, there is room for bias and variability on the UR side. Thus, a third level of evolution is necessary.

Utilization Review as a Set of Quantified Clinical Dimensions

A managed care company's idea, or worse yet, a managed care company employee's idea about what these relevant clinical dimensions mean in a given case can lead to bias, the implications of which include stress for providers and reviewers, lawsuits, and poor patient care. There must be a well-quantified system (see Figure 13–2) to apply these clinical dimensions to a review situation. The initial efforts to reach this third level are currently under way in some managed care organizations. The essential feature of a criteria set composed of quantified clinical dimensions is that behavioral descriptors anchor the dimensional scales. It is not enough to say that a clinical dimension (e.g., severity of illness) is mild, moderate, or severe. There must be easily measurable, behaviorally based indicators that correlate with pathology and treatment intensity. Such anchor points should define the clinical dimensions in a way that allows utilization reviewers as well as practitioners to agree among themselves on a rating of a given case.

There have been few published reports of such an effort in the managed mental health care literature. A concurrent review scale for psychiatric hospitalization has demonstrated intraclass coefficients mostly above .70 (Glazer et al. 1992). This was the first and only effort to study the reliability of a UR tool in a managed care environment. The problem with this research was that the content of the scales has remained proprietary, and no attempt to validate the data has been made. The paucity of such data reflects the lack of effort to quantify the clinical dimensions that constitute the foundation of mental health UR.

Utilization Review as a Treatment Allocator

None of the first three evolutionary levels mentioned above constitute UR in any real sense inasmuch as they do not provide reliable and valid guidelines for assigning level of treatment. One assessment instrument developed by Bengelsdorf et al. (1984) for UR in emergency department settings provided guidelines for level-of-care assignment. The focus of this scale was on three domains: dangerousness, support system, and motivation or ability to cooperate. Each of these three areas was rated on a scale of 1 to 5. A score of <9 was associated with hospitalization. Chemical dependency cases were excluded from the study. In an initial study of 300 patients, it was found that predictions of disposition decision by Crisis Triage Rating Scale (CTRS) scores were concordant with the clinical judgment in 291 of 300 cases. This impressive predictive capacity held in a prospective validation study. It is important to note, however, that the personnel performing the scale ratings were also making the clinical decisions. Thus, it is not surprising that the actual treatment decisions paralleled the logic of the scale. Another important feature of this group's work was that it was the first (and only) group of investigators to publish the interrater reliability of a precertification UR scale. Kappas for interrater reliability were .35 for dangerousness, .42 for support, .55 for motivation, and .42 for the total scale—hardly acceptable for clinical application under current standards. Stepwise discriminant analysis found motivation to be a weak predictor compared with dangerousness and support system. This study was important because it was the first (and only) effort to demonstrate both reliability and validity of a UR tool. The main problem with the study was that the CTRS scores influenced the treatment decision—the raters were the treaters. UR scales must rely on the treating mental health professional to generate the reality of the conclusions. The inability of raters to agree on patients' motivation was clearly demonstrated from this work.

In addition to methodological concerns, the major shortcoming of UR tools is that they are too simplistic for the demands of contemporary managed care practice. The Whittington Scale and its derivatives as well as the CTRS were not developed to support decisions in which patients are assigned to *multiple levels* of treatment (i.e., they were designed for the old dichotomy of "admit or not"). The decision to assign treatment in a comprehensive continuum of care is a *multidimensional* decision (i.e., several domains or dimensions must be considered individually in every case, and these domains influence the decision variably, depending on the clinical circumstance).

The Components of Utilization Review

As Flynn and Henisz (1975) commented two decades ago, "the patient's path to the mental hospital is complexly determined by a large number of behavioral, familial, social, and situational variables rather than simply by the patient's symptoms, diagnosis, or degree of distress" (p. 847). Thus, without an objective validator, care can be driven by forces that are not associated with the illness. Until the biological validators for nervous and mental conditions are identified, the field needs a system that provides systematic guidance (i.e., an objective structural map to guide treatment determinations). Such a system must

- in the initial stages reflect the normative clinical judgment of mainstream mental health professionals but also "draw on knowledge from decision theory, social judgement theory and information processing theory" (Marson et al. 1988 p. 924). Later in the process guidelines must be linked (and informed) by outcomes.
- consist of multiple dimensions or domains that drive treatment decisions.
- quantify the severity of these dimensions and correlate them with the appropriate and effective level of care.
- be reliable in the hands of the users.
- be valid in the hands of the users.
- be independent of the benefit design (i.e., be applicable to the complete range of mental and substance abuse benefit designs).

- be applicable to vertically integrated systems of care that use multiple levels of treatment in a continuous and integrated fashion.

A Model Utilization Review Tool

We developed a UR tool (Glazer and Gray 1993; Gray and Glazer 1994) to ensure reliable and valid clinical guidelines for assigning treatment levels for acutely ill psychiatric patients. This tool, called PsychPro, offers a model approach for allocating the appropriate level of care for an acutely ill person. It ensures that decisions are supported by a rational, nonbiased database.

From an extensive review of the literature as well as hundreds of clinical cases in a psychiatric department of a Connecticut-based HMO, five key clinical dimensions that drive the decision for psychiatric treatment were identified: 1) the occurrence of dangerous behavior; 2) the provider's opinion about the patient's risk to be dangerous or relapse into chemical dependency or both; 3) social performance (i.e., the patient's recent capacity to work and love); 4) the availability of social and environmental resources; and 5) the likelihood that the patient is about to undergo serious medical complications from substance use. These five clinical dimensions are rated on a 3-point scale with a 3 rating consistent with acute inpatient care; a 2 rating consistent with diversion care (i.e., a range of crisis intervention programs designed to avoid or divert acute inpatient hospital care); and a 1 rating consistent with standard outpatient treatment. *Anchor points*—behavioral descriptors that would distinguish these levels of care among the five components—were developed in a multidisciplinary team using a systematic format. Together, these five dimensions constitute a clinical profile for a given patient in a specific clinical condition. Each patient is rated on a scale from 1 to 3 on each of the five dimensions so that there are 3 to the 5th power, or 243, discrete possibilities. Each possibility describes a different configuration of behavioral disturbance that is empirically tied to a treatment intensity. These treatment intensities have been based on consensus standards of care of practicing psychiatrists.

The Future of Utilization Review

If the paradigm shift mentioned above means that providers will be working in integrated systems at financial risk, then it is predictable that UR as it currently exists in most venues will not be necessary. Figure 13–3 displays yet another theme of the paradigm shift. As payers recognized the need to rein in costs, they became the driving force behind UR, for they recognized correctly that it was the allocation-of-care decision that was the linchpin in cost containment. As UR intruded into decision making, the autonomy of physicians was challenged as authority for deciding how care was delivered was shifted to reviewers. The ascendancy of UR has resulted in *micromanaged* case review targeted at overutilization (false positives), the inevitable consequence of fee-for-service medicine. With the arrival of capitation, the logic of UR no longer holds. With costs contained under capitation, the problem is no longer one of preventing overutilization, it is guarding against underutilization, the natural consequence of capitation.

However, detecting underutilization is more difficult than spotting overutilization. In most care settings the cases that must be reviewed are those that require high-intensity (costly) services. Those that do not require such services are typically not reviewed. With capitation, the tendency would be for fewer patients to be referred for high-intensity services. If traditional UR were applied, then patients in need of treatment would never come to the fore! Thus, the challenge is detecting those patients in need of higher intensity services who are not so identified (false negatives). To create a mechanism to accurately and efficiently identify these patients, an assessment system that issues guidelines for allocation of care must be built into the process of care itself. The meta-assessment that is UR is too inefficient and must be transformed so that it becomes part of the direct assessment performed by the provider. Put otherwise, UR must give way to *decision support*, the fifth and final evolutionary level (Figure 13–2).

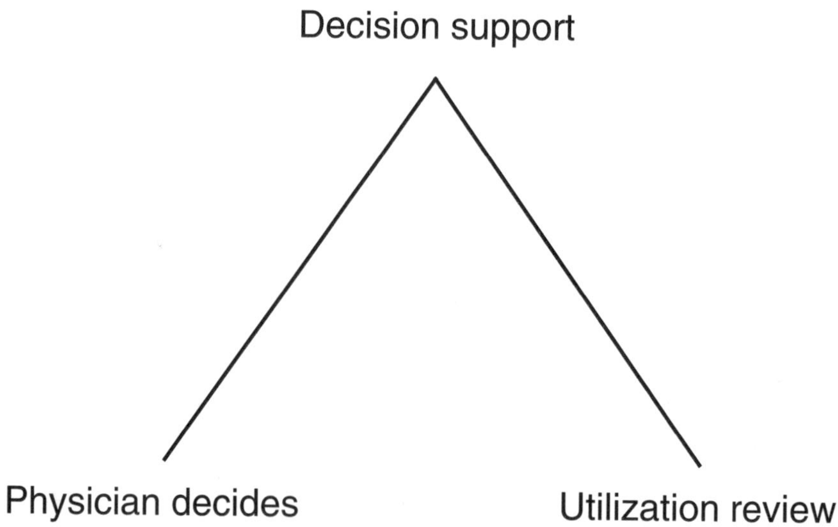

Figure 13–3. Paradigm shift in utilization review.

Utilization Review as a Decision Support Tool

Will the innovation of capitation render external UR obsolete? We think so. In capitated systems the UR function will be owned by the providers who are at risk. UR's primary goal will be to ensure that patients are treated at the appropriate level of intensity and that undertreatment does not pervade the delivery system. UR will take on a decision support function and will no longer be perceived as an outside force. Rather, providers will welcome the results of *decision analyses* to guide them in their decision-making task.

Here is how the model UR tool described could provide the application of decision support methodologies. As described, this tool allocates treatment based on observable behaviors rated by trained UR specialists. However, in the hands of providers, this tool makes continual improvement of the clinical decision-making process possible. Providers in managed care settings will be motivated to measure the quality of their work because it will strengthen their ability to win contracts from payers. One way providers can accomplish this continuous quality improvement goal is to apply signal detection theory (Swetts 1988), which eliminates *noise* (false negatives and false positives), that is, irrelevant criteria, and enhances *signal,* that is, criteria that accurately predict outcome. When signal detection theory is applied in the clinical setting, the focus is on the decision to allocate care, which yields a treatment and a subsequent outcome. The outcome is either accurate (a *hit*) or inaccurate (a *miss*). An example of a relevant outcome measure would be readmission to the same or greater treatment within 30 days after discharge from that treatment. A *hit* would be a treatment that did not result in such a readmission. Over time, with enough cases involving different patient populations, the ability of this scale to predict hits will improve. Such a quality improvement process will strengthen the practitioner's decision-making ability. Note that to apply an approach such as signal detection theory, the UR tool must have evolved to the fourth level depicted in Figure 13–2.

Conclusion

We have found very few studies that help answer the question, "How effective is utilization review?" Perhaps this lack of research effort reflects the difficulty of separating UR from the reimbursement mechanism, benefit design, and provider network that it serves.

To date, many UR applications are still in prototypical forms (levels 1–3 of Figure 13–2), not having been subjected to the rigors of psychometric validation. More important, most mental health UR applications do not accurately allocate treatment intensity levels correlated to the presentation of the patient's condition (level 4 of Figure 13–2).

In this chapter, we have offered a blueprint and a model UR tool to delineate current and future directions for UR. We have suggested that UR *has* been effective as a facilitator of the managed care movement in this country. In business, management follows risk. As risk is shifted to providers in the form of capitation, the management functions follow, including that of UR. UR in capitated systems will not be external to the care but will be integrated into the process of care itself. Thus, an essential component of the paradigm shift will occur when UR is no longer a meta-assessment, but rather an internalized process, fully owned by providers. At that point, UR will have been transformed into a decision support function where it will provide a means for internal continuous quality improvement by linking guidelines to outcomes (level 5 of Figure 13–2).

References

Allen JG, Scovern AW, Logue AM, et al: Indications for extended psychiatric hospitalization: a study of clinical opinion. Compr Psychiatry 29:604–612, 1988

Anderson DF: How effective is managed mental health care? Bus Health 7(9):34–35, 1989

Bengelsdorf H, Levy LE, Emerson RL, et al: Brief dispositional assessment of patients at risk for hospitalization. J Nerv Ment Dis 172:424–430, 1984

Blackwell B, Gutmann M, Gutmann L: Case review and quantity of outpatient care. Am J Psychiatry 145:1003–1006, 1988

Costello AJ, Dulcan MK, Kalas R: A checklist of hospitalization criteria for use with children. Hosp Community Psychiatry 42:823–828, 1991

Feldman SE, Rundall TG: PROs and the health care quality improvement initiative: insights from 50 cases of serious medical mistakes. Med Care Rev 50(2):123–151, 1993

Flynn HR, Henisz JE: Criteria for psychiatric hospitalization: experience with a checklist for chart review. Am J Psychiatry 132:847–850, 1975

Glazer W: Medical necessity and psychiatry. Psychiatric Annals 22:362–366, 1992

Glazer W, Bell N: Mental Health Benefits: A Purchaser's Guide. Brookfield, WI, International Foundation of Employee Benefit Plans, 1993

Glazer W, Gray G: A decision support system for psychiatric care in an HMO setting. Medical Interface 6(6):111–114, 1993

Glazer W, Kramer R, Montgomery J, et al: Medical necessity scales for inpatient psychiatric concurrent review. Hosp Community Psychiatry 43:935–937, 1992

Goldman RL: The reliability of peer assessments of quality of care. JAMA 267:958–960, 1992

Goodman M, Brown J, Dietz P: Managing Managed Care. Washington, DC, American Psychiatric Press, 1992

Gotowka TD, Smith RB: Focused psychiatric review: impacts on expense and utilization. Benefits Q 7(4):73–81, 1991

Gray GV, Glazer WM: Psychiatric decision-making in the 90s: the coming era of decision support. Behavioral Healthcare Tomorrow 3(1):47–54, 1994

Grossman J: The psychiatric, alcohol, and drug algorithm: a decision model for the nurse reviewer. QRB Qual Rev Bull 13(9):302–308, 1987

Henisz JE, Etkin K, Levine MS: Criteria for psychiatric hospitalization: a checklist approach. Behavior Research Methods and Instrumentation 13:629–636, 1981

Institute of Medicine Committee on Utilization Management by Third Parties: Controlling Costs and Changing Patient Care? The Role of Utilization Management. Edited by Gray BH, Field MJ. Washington, DC, National Academy Press, 1989

InterQual: 15D-A Inpatient Psychiatric Criteria and Instructions. Westborough, MA, InterQual, 1987

Marson DC, McGovern MP, Pomp HC: Psychiatric decision making in the emergency room: a research overview. Am J Psychiatry 145:918–925, 1988

Mechanic D, Aiken LH: Capitation in mental health: potentials and caution, in Paying for Services: Promises and Pitfalls of Capitation. Edited by Mechanic D, Aiken LH. San Francisco, CA, Jossey-Bass, 1989, pp 5–18

Neuwirth E, Noone D: A five-year case study: the effect of managed health on utilization patterns. Medical Interface 5(5):38–45, 1992

Newmark CS, Gentry L, Goodman M: Validation of criteria for psychiatric hospitalization checklist. J Clin Psychol 33:156–159, 1977

Rogers WH, Wells KB, Sturm MR, et al: Outcomes for adult outpatients with depression under prepaid or fee for service financing. Arch Gen Psychiatry 50:517–525, 1993

Sederer LI, Summergrad P: Criteria for hospital admission. Hosp Community Psychiatry 44:116–118, 1992

Strumwasser I, Paranjpe NV, Udow M, et al: Appropriateness of psychiatric and substance abuse hospitalization. Med Care 29 (suppl):AS77–AS90, 1991

Swetts JA: Measuring the accuracy of diagnostic systems. Science 240:1285–1294, 1988

Tischler GL: Utilization management of mental health services by private third parties. Am J Psychiatry 147:967–973, 1990

Warner SL, Fleming B, Bullock S: The Philadelphia program for home psychiatric evaluations, precare, and involuntary hospitalization. Am J Public Health 52:29–38, 1961

Whittington HG: Intake and evaluation, in Psychiatry in the American Community. New York, International Universities Press, 1966, pp. 206–207

Wickizer TM, Wheeler JRC, Feldstein PJ: Does utilization review reduce unnecessary hospital care and contain costs? Med Care 27:632–647, 1989

Wilson AS, Scheibner IH, Winslow CM: Designing a guideline-based utilization management program. Benefits Q 7(4):42–47, 1991

Wilson GF: An evolution of cost-control approaches to health care, in Manual of Psychiatric Quality Assurance: Report of the APA Committee on Quality Assurance. Edited by Mattson MR. Washington, DC, American Psychiatric Press, 1992, pp 3–6

Section IV

Research and Training

Chapter 14

Can Research on Managed Care Inform Practice and Policy Decisions?

David Mechanic, Ph.D.

There is much confusion, misinformation, rhetoric, and controversy surrounding managed care, yet few areas in health care need disinterested and careful evaluation more. Managed care is a vague and ambiguous designation incorporating a great variety of organizational arrangements, financial mechanisms, and review processes (Mechanic 1994). Researching managed care requires that we be clear about the specific arrangements under study. Unfortunately, the field abounds with vague assertions, anecdotes, inflated claims, and exaggerated concerns. Systematic evidence would be helpful both for practice and for policy decisions.

In the mental health field, the term *managed care* is used to refer to three strategies that may overlap but are quite distinct (Mechanic et al. 1995). Perhaps most controversial are a variety of review mechanisms, usually part of a utilization management (UM) program, that are motivated by utilization and cost-control needs (Hodgkin 1992). The most commonly used mechanisms are precertification for inpatient admission, concurrent review of inpatient care, and case management of high-cost cases. UM of outpatient psychotherapy is also increasingly common. Such UM strategies might be combined with particular benefit design features, employee assistance plans, and other insurance variations such as preferred provider organizations. This complexity makes comparisons across varying UM programs difficult. Even within comparable programs there may be significant differences in the training and qualifications of the persons carrying out UM functions, the quality of the protocols used, or how the UM process is carried out. Factors such as ease of access, quality of communication, responsiveness to feedback, and appeals opportunities affect the degree to which hospital admission personnel and physicians feel harassed and the costs they incur.

Managed care also refers to health maintenance organization (HMO)–type arrangements that function on a prospective basis and in which professionals are required to practice within a budget, balancing to some degree patients' needs against one another. In respect to mentally ill persons, such capitation models may involve mainstreaming into generic HMOs or encompass special demonstrations or experiments capitating persons with mental illness within specialty mental health organizations such as community mental health centers (Mechanic and Aiken 1989). In each case, the specific arrangements that characterize the program, including particularly the financial incentives affecting professionals, may be much more important than the organizational designation. Knowing that an entity is an HMO does not reveal a great deal about its capacity to deliver mental health services, the professional mix, the facilities available, the attitudes and commitment toward mentally ill persons, and many other key features of the program.

A third approach, sometimes confused with managed care, involves organized intensive case management systems for persons with severe and persistent mental illness such as the Program in Assertive Community Treatment (Stein and Test 1985). As in many public and nonprofit programs, care is provided in the context of a budget, and program survival depends on balancing clinical efforts against budgetary concerns. A major goal in such programs is to reduce inpatient care as a way of garnering needed resources for outpatient and rehabilitation programs. Although responsibility typically is defined in terms of a catchment area population, and not on a capitated basis, the incentives are often similar to those in capitated programs (Stein 1989).

Any and all of the managed care approaches described above can be combined; for example, an HMO can use UM strategies or develop specialized case management for particularly difficult or expensive clients. In some UM programs within indemnity insurance programs, case managers of high-utilization cases may offer substitute services that extend beyond those covered by the patient's insurance plan, allowing the benefit flexibility more typical of capitated programs. In short, understanding research on managed care requires considerable attention to the details of financing, incentives, structures, and implementation processes.

The Research Process: Experiments

The study of managed care poses formidable problems for researchers who wish to conform to acceptable research requirements. The gold standard is the randomized, controlled trial in which patients are assigned to different delivery systems in an unbiased way allowing the possibility of conclusions that differences observed are the result of financial and organizational arrangements and not selection effects. Unlike studies of drugs or surgical interventions, it is difficult in studies of managed care to assess how representative the managed care entities studied are of the generic form researchers wish to make inferences about.

The most ambitious study involving one form of managed care was the RAND Corporation Health Insurance Experiment (HIE), an $80 million effort to study the effects of co-payment on utilization, cost, and health status outcomes (Newhouse and Insurance Experiment Group 1993). Carried out between 1974 and 1982, this experiment randomized 6,970 respondents in six areas of the country for 3–5 years. As one aspect of the study, families were randomized into the Group Health Cooperative of Puget Sound in Seattle, a staff-model HMO. Much of what we know with confidence about HMOs relative to fee-for-service practice comes from study of this single site. Because many of the findings confirmed nonexperimental studies of the performance of other prepaid group practices (Luft 1987), they provide greater confidence for generalizations about such entities than any single study ordinarily would.

In many respects, however, the Group Health Cooperative differs from other prepaid group practices and certainly a great deal from other HMOs. An analysis of the effects of prepaid care on health status in the RAND Corporation HIE suggested that the poor, sick patients randomized into prepaid practice did less well than those assigned to the fee-for-service condition with no co-payment (the appropriate comparison group). This may have been a result of the absence of well-designed outreach efforts later introduced in the Group Health Cooperative (Manning et al. 1984). The point here is that outcomes may depend as much on the specific programs in place in any organization as on the generic definition of the delivery system. Global generalizations are likely to miss important financial, organizational, and managerial subtleties of great importance for policy and practice.

In respect to mental health services, the RAND researchers found that more prepaid enrollees used mental health services than persons in the comparable fee-for-service plan, but services were provided much less intensively. Prepaid enrollees were more likely to receive mental health services from a general medical provider than from a mental health specialist, and when they saw a mental health provider, they had only one-third the number of mental health visits of the comparable fee-for-service group. Group Health relied more on social workers and group or family therapies than fee-for-service contexts did. Overall, prepaid mental health expenditures were only one-third those in the comparable fee-for-service plan (Wells et al. 1986, 1987). These findings generally supported observations from nonexperimental studies.

The RAND experiment found no significant differences in mental health outcomes between those individuals treated in prepaid and comparable fee-for-service contexts despite the lower intensity and lower costs of care (Wells et al. 1990). The outcome measures used, however, were of a very general kind, and it is unclear whether significant qualitative differences were missed by such general measures. More important, the RAND experiment included few persons with serious and persistent mental illness. Thus, it tells us relatively little about how such vulnerable clients are likely to fare in the lower intensity of service characteristic of prepaid arrangements.

There have been several efforts to randomize mentally ill Medicaid enrollees into capitated versus fee-for-service arrangements, and a number of such new experiments are in process or are now being initiated in California, Utah, and Colorado. An earlier effort in Minnesota to randomize Medicaid enrollees, including mentally ill and disabled persons, suggests the potential but also the difficulties of such experimental demonstrations (Christianson et al. 1989). Initially, four prepaid plans were enlisted to provide care for mentally ill clients, but the largest provider, a Blue Cross/Blue Shield–sponsored plan, announced its withdrawal from the demonstration only 7 months after it began. The state of Minnesota was concerned about the capacity of the other three plans to accommodate the Blue Cross/Blue Shield enrollees and thus withdrew all disabled enrollees from the demonstration after the first year. Thus, the data from this experiment cover less than a year, although a subpopulation of clients with schizophrenia were followed up 11 months after withdrawal from the demonstration.

Even had the Minnesota program continued, it would have been difficult to generalize results to other capitated programs. Advocates for disabled people had many concerns about access to services under this demonstration, and they successfully negotiated arrangements that weakened the utilization controls associated with capitation. Participating plans, for example, could not require that referral to nonphysician mental health providers be made only through a primary care physician, and this limitation ensured that patients could continue earlier patterns of service utilization if they wished. Nevertheless, the Minnesota demonstration provided important new insights. There was little difference in how prepaid and fee-for-service enrollees used services, but enrollee use of community services was less likely to be reimbursed for prepaid patients (Christianson et al. 1992). In essence, the HMOs were cost shifting to the public and nonprofit sectors.

In the Minnesota demonstration, the prepaid group had less outpatient physical care, fewer visits, and fewer inpatient admissions than fee-for-service clients, and they were less likely to receive chemical dependency treatments on either an inpatient or outpatient basis (Lurie et al. 1992). There were no differences in the number of inpatient mental health admissions, but prepaid patients had shorter stays (1.56 versus 4.3 days) and were more likely to report refusal of care during the prior year primarily at the emergency department, but this relationship was not statistically significant (17% versus 12%; $P = .06$). Ironically, only 15% of these clients had changed their previous providers (because clients were permitted to stay with their previous mental health providers), but many of these providers were now functioning under new financial constraints. Efforts to assess outcomes were made using measures of health status, physical and social functioning, and psychiatric symptoms. These measures were obtained both at baseline and follow-up, but there were few significant measures differentiating prepaid and fee-for-service groups. Among schizophrenic patients in prepaid care there was a nonsignificant decline in global assessment scores between baseline and time 1, but the decline continued and reached statistical significance at time 2, 11 months after the demonstration was discontinued. At the end of the demonstration, prepaid enrollees had a significant decrease in the likelihood of being assaulted, raped, or robbed, but they also were more likely to report suicide attempts. It is difficult to explain these observations in a clear-cut fashion because the results may be in substantial ways a product of the instability of the demonstration. The data do show, however, a lower intensity of care among prepaid enrollees and suggest the possibility that this may have had negative consequences for those who are most severely mentally ill.

There have been a number of efforts in health services research to randomize clients with mental illness to different service arrangements, but true random assignment is commonly compromised. In an ambitious capitation demonstration in Rochester, New York, participating mental health centers were allowed to reject clients, and high attrition also contributed to biased selection (Babigian et al. 1992). In many efforts to randomize patients, the number of patients lost through attrition often compromises the results. In other demonstrations and experiments, as in the Minnesota study discussed above, the compromises often necessary to gain acceptance of the demonstration require changes in design features that make it difficult to generalize to contexts where design features may be different. Confidence in particular patterns of results can only come with findings that persist across a range of studies and contexts.

Experiments are more common and more easily executed in comparing case management models to one another or to conventional care. In a classic study in Dane County, Wisconsin, Stein and Test (1980a, 1980b) randomly assigned an unselected group of patients seeking mental hospital admission to experimental and control groups. Subsequent analysis showed that successful randomization had been achieved. The researchers compared an assertive team treatment and psychoeducational model with a control group receiving hospital treatment linked with community aftercare services and found that the experimental treatment resulted in reduced hospital use and higher function and quality of life. This was a highly complex set of interventions with many components. Although one can say that the service system had positive effects when compared with traditional care, it is impossible to identify the efficacious elements. A number of other studies are also based on the same assertive treatment model, but none are true replications (Stein and Test 1985). Almost all such studies of assertive community treatment show that hospitalization can be significantly reduced, but few replicate the advantageous psychosocial outcomes reported by Stein and Test (Olfson 1990). Because all the components of service programs are rarely adopted in new settings, it is essential to understand the contributions of varying components to effectiveness. For example, the effort in Australia to replicate the Stein and Test model had comparable favorable outcomes but achieved these outcomes with lower staff intensity (New South Wales Department of Health 1983). Learning the tolerance for reduced staffing in such programs has obvious significance.

Studies of case management models suggest that there is a threshold of service intensity needed to achieve favorable outcomes, but intensity of service is not associated with positive outcomes in a linear way (Dietzen and Bond 1993). Much of the controversy associated with case management experiments concerns the content of the clinical model and its appropriateness. Varying strategies and approaches are described by such generic terms as *case management* and *utilization management*. However, it is essential to get beyond these general terms to understand the specific management components and their interrelations. Similarly, the quality of treatment personnel, their training and experience, and supervision are all likely to have an important role in the results achieved. Conclusions about case management or about any of these other strategies, independent of a careful description of the contents of the program, are not likely to be informative.

The Research Process: Multivariate Studies

Randomized studies are still relatively rare in the mental health services field, and no such studies have been attempted in the field of UM of mental health services. (Randomized studies have been carried out in the area of second surgical opinions.) In the real world, of course, selection effects are pervasive and typically highly influential. Patients sort themselves into varying types of health care plans in accord with their means, needs, and expectations. Physicians also sort themselves over time into practice settings they find compatible. Employers who seek out UM services are not a random draw but typically are firms with higher-than-average costs or sharply increasing expenditures. The challenge to any research, thus, is to use analytical and statistical tools to reduce the chances that any performance differences observed are the result of selection biases as opposed to programmatic effects. In mental health managed care, where developments are proceeding rapidly, even careful multivariate studies are relatively unusual.

One such ambitious effort is the Medical Outcomes Study, an observational study of more than 12,000 patients cared for in group practice and 10,000 cared for in solo practice with the purpose of examining differences in care under various organizational arrangements (Rogers et al. 1993). The study focuses on persons with various chronic conditions in Chicago, Boston, and Los Angeles, and depression was one of the conditions studied. A representative sample of providers was selected at each site, and patients sampled from these providers completed an initial questionnaire supplemented by visit report forms completed by the clinician.

Patients with depression were identified in a two-stage process. Those who met the established threshold on the initial screening were then interviewed by telephone with the depression section of the National Institute of Mental Health's Diagnostic Interview Schedule. As part of this large study, 507 patients with current depression and 469 patients who did not meet diagnostic criteria but had depressive symptoms were followed up for periods of 1 or 2 years after the initial telephone interview to assess symptoms and functional status. Among the selective factors controlled were age, sex, race, income, education, study site, and seasonal effects. Prepaid providers were less likely to talk to patients about depression during the screening visit for more than 3 minutes (59% versus 74%), and their patients were less likely to be using antidepressants at the 2-year follow-up (15% versus 27%).

As one might anticipate, psychiatrists in all settings treated patients with the most serious depressions. However, those patients treated by psychiatrists in prepaid settings developed new limitations in role and physical functioning over time. Such deterioration was not evident in patients treated in fee-for-service settings. Although psychiatrists in all settings were more likely to prescribe antidepressant medication than other clinicians, there was a significant decline in patients' continuity of medication in prepaid settings. Therapists or clinicians other than psychiatrists did equally well in both settings in relation to patient outcomes.

This study provides useful insights but also contains many ambiguities. Despite its large size and scope, the number of patients treated by psychiatrists included only 41 in prepaid practice and 82 in fee-for-service practice. With attrition on outcome measures at the 2-year follow-up, the numbers become even smaller (29 and 69, respectively). Prepaid practice involves different structures, and the researchers examined effects in independent practice associations versus other HMOs. Patients in independent practice associations did significantly worse on outcomes than fee-for-service patients; patients in other HMOs also did less well than fee-for-service patients, but the differences were not statistically significant. There was also a site effect, with two of the sites largely responsible for the finding.

The authors reported that once patients were given antidepressant medication, there were no differences in dosage between practice settings. Thus, the differences must be attributed to the lower probability of medication use by psychiatrists in prepaid settings. Because HMOs are less likely to refer patients to psychiatrists than fee-for-service practitioners, one would anticipate that patients seen by psychiatrists in prepaid practice are more severely ill. Thus, it is especially puzzling that patients are less likely to be on antidepressant medication. The fact remains that the system of care continues to be a "black box," and we lack clear understanding of the observed differences. Moreover, the prepaid practice arrangements representative of the prepaid designation are too heterogeneous to give guidance on what is wrong or how to intervene.

Despite these ambiguities, the literature on prepayment is more rigorous than the literature on UM, where selective descriptive data are typically presented to make an argument for or against. There are some efforts, however, that meet higher research standards and are informative. One such set of studies at Aetna (Gotowka and Smith 1991; Smith 1991, 1992) compared a telephone-based precertification and concurrent review program of inpatient care (called *focused psychiatric review*) with a complex combination of strategies, including a comprehensive employee assistance program, counseling and referral program, networks of preferred providers, precertification of services, case management, and benefits counseling (called *managed mental health care*). Careful multivariate analyses with sophisticated controls were used to analyze nine quarters of data. During this period, both forms of UM achieved savings relative to no intervention, but the more comprehensive program was superior. Because of the complexity of program design, however, it is impossible to identify which aspects of the intervention made a difference. Furthermore, no data are available allowing assessment of patient outcome or cost shifts to providers, patients, their families, and the community. Also, firms are not assigned to managed care programs, and those who have higher-than-average utilization will be more likely to seek out managed care programs. Thus, it is difficult to generalize to firms with average or lower initial utilization. Although firms with higher utilization showed savings under managed care, some nevertheless continued to have higher costs than firms outside UM programs.

In another analysis, Brookmeyer and Frank (R. Brookmeyer and R. G. Frank: Cost sharing, managed care and inpatient psychiatric utilization in private insurance, unpublished manuscript, Baltimore, MD, Johns Hopkins University, 1993) used MEDSTAT claims data on the experiences of 25 self-insuring firms focusing on some 13,000 individuals with at least one hospital admission for depression. Outcomes measured included length of stay for an episode and number of admissions in a 2-year period. Although the multivariate analysis applied to these data was sophisticated, the complex variations in benefit design and UM strategies make it difficult to interpret the meaning of results. Firms, for example, varied on cost-sharing and day limits, the use of preferred providers, and requirements for precertification and concurrent utilization review. The researchers found no effects at all on length of stay for precertification or concurrent review. Precertification, however, was associated with a significantly lower rate of hospital admissions. Concurrent review had the opposite effect, and the use of preferred provider organizations had no effect. Although one can imagine a scenario that makes these results intelligible, such post hoc interpretations would not be particularly convincing.

Case Management

I have not been able to find published studies of high-cost case management as the concept is used in the UM literature. However, case management of patients with severe and persistent mental illness is a common theme in the services literature, although the emphasis is more on public than private sector programs and more on the quality of care and patient outcomes than on cost savings. In this literature the focus is on the effective integration of services in relation to patient need as orchestrated by a case manager or a team that performs case management functions. The definitions of the role of case management, the resources commanded, and the systems in which they are embedded may vary widely, leading to controversy on how results should be interpreted.

In one often cited but controversial study done in Texas by Franklin and associates (1987), 417 patients with chronic mental illness were assigned randomly to experimental and control groups. All the patients had a history of at least two admissions to state or county hospitals within approximately a 2-year period. The control group could receive any service other than case management, while the experimental patients were assigned to case management services staffed by an experienced supervisor and seven case managers. In the course of the experiment staff members spent about half their time providing nonclinical services to patients and two-fifths of their time brokering services. After 1 year, the case management group had received more services, were admitted to mental hospitals more often, and accrued higher costs. Although there were tendencies in favor of the experimental group on quality of life measures, they were small and not statistically significant.

Case management is a vague concept, and there is much room to debate the content of the service itself. In the experiment described above, case managers functioned in a relatively open-ended context. More typically, they must function within tightly constrained budgets and high caseloads. In some situations, case managers function primarily as patient advocates; in others they function more like bureaucratic gatekeepers seeking to protect limited agency funds. Serious evaluation of case management experience, requires knowing a great deal about the system in which the case manager is operating; the organizational incentives, workload, and patient responsibility; and the available resources. Attention must also be given to the training and experience of the case managers and the support services available to carry out their functions. Research in the general medical sector found consistently that adding services outside a controlled system of care almost always increases costs (Lewis and Keairnes 1970).

Measurement of Costs and Benefits

In discussions of managed care strategies the emphasis is on cost savings. Costs, however, are typically construed quite narrowly, and savings usually refer to those gained by the employer or insurance plan. Most reasonable studies factor in the cost of administering the UM program, but consideration of costs frequently stops here. If managed care is considered not simply as a product marketed to employers but also as a community strategy for allocating medical resources, then costs must be considered more broadly.

Among the costs are the administrative personnel required in hospitals, clinics, and physicians' offices to deal with UM issues and the time such items take from the clinician's daily schedule. Although some of these costs might be thought of as a quality enhancement by inducing physicians to think more carefully about the treatment plan, no one doubts that there are significant unmeasured costs involved. These might also include the feelings of harassment, frustration, and loss of autonomy many physicians report, as well as the effects these feelings have on morale and performance. The difficulty of measuring such costs makes them no less important.

Probably more significant are the costs for patients and families when needed treatment is denied or when patients are returned home or to other community settings prematurely. Such costs are easily transferred and often invisible to all but the family who must take on new burdens and disruptions of family life. Secondary effects include work absenteeism and effects on the health and welfare of other family members. Patients prematurely discharged may suffer long-term consequences in terms of unsatisfactory community adjustment and loss of employment. Other costs may include higher rates of victimization and increased use of social services. The community also may incur costs through disruptive and dangerous behavior and involvement of the criminal justice system. Every study need not consider all such costs, but broad consideration of costs and cost shifting enhances the value of research and its usefulness in policy considerations.

Managed care, of course, also may impose barriers on patients, requiring them to report their personal histories and symptoms to screening clinicians who then decide on the necessity of care. The patient then may have to initiate contact with a new clinician and again report the history and symptoms, a process he or she may find aversive with unfamiliar clinicians. Indeed, some patients ambivalent about treatment may be diverted from seeking care, and others may choose services outside their insurance plan to protect confidentiality or avoid hassles. At the very least, cost evaluations must take into account outside utilization or other obvious types of cost shifting.

Another category of costs and benefits includes offsets between physical and mental health services. Timely and attentive treatment of psychiatric conditions may affect the course of comorbid physical conditions and overall medical utilization. Persons with unrecognized depression, anxiety, and other psychiatric conditions often use more general medical services and are the recipients of diagnostic and treatment interventions that involve risk as well as cost. Some assessment of such cost shifts or cost offsets adds to the value of evaluations of managed care.

Where Does Research on Managed Care Lead Us?

There is little likelihood that research on managed care will be able to adjudicate the polarized discussion that surrounds managed care practices, although well-executed projects help in important ways to clarify the issues, identify valuable innovations, and throw light on particularly harmful practices. A major challenge facing researchers is the rapidly changing character of managed care and its customized format with little consensus on generic models or standards. Moreover, many existing programs in the private sector are proprietary and are not easily accessible to researchers. Although there are increasing efforts to apply the methodology of the controlled trial to this arena, particularly in the public sector, programs vary so much in details that it is difficult to generalize beyond the individual research setting.

It would be naive, however, to expect a small number of studies to resolve contentious ideological disagreements among proponents and detractors of various managed care alternatives. Unlike the testing of a drug or even a surgical procedure, the application of which may be more variable as a result of differences in the expertise of the surgical team, the evaluation of managed care depends as much on context and implementation as on the generic form of the intervention. The cumulation of consistent results across some of these various situations gives observers more confidence in the credibility of the results. In the final analysis, it is credibility that counts, and this depends on the weight of the evidence and its consistency across settings and over time.

The literature on cost savings of HMOs provides a good example. A substantial amount of literature developed over several decades showing that prepaid group practices could reduce costs by 20% to 40%, largely by reducing the rate of inpatient admissions and surgical interventions (Luft 1987). Although some studies controlled for sociodemographic and other risk factors in efforts to assess results independent of selection effects, much skepticism remained because of the belief that prepaid groups were attracting or selecting more favorable risks that accounted for observed cost advantages. The difficulties of conceptualizing, measuring, and predicting risk reinforced the view that multivariate controls were not sufficiently sensitive to partial out such biases. This research area, and the conclusions about cost savings, became more plausible and more widely accepted when the RAND Corporation HIE replicated the general finding within a randomized design.

Randomized trials are becoming more common in the prepaid care sector, although the studies are typically too small to inform us about the organizational variables that are particularly important for various outcomes. Although such studies have not been carried out in UM of mental health services, theoretically it would not be difficult to randomly assign patients to well-designed managed care programs and compare experience and outcomes with those of conventional practice. Such trials raise ethical and legal issues, and it is not easy to enlist cooperation or informed consent for such endeavors. The RAND Corporation HIE faced similar issues, and researchers developed an ingenious methodological approach to assure patients that they would not be disadvantaged if they consented to be randomized into programs that were more restrictive than the ones in which they were presently enrolled (Newhouse and the Insurance Experiment Group 1993).

The weakest link in the managed care literature is the absence of trustworthy data that speak to the quality issue. Most typically, assessments of patient need are made by the same individuals who carry out UM functions, making such data highly suspect. Moreover, even if diagnostic descriptors are reliable, diagnosis itself is inadequate as a measure of need for care or resource intensity. Patient populations undergoing varying types of UM need to be carefully described using standard and reliable assessment tools, and measures of change of status require assessment by researchers independent of UM (Thompson et al. 1992). To be complete, such assessments should include measures of impact beyond the patient to include family and community burdens.

Conclusion

Generalizations about managed care are more difficult and less conclusive than assessments of the effectiveness of a well-tested drug or surgical procedure. The conditions of managed care can vary widely in ways that affect all relevant outcomes, and the same strategy may function differently depending on the implementation procedures, the personalities and communication skills of utilization reviewers, and the quality of the protocols used. Research on managed care, however, alerts practitioners and policymakers to important considerations, and over time robust generalizations emerge across settings and provide policy guidance. The process of examining UM closely also sharpens thinking about the criteria for using various mental health interventions. Thus, studies of managed care not only enrich decision making but help define the dimensions of quality and how they might be assessed.

References

Babigian H, Mitchell O, Marshall P, et al: A mental health capitation experiment: evaluating the Monroe-Livingston experience, in Economics and Mental Health. Edited by Frank R, Manning W. Baltimore, MD, Hopkins University Press, 1992, pp 307–331

Christianson JB, Lurie N, Finch M, et al: Mainstreaming the mentally ill in HMOs, in Paying For Services: Promises and Pitfalls of Capitation. Edited by Mechanic D, Aiken L. San Francisco, CA, Jossey-Bass, 1989, pp 19–28

Christianson JB, Lurie N, Finch M, et al: Use of community-based mental health programs by HMOs: evidence from a medicaid demonstration. Am J Public Health 82:790–796, 1992

Dietzen LL, Bond GR: Relationship between case manager contact and outcome for frequently hospitalized psychiatric clients. Hosp Community Psychiatry 44:839–843, 1993

Franklin JL, Solovitz B, Mason M, et al: An evaluation of case management. Am J Public Health 77:674–678, 1987

Gotowka TD, Smith RB: Focused psychiatric review: impacts on expense and utilization. Benefits Q 7(4):73–81, 1991

Hodgkin D: The impact of private utilization management on psychiatric care: a review of the literature. J Ment Health Adm 19:143–157, 1992

Lewis CE, Keairnes HW: Controlling costs of medical care by expanding coverage: study of a paradox. N Engl J Med 282:1405–1412, 1970

Luft H: Health Maintenance Organizations: Dimensions of Performance. New Brunswick, NJ, Transaction Publishers, 1987

Lurie N, Moscovice IS, Finch M, et al: Does capitation affect the health of the chronically mentally ill: results from a national trial. JAMA 267:3300–3304, 1992

Manning WG, Leibowitz GA, Goldberg A, et al: A controlled trial of the effect of a prepaid group practice on use of services. N Engl J Med 310:1505–1510, 1984

Mechanic D: Managed care: rhetoric and realities. Inquiry 31:124–128, 1994

Mechanic D, Aiken L (eds). Paying For Services: Promises and Pitfalls of Capitation. San Francisco, CA, Jossey-Bass, 1989

Mechanic D, Schlesinger M, McAlpine D: Management of mental health and substance abuse services: state of the art and early results. Milbank Q 73:19–95, 1995

Newhouse JP, The Insurance Experiment Group: Free For All?: Lessons from the RAND Health Insurance Experiment. Cambridge, MA, Harvard University Press, 1993

New South Wales Department of Health: Psychiatric Hospital Versus Community Treatment: A Controlled Study (HSR 83–046). Sidney, Australia, New South Wales Department of Health,1983

Olfson M: Assertive community treatment: an evaluation of the experimental evidence. Hosp Community Psychiatry 41:634–641, 1990

Rogers WH, Wells KB, Meredith LS, et al: Outcomes for adult outpatients with depression under prepaid or fee-for-service financing. Arch Gen Psychiatry 50:517–525, 1993

Smith RB: Managed Mental Health and Focused Psychiatric Review: Evaluation of Effects on Inpatient Utilization and Expense. Hartford, CT, Aetna Health Plans, Research and Evaluation Unit, 1991

Smith RB: Evaluations of Managed Mental Health Care. Hartford, CT, Aetna Health Plans, Research and Evaluation Unit, 1992

Stein LI: Wisconsin's system of mental health financing, in Paying For Services: Promises and Pitfalls of Capitation. Edited by Mechanic D, Aiken L. San Francisco, CA, Jossey-Bass, 1989, pp 29–41

Stein LI, Test MA: Alternatives to mental hospital treatment, I: conceptual model, treatment program and clinical evaluation. Arch Gen Psychiatry 37:392–397, 1980a

Stein LI, Test MA: Alternatives to mental hospital treatment, III: social cost. Arch Gen Psychiatry 37:409–412, 1980b

Stein LI, Test MA: The Training in Community Living Model. San Francisco, CA, Jossey-Bass, 1985

Thompson JW, Burns BJ, Goldman HH, Smith J: Inital level of care and clinical status in a managed mental health program. Hosp Community Psychiatry 43:599–603, 1992

Wells KB, Manning WG Jr, Benjamin B: Use of outpatient mental health service in HMO and fee-for-service plans: results from a randomized controlled trial. Health Serv Res 21:453–474, 1986

Wells KB, Manning WG Jr, Benjamin B: Comparison of use of outpatient mental health services in an HMO and fee-for-service plans. Med Care 25:894–903, 1987

Wells KB, Manning WG Jr, Valdez RB: The effects of prepaid group practice on mental health outcomes. Health Serv Res 25:615–625, 1990

Chapter 15

Does Managed Mental Health Care Offset Costs Related to Medical Treatment?

Nicholas A. Cummings, Ph.D., Litt.D.

The renewed interest in medical cost offset belies the fact that the phenomenon was first discovered 35 years ago at the Kaiser Permanente health maintenance organization (HMO) (Cummings et al. 1962). Defined as the "reduction of medical/surgical utilization following the provision of mental health and chemical dependency (MH/CD) services," *the medical cost offset effect* persuaded the Kaiser Permanente Health Plan to write the nation's first comprehensive prepaid psychotherapy benefit. For two decades, medical cost offset remained the single most powerful argument for the inclusion of MH/CD benefits in health insurance (Cummings 1991a).

For medical cost offset to be credible, the savings in medical utilization must exceed the cost of providing the MH/CD services, yielding a net savings in overall health costs. In the early 1980s, when mental health costs skyrocketed and became one of the most significant contributors to the health care inflation spiral, interest in medical offset disappeared. Instead, the health industry turned its attention to tethering MH/CD costs themselves as they were rising faster than medical-surgical costs. Now that managed care has succeeded in removing most of the unnecessary MH/CD expenditures, there is an intense, renewed interest in medical cost offset within the health care industry.

The medical cost offset effect has not been demonstrated in every setting in which it has been tested. The literature is extensive and has only recently begun to reveal under what circumstances this effect occurs. When it does occur, research has attempted to elucidate the kinds of services and interventions that result in the greater net cost savings. In this chapter I briefly present the history of the medical cost offset effect, review the salient research, discuss why medical cost offset occurs and why it does not, delve into the richness of the literature and tantalizing doors that have been opened, and finally demonstrate how it can be one of the most powerful, if not *the* most powerful tool in MH/CD outcomes research. I will examine why, when medical cost offset is so widely recognized, especially by employers, policymakers within government and the insurance industry have generally ignored the phenomenon in health planning.

Medical Cost Offset and Somatization

The history of the discovery of the medical offset effect has been extensively reviewed (Cummings 1991c; Cummings and VandenBos 1981) and will be only briefly discussed here. Immediately following World War II capitated health care was seen as revolutionary. The newly established Kaiser Permanente Health Plan grew rapidly because it eliminated all of the exclusions, co-payments, and deductibles that characterized indemnity insurance of that time. By the late 1950s Kaiser Permanente had grown to 2.5 million enrollees and had firmly established itself as the prototype of the HMO. It had also discovered to its dismay that 60% of all physician visits were by patients who had no obvious physical diseases. The relationship of stress to physical symptomatology was not clearly understood at that time, and it was believed that the propensity of healthy HMO patients to seek medical treatment was the result of the removal of all financial barriers to access. In keeping with the medical parlance of that period, many of these patients were diagnosed as *hypochondriacs* and that term was entered into their charts.

I found the diagnosis of hypochondriasis to be distasteful because physicians often neglected patients with multiple physical complaints. I made several attempts to replace the term, all of which met with resistance until the term *somatization* was proffered. Physicians readily accepted that term because it sounded medical. Patients who manifested emotional distress through physical symptoms were termed *somaticizers*, which was later shortened to *somatizers*. It must be recalled that these events were long before Paul Ellwood, M.D., coined the term *worried well*.

Estimates as to the scope of somatization vary, but there is general agreement that these patients account for a disproportionate share of the nation's medical bills. They repeatedly go to physicians in a fruitless search for medically based diagnoses and treatment and have yearly medical costs 10 to 14 times higher than the national average (Cummings 1993, p. 225). The American Academy of Physicians estimates that between $20 to $30 billion a year is spent on unnecessary care for somatizers (Ford 1983, 1986). The prevalence of somatization in our society was made clear in 1976 when the American Medical Association testified before the U.S. Senate Committee on Health that "in the United States on any given day, 60 to 70 percent of the patients who are waiting to see the physician either have no physical disease but are somatizing stress, or stress is impeding the treatment and healing of a physical condition" (Cummings 1993, p. 224).

Challenging the Frontiers of Medicine

There are several theories why somatization occurs. The most common theory holds that somatizers are not able to express their feelings in words but instead express them as somatic perceptions. It is possible that neuropeptides, chemicals that are active both in the brain's emotional centers and in organs throughout the body, orchestrate the connections between emotional distress and its expression in physical symptoms.

A somewhat different theory holds that the failure of parents to attune and respond to an infant's needs makes the child unable to distinguish between internal states, such as differentiating between anger and sadness. In later life this inability interferes with social connections, and physical symptoms become the means by which these people reach out for care and contact. In a third variation, parents of the somatizer are seen as having inadvertently rewarded a child for having symptoms, for example, paying attention to recurrent stomachaches and letting a child stay home from school. In any case, physical symptoms come to represent a deep emotional need to be nurtured.

It should be noted that the somatizer is not a malingerer because there is no obvious benefit derived from having the condition. A somatizing patient is manifesting a form of psychological denial for which psychotherapy is the treatment of choice to break through the unconscious process. A physician's reassurance that nothing is wrong is seldom, if ever, effective. Somatization as used in medical cost offset research is defined as the automatic substitution of physical symptoms for emotional distress or the exaggeration of physical symptoms in an actual disease because of underlying emotional distress. As used for medical research purposes, the concept of somatization usually has a broader application than the actual DSM-IV (American Psychiatric Association 1994) diagnosis of somatization disorder.

The unconscious *choice* of illness is influenced by many factors. In some cases, a patient chooses a particular malady because it best symbolizes his or her plight. For example, romantic disillusionment may be expressed through an imagined heart ailment, or the inability to *stomach* a bad life situation finds its expression in recurrent stomachaches or even the inability to swallow. More often, however, the somatizer selects a symptom that challenges the frontiers of medicine.

In the late 1950s, when the concept of somatization was "discovered," cardiologists lacked their current diagnostic acumen, and the most frequent form of somatization was hyperventilation syndrome in a sufferer who was convinced that he or she had heart disease. As the field of cardiology became more sophisticated, *cardiac neurosis* gave way to an epidemic of low back pain. However, as back centers developed more precise diagnostic methods, low back pain yielded to hypoglycemia, chronic fatigue syndrome, and strange and rare allergies that continue to baffle physicians.

The manner in which health care is dispensed inadvertently encourages somatizing. In our litigious society, physicians cannot risk missing a diagnosis, and when a patient complains of discomfort, physicians may order numerous consultations and laboratory tests in search of a physical cause. Reassurance does not satisfy the patient's anxiety, and medical attention only serves to increase the conviction that a physical cause has yet to be found. The patient continues to channel emotional conflicts into physical symptoms, seeking a new physician after previous ones have been exhausted. Meanwhile, the suffering continues.

Some somatizers seem to choose a particular symptom because it is an actual extension of a physical problem they already have, but it is now complicated by stress. For example, somatizers with baffling allergies have usually suffered from known allergies to a lesser extent. As their stress escalated, mysterious allergies became an available route for expressing the effects of stress.

The First Generation of Medical Cost Offset Studies

Following the seminal research of Follette and Cummings (1967) and Cummings and Follette (1968, 1976), there were 28 medical cost offset studies reported in a wide variety of settings. These studies were summarized by the federal Alcohol, Drug Abuse, and Mental Health Administration in a special report (Jones and Vischi 1979) that was followed by the Bethesda Consensus Conference in 1980. That conference noted that all but one study demonstrated medical cost offset, but more important, the medical cost offset obtained in the array of studies varied from savings that were highly significant to those that were not sufficient to cover even the cost of providing the MH/CD services. Despite these difficulties, the leading researchers in the field concluded at the Bethesda Conference that the health care system is burdened by patients with no real physical disease whose symptoms are caused by stress. Without psychotherapy, it was believed that these persons would suffer needlessly.

The report by Jones and Vischi (1980) was never widely disseminated, because the Bethesda Conference was convened only a few weeks before the end of the Carter administration and the government scientists who convened it were swept out of office by the electorate, but that report directed several important conclusions toward the second generation of medical cost offset studies. Noting that medical cost offset is more likely to occur in organized settings, it was recommended that future research determine what factors increase medical-surgical cost savings and what factors mitigate such savings. It was further noted that most of the findings were based on retrospective studies (prospective studies would require denial of MH/CD services to a control group). To overcome the limitations of past studies it was recommended that a way be found to conduct controlled experiments and to address the problem of how medical cost offset research could aid in program planning and in clinical service delivery (Jones and Vischi 1980).

The succeeding generation of studies numbered more than 80, and along with merely replicating many of the previous findings, the studies addressed several of the issues discussed at the Bethesda Conference. Suddenly, as the mental health industry turned its attention to controlling the escalation of MH/CD costs, medical cost offset research entered a relatively dormant period from which it is now emerging.

The Difficulty of Doing Medical Cost Offset Studies: The Second Generation

The health insurance industry has three primary functions: 1) collect money, 2) maintain data (records), and 3) dispense money. Those outside the industry are startled to learn that historically only the first of these functions has been conducted with any noteworthy efficiency. The second generation of medical cost offset research was severely hampered by the fact that most settings did not possess the information systems needed to conduct such studies. Embarrassed by this, actuaries found it easier to ignore the medical offset phenomenon than to acknowledge their data processing shortcomings. The current emphasis on outcomes research and accompanying drives toward sophisticated medical informatics have heralded a brighter future for researchers.

A second major difficulty in conducting medical offset research stems from practice disparity among psychotherapists. Whereas there may be only a limited number of ways to perform an appendectomy, psychotherapists display a seemingly infinite number of competing and warring approaches to treatment. Unfortunately, most medical cost offset studies have based their findings on a "lumping" of practitioners who may be canceling each other out. The more organized and homogeneous the practitioners, the more likely is the positive outcome. For example, in HMOs in which the practitioners are trained to perform effective short-term psychotherapy, brief psychotherapy—even a single session—has been shown to result in medical cost offset (Cummings and Follette 1968, 1976; Goldberg et al. 1970, 1979). On the other hand, in a fee-for-service setting, in which practitioners characteristically practice longer term therapy, a dosage effect seems to prevail (Schlesinger et al. 1983). In the latter study, the greatest savings occurred with hospitalization, inasmuch as the higher costs of longer term therapy seemed to subtract from the potential savings in ambulatory medical care. Thus, there needs to be greater specificity in selecting providers and treatment.

Medical offset studies need to be prospective and controlled, in contrast to most previous studies, which relied on retrospective data and multiple regression analyses. Such studies are subject to selection bias and do not answer the question of whether so-called positive results are a statistical regression to the mean (Fiedler and Wight 1989). As previously mentioned, prospective studies would have to include a randomly selected group of somatizers who do not receive psychotherapy. The denial of services is generally contractually not permitted by the third-party payer and constitutes an ethical dilemma for the practitioner. One way of addressing this problem is to phase in a new psychotherapy benefit. A random phase-in could include the required control group, at least until the implementation of new psychotherapy benefits is completed.

Most somatizers are not referred for psychotherapy, and the nonpsychiatric physicians who see them recognize less than one-fourth of those with emotional distress or chemical dependency (Glazer 1993; Glazer and Bell 1993). In a study by the RAND Corporation (1987), physicians who were capitated were more likely to refer patients for psychotherapy than were fee-for-service physicians, and the likelihood of referrals markedly decreased in geographical areas where there was a surplus of physicians. One physician was quoted as saying, "One good somatizer is worth at least 9 to 10 patients" (RAND Corporation 1987, p. 23). Some studies have sought to train nonpsychiatric physicians to recognize the somatizer and to appropriately refer him or her for psychotherapy. Even screening with computer printouts to primary care physicians has been utilized (Cummings and Follette 1968). However, to maximize referral to a psychotherapist, in addition to increasing physician cooperation, an outreach program directed at the somatizer may be necessary.

A large number of second-generation studies have helped to clarify the roles of stress and unhealthy lifestyles in relation to medical utilization and to identify and promote issues of wellness. This body of literature is extensive and beyond the scope of this chapter, but it should be noted that somatization as a lifestyle has been reviewed by Ford (1983) and Pelletier (1993). The relationship between stress and somatization, which was not well understood when Kaiser Permanente dealt with the problem in the 1950s, will continue to occupy a significant sector of the health field. Medical overutilization can be affected by programs designed to promote healthy lifestyles (Ford 1983, 1986).

The Reverse Medical Offset Threat

When the medical cost offset phenomenon was first demonstrated, a frequent criticism from traditional psychotherapists was that psychological symptoms would replace physical symptoms in remission (symptom substitution). However, an 8-year follow-up study showed otherwise; not only had the somatizing abated, but patients had actually resolved the underlying stress that had resulted in their original physical symptomatology (Cummings and Follette 1976). This findings seemed to put an end to the criticism called *transfer of equivalence* by more traditional psychotherapists. Less clear was the relationship between medical and psychiatric hospitalization.

Several studies have shown that hospitalized medical patients with psychiatric comorbidity have longer hospital stays and that psychotherapeutic consultation in the hospital can reduce the length of stay (Fulop et al. 1989; Hengeveld et al. 1988; Levenson et al. 1986). However, what is the fate of a patient who presents for psychiatric hospitalization and is denied admission? Does that patient have a greater incidence of medical hospitalization? Such a finding would clearly be a *reverse* medical cost offset effect. For 1 year, Pallak and Cummings (1992) followed every patient who presented for psychiatric hospitalization within a 6-month period in a managed care program and who was either admitted to a psychiatric hospital or was diverted to outpatient psychotherapy. They were interested in whether patients who presented for psychiatric hospitalization and were denied admission were more likely to be admitted for medical and surgical hospitalization for ostensibly a nonpsychiatric diagnosis. Patients who responded to outpatient psychotherapy either in lieu of psychiatric hospitalization or subsequent to discharge from a psychiatric unit, whether they were diverted or hospitalized psychiatrically, were not likely to be admitted to a medical or surgical unit. Both psychiatrically diverted *and* hospitalized patients who did not accept outpatient psychotherapy were more likely to be medically or surgically hospitalized during the subsequent year. The critical variable determining hospitalization was whether patients received outpatient psychotherapy.

Challenging the Frontiers of Psychiatry and Psychology

Similar to the somatizer who can display many physical symptoms in the service of an underlying need for attention and caring is the *psycholyser,* who can increase health costs by mimicking any emotional or mental condition. This trend has been aided by providers who have broadened the definition of psychiatric syndromes to include behavior that is within normal limits and by the media who have popularized tentative psychological findings into fads. When depression is redefined so as to encompass 60% of adults, or attention-deficit/hyperactivity disorder is said to affect 35% of all males in grammar school, it is questionable whether these are any longer valid syndromes with pathognomonic features.

More dramatic is the mimicry of the psycholyser who reflects the latest psycho-fad. However, it is important to stress that the follower of that psycho-fad must first be the provider, who then inadvertently encourages the needy patient to mimic that condition. Borderline personality disorder is particularly vulnerable to becoming whatever the psychotherapist is looking for, and even more adept at mimicking it. Multiple personality disorder is far more iatrogenic than real, with the incidence closely allied to the number and location of practitioners who overdiagnose the "disorder" in their patients (Bloom 1991). Similarly, the scandal of false memory syndrome is following closely by the overdiagnosis of childhood sexual abuse and the highly suspect satanic ritual abuse (Loftus 1993). It will be imperative in medical cost offset research in the future that the setting be organized so as to control for questionable psychiatric syndromes and overzealous providers.

The Third Generation: Managed Care Outcomes Research

The unprecedented growth of managed behavioral health care plans over the past several years has provided large organized settings that have shown a revitalized interest in medical cost offset research. These companies are under considerable pressure to empirically demonstrate claims of quality, efficiency, and effectiveness. Outcomes research is experiencing a surge of activity, with contract research organizations springing up to meet the demand. Today, most of the unnecessary costs in delivering behavioral health care have been eliminated, and managed care organizations are turning to answer whether, how, and when such services can have an effect on unnecessary medical and surgical costs.

The forerunner and prototype of this new medical cost offset research is the Hawaii Medicaid Study (Cummings et al. 1993; Pallak et al. 1994), conducted during a period of 7 years with the entire Medicaid population of the Island of Oahu (Honolulu) and in a managed behavioral care setting specifically organized for that purpose under the auspices of the federal Health Care Financing Administration (HCFA). The study was designed to meet several scientific criticisms delineated in the second generation of medical cost offset research.

Under waivers obtained from HCFA, this is a prospective study with experimental and control groups randomly assigned to keep recipient families intact. A managed behavioral health care delivery system was specially created on a closed-panel staff model with the main center in Honolulu and with satellites in outlying areas of heavy Medicaid concentration. Every month the top 15% of users of health services, who accounted for 80% of the Medicaid costs, were outreached by mail, telephone, and, for patients that responded to neither of these, by a house call from a registered nurse. Programs were instituted to elicit cooperation from physicians, welfare department social workers, and other health care professionals, but the outreach program consistently elicited the greatest number of referrals.

The most ambitious part of the Hawaii Medicaid medical cost offset project was the 6-month half-time advance training of the practitioners who subsequently became the half-time staff who provided the services in a 3-year period. During those 3 years of service these practitioners spent 15% of their salaried time in ongoing quality assurance and in the monitoring of adherence to the protocols in which they were trained. Thus, the highest probable level in standardization of practitioners and treatment was achieved.

Interestingly, this controlled prospective study confirmed years of retrospectively derived results. Overall, the cost of creating the managed behavioral health care system was recovered by medical-surgical savings within 18 months, and the significant reduction in medical utilization continued thereafter with no additional behavioral care required to maintain the cost savings. These were estimated to be $8 million per year in constant dollars, with the greatest savings attributed to the group with a chronic medical diagnosis. This group consisted of high utilizers who suffered from diabetes, hypertension, chronic airway and respiratory diseases, and ischemic heart disease and who accounted for 40% of all Medicaid costs in Hawaii.

In contrast, the control group, which was seen in the fee-for-service private sector for psychotherapy, revealed a 17% increase in medical and surgical utilization, which was not statistically different from the 27% increase in control group patients who received no MH/CD services whatsoever. It must be emphasized that Hawaii was chosen for its liberal Medicaid benefit of up to 52 sessions per year with a psychiatrist or psychologist in the community of the patient's own choosing. Thus, this study yielded data on no less than three groups: 1) those seen in the private fee-for-service sector, 2) those seen in a highly organized managed care setting, and 3) those who were not seen by any MH/CD practitioner at all. The findings confirmed the conclusion reached at the Bethesda Consensus Conference that medical cost offset is less likely to occur in traditional, nonmanaged care settings.

Medical Cost Offset in Programmatic Planning

One of the problems associated with outcomes research is the "soft" nature of the criteria for improvement, often referred to as *happiness variables*, relying heavily on the patient's self-report (Luborsky et al. 1988). The following example, which has been published elsewhere (Cummings 1994), demonstrates how reduction in medical utilization is an objective measure of successful outcome in psychotherapy and how this can be useful in program planning. In our society persons in emotional distress very often have somatic symptoms, and reduction in somatization is a reliable measure of diminution of emotional distress in that group of people.

The researchers at Kaiser Permanente intuitively observed that certain conditions seemed to respond better to dynamically oriented therapy, others to behavior therapy, and still others to systems approaches. Within the school of therapy, some conditions were more effectively treated in individual therapy, others in group therapy, and still others in psychoeducational programs. The researchers tentatively accepted the premise that all schools and modalities had truth, but none had ultimate truth. The optimal specific treatment could well be an admixture of several approaches, and they set about to test this hypothesis through outcomes research using medical offset as the criterion of efficacy. Because in society persons under stress somaticize their stress, a greater reduction of medical utilization in an aggregate group receiving one type of psychotherapy intervention compared with another aggregate group receiving a different intervention would be a measure of the effectiveness of the intervention.

The cost-therapeutic effectiveness ratio, also known as the efficiency-effectiveness ratio, was derived by dividing the average (mean) medical utilization for the entire group for the year prior to the intervention by the average (mean) medical utilization plus average (mean) psychotherapy visits for that same group in the year after the intervention:

$$r = \frac{\text{Mean medical utilization year before}}{\text{Mean medical utilization year after + mean psychotherapy sessions}}$$

Differentially weighting by cost the various kinds of medical utilization, such as giving an outpatient visit a value of 1 and a day of hospitalization a value of 10, only complicated our computations and neither added precision nor altered outcome. However, weighting individual therapy, group therapy, and psychoeducational programs did add precision. The formula adopted was based on psychotherapist time to accomplish a unit. Thus, individual therapy (1 therapist with 1 patient for 45 minutes) received a value of 1, while group therapy (1 therapist with 8 patients for 90 minutes) received a value of 0.25, and a psychoeducational group (1 therapist with 12 patients for 90 minutes) was given a value of 0.08. To clarify further, 10 sessions of individual therapy equals 10, the same number of group therapy sessions equals 2.5, and finally 10 sessions of psychoeducational programming yield less than 1. Emergency department visits were weighted 2, which means that 10 emergency department visits had a total value of 20.

To illustrate from actual research, a group of 83 borderline personality disorder patients were placed in individual psychotherapy, with the result that medical utilization declined slightly, but at an enormous expenditure of both individual sessions and emergency department visits.

$$r = \frac{163}{141 + 68} = 0.8$$

The ratio is low, indicating that interventions were neither therapeutically effective (reduction in medical utilization) nor cost efficient (number of mental health units). Over time the staff created a focused set of interventions within individual therapy with some improvement in cost efficiency but little impact on therapeutic effectiveness with another group of 73 borderline personality patients:

$$r = \frac{167}{148 + 51} = 0.7$$

The overall effectiveness-efficiency ratio actually declined. With another population of 76 patients with borderline personality disorder, a great deal of care and effort were expended in designing a program with 20 group therapy sessions, augmented with 10 sessions of individual therapy and then with monthly follow-up sessions. Emergency department visits were virtually eliminated and the ratio rose dramatically:

$$r = \frac{166}{27 + 31} = 2.8$$

Learning a great deal from this group of patients, we sharpened the group therapy to 15 group therapy sessions, followed by 10 psychoeducational sessions and subsequent monthly follow-up individual sessions, yielding a ratio and a program that was adopted as both effective and efficient:

$$r = \frac{171}{11 + 12} = 7.8$$

The research team continued to experiment with honing the program even further, but the work with borderline personality disorder patients, a category of patients with a high degree of resistance and acting out, never achieved the ideal ratio of 9.0 or higher, which became the goal or standard.

In this way, using medical offset, 68 focused, targeted interventions for 68 psychological or psychiatric conditions were designed. The methodology was described as brief, intermittent psychotherapy throughout the life cycle (Cummings 1991b), an approach that concentrates on solving the problem in the here and now while also giving the patient a greater repertoire of responses to stress. These findings were the backbone of the clinical training and service delivery, early at Kaiser Permanente and later at American Biodyne (Cummings and Sayama 1995).

Conclusion

Medical offset as a type of outcomes research has been employed effectively in both programmatic planning and the development of clinical service models for more than 35 years. The first generation of research established that no health plan is complete without a comprehensive mental health benefit because its absence will result in the overutilization of medical-surgical facilities by persons who are somatizing stress. The Bethesda Consensus Conference on Medical Offset concluded that medical offset can be used to improve the delivery of mental health services and that improved services result in greater medical offset, defined as savings in medical-surgical costs over and above the cost of providing the mental health services.

The second generation of medical cost offset research identified problems from retrospective research. It also revealed that most health plans do not collect data in a way that renders medical offset research possible. These criticisms have in large measure been answered by the HCFA–Hawaii–Medicaid Study, a 7-year prospective medical offset study, which may be the prototype of the third generation of research. Medical cost offset research parachuted into a traditional setting cannot be expected to yield positive outcomes. Savings are found in organized (managed) care settings and not in the private fee-for-service sector, explaining the contradictory findings of many past studies.

The current resurgence of interest in medical cost offset reflects the success of managed behavioral care that, having controlled psychiatric costs, now is in a position to curb medical-surgical costs incurred by somatizers who overload our health system. In addition, medical cost offset is an objective measure in outcomes research that can aid in treatment planning, empirical derivation of treatment protocols, and practitioner training, all of which are keen interests in today's highly competitive environment.

References

American Psychiatric Association: Diagnostic and Statistical Manual of Mental Disorders, 4th Edition. Washington, DC, American Psychiatric Association, 1994

Bloom BL: Planned Short-Term Psychotherapy: A Clinical Handbook. Boston, MA, Allyn & Bacon, 1991

Cummings NA: Arguments for the financial efficacy of psychological services in health care settings, in Handbook of Clinical Psychology in Medical Settings. Edited by Sweet JJ, Rozensky RG, Tovian SM. New York, Plenum, 1991a, pp 113–126

Cummings NA: Brief intermittent psychotherapy throughout the life cycle, in Psychotherapy in Managed Health Care: The Optimal Use of Time and Resources. Edited by Austad CS, Berman WH. Washington, DC, American Psychological Association, 1991b, pp 35–45

Cummings NA: The somatizing patient, in Psychotherapy in Managed Health Care: The Optimal Use of Time and Resources. Edited by Austad CS, Berman WH. Washington, DC, American Psychological Association, 1991c, pp 234–247

Cummings NA, Somatization: when physical symptoms have no medical cause, in Mind-Body Medicine. Edited by Goleman D, Gurin J. Yonkers, NY, Consumer Reports Books, 1993, pp 221–232

Cummings NA: The successful application of medical offset in program planning and in clinical delivery. Manag Care Q 2(2):1–6, 1994

Cummings NA, Follette WT: Psychiatric services and medical utilization in a prepaid health plan setting: part 2. Med Care 6:31–41, 1968

Cummings NA, Follette WT: Brief psychotherapy and medical utilization: an eight-year follow-up, in The Professional Psychologist Today. Edited by Dörken H, et al. San Francisco, CA, Jossey-Bass, 1976, pp 126–142

Cummings NA, Sayama M: Focused Psychotherapy: A Casebook of Brief, Intermittent Psychotherapy Throughout the Life Cycle. New York, Brunner-Mazel, 1995

Cummings NA, VandenBos GR: The twenty year Kaiser-Permanente experience with psychotherapy and medical utilization: implications for national health policy and national health insurance. Health Policy Q 1(2):159–175, 1981

Cummings NA, Kahn BI, Sparkman B: Psychotherapy and Medical Utilization: A Pilot Study. Oakland, CA, Annual Reports of Kaiser Permanente Research Projects, 1962

Cummings NA, Dörken H, Pallak MS, et al.: The impact of psychological intervention on health care costs and utilization, in Medicaid, Managed Behavioral Health and Implications for Public Policy. Healthcare Utilization and Cost Series, Vol 2. Edited by Cummings NA, Pallak MS. South San Francisco, CA, Foundation for Behavioral Health, 1993, pp 1–23

Fiedler JL, Wight RB: The Medical Offset Effect and Public Policy. New York, Praeger, 1989

Follette WT, Cummings NA: Psychiatric services and medical utilization in a prepaid health plan setting. Med Care 5:25–35, 1967

Ford CV: The Somatizing Disorders: Illness as a Way of Life. New York, Elsevier, 1983

Ford CV: The somatizing disorders. Psychosomatics 27:327–337, 1986

Fulop G, Strain JJ, Fahs MC, et al: Medical disorders associated with psychiatric comorbidity and prolonged length of stay. Hosp Community Psychiatry 40:80–82, 1989

Glazer W: Approaching hidden psychiatric illness in PPOs: the "medical offset" effect. AAPPO Journal June-July: 1993, pp 15–21

Glazer W, Bell N: Mental Health Benefits: A Purchaser's Guide. Brookfield, WI, International Foundation of Employee Benefits Plans Press, 1993

Goldberg ID, Krantz G, Locke BZ: Effect of a short-term outpatient psychiatric benefit on the utilization of medical services in a prepaid group practice medical program. Med Care 8:419–428, 1970

Goldberg ID, Krantz G, Locke BZ: Effect of short-term outpatient benefit and the utilization of health care. Med Care 17:118–124, 1979

Hengeveld MW, Ancion FAJM, Rooihans HMG: Psychiatric consultations with depressed medical inpatients: a randomized controlled cost-effectiveness study. Int J Psychiatry Med 18:33–43, 1988

Jones KR, Vischi TR: The impact of alcohol, drug abuse, and mental health treatment on medical care utilization: a review of the research literature. Med Care 17 (suppl):43–131, 1979

Jones KR, Vischi TR: The Bethesda Consensus Conference on Medical Offset. Alcohol, Drug Abuse, and Mental Health Administration Report. Rockville, MD, Alcohol, Drug Abuse, and Mental Health Administration, 1980

Levenson JL, Hamer R, Silverman JJ: Psychopathology in medical inpatients and its relationship to length stay: a pilot study. Int J Psychiatry Med 16:231–236, 1986

Loftus EF: The reality of repressed memories. Am Psychol 48:518–537, 1993

Luborsky L, Crits-Christorph P, Mintz J, et al: Who Will Benefit From Psychotherapy: Predicting Therapeutic Outcomes. New York, Basic Books, 1988

Pallak MS, Cummings NA: Inpatient and outpatient psychiatric treatment: the effect of matching patients to appropriate level of treatment on psychiatric and medical–surgical hospital days. Applied and Preventive Psychology 1:83–87, 1992

Pallak MS, Cummings NA, Dörken H, et al.: Medical costs, Medicaid, and managed mental health treatment: the Hawaii study. Manag Care Q 2(2):64–70, 1994

Pelletier KR: Between mind and body: stress, emotions and health, in Mind-Body Medicine. Edited by Goleman D, Gurin J. Yonkers, NY, Consumer Reports Books, 1993, pp 19–38

RAND Corporation: A Report on the Changing Practice Patterns of Primary Care Physicians in Geographical Areas with Too Many Physicians. Santa Monica, CA, RAND Corporation, 1987

Schlesinger HJ, Mumford E, Glass GV, et al.: Mental health treatment and medical care utilization in a fee-for-service system: outpatient mental health treatment following the onset of a chronic disease. Am J Public Health 73:422–429, 1983

Chapter 16

Can Psychotherapy Be Conducted Effectively in Managed Care Settings?

Carol Shaw Austad, Ph.D.

Can psychotherapy be conducted effectively in managed care settings? This question has polarized opinions of mental health professionals and generated considerable controversy. Before attempting to answer the question, however, it is crucial to identify, define, and discuss the central issues and concerns underlying the question of whether psychotherapy of high quality can exist in managed care environments.

Elements of the Controversy

Adversaries of managed care echo the fact that the "golden age of medicine," when physicians could practice in an unfettered manner, is ending. Insurance and government interference in the practice of medicine is growing at an unprecedented rate. Opponents see managed mental health care as an unwelcome third party intruding on the sanctity of the psychotherapist-patient relationship (Feldman 1992; Sammons 1991). Their criticisms are that managed mental health 1) uses cost rather than need to deny care, 2) blocks access to and erects barriers to needed care, 3) threatens the security of the patient-therapist relationship, 4) violates patient-therapist confidentiality, 5) decreases freedom of provider choice, 6) forces the use of short-term models of therapy that produce only superficial change and discourages the use of long-term models that produce long-term change, and 7) excludes providers from networks. To bolster opposition to managed care, opponents cite the fact that some professionals who initially believed in the positive potential of managed mental health care are now disappointed in what they perceive to be a failure to fulfill its promise. Antagonists also cite examples of patients who have suffered damage as a result of undertreatment, contending that managed care's overall effect on quality of care and the evolution of psychotherapy is negative (Bennett 1988; Kohrman 1986; Starr 1982).

Supporters of managed care assert that managed care has ushered in an age of accountability in which practitioners confront and deal with the reality of runaway costs and limited resources. They praise managed care because it 1) is a tool to decrease inflationary mental health costs; 2) distributes care equitably so that instead of a few people receiving much therapy, many people receive some therapy; 3) demystifies the therapeutic relationship by subjecting it to scrutiny and evaluation; 4) increases clinician accountability for treatment decisions; 5) encourages patient involvement in and responsibility for treatment; 6) stimulates the use of cost-effective short-term interventions; 7) makes therapy goals more realistic; and 8) spurs outcome research (Cummings 1986; Flinn et al. 1987; Pearson 1992). To bolster support for managed care, proponents cite examples of patients who have suffered the iatrogenic effects of treatment and overtreatment, contending that managed care's net effect on the quality of care and the evolution of psychotherapy is positive (Austad and Hoyt 1992; Bloom 1990; Sederer and St. Clair 1990; Truscott 1992).

From whence do these vastly different viewpoints come? Although the argument that managed care jeopardizes quality of care is primarily based on humanitarian and professional concerns, some chagrin may be related to economics, professional or personal self-preservation, theoretical loyalties, and miscommunication.

Theoretical, Professional, and Economic Issues

Payers (insurance companies, the government, employers, and individuals) are asking, "What type of therapy performed by what type of therapist is most effective?" and "What is the advantage of paying one profession higher fees than another for rendering the same service?" Payers want assurance that treatment decisions will enhance patient welfare and not provider income.

As the health care status quo changes, two traditional assumptions are being questioned: 1) Is long-term therapy superior to short-term therapy (Hoyt 1991)?, 2) Do some professions, by virtue of their superior training, deserve to earn greater fees for performing psychotherapy? Because many forms of psychotherapy are rendered by experienced psychiatrists, psychologists, nurses, and social workers (Lambert 1991; VandenBos 1986; VandenBos and DeLeon 1989), some payers want to reimburse providers according to current procedural terminology code, especially with the lower paid professions lobbying with a cry of "equal pay for equal work" (Carter 1993). As the mental health professions compete for the same health care dollars, they each also vie for the right to expand services (e.g., evaluations, hospital privileges, prescriptive privileges, licensing, testing, and biofeedback). Each profession jealously guards its turf, protecting itself by defining responsibilities it is uniquely qualified to perform. This protecting of territory can sometimes be based on economic concerns. In addition, providers are reluctant to support the use of systems that do not financially support the familiar, neutral, safe, and predictable treatment models that they customarily use. Thus, they may find it easier to cling to the commonplace rather than reexamine the basic premises of familiar treatment models (Berlin 1969; Hoyt 1985; Zimet 1989).

An objective review of empirical studies of psychotherapy shows that there is no absolute proof that one profession can perform psychotherapy better than another or that long-term psychotherapy is superior to short-term psychotherapy.

It may not be a coincidence that disciples of long-term psychotherapies and practitioners who have income to lose are among managed care's greatest enemies. Mental health professionals may unwittingly base some of their views about managed care on self-interest. Controversy may mask motives that have at their base turf wars around acquisition of diminishing and ever-shifting resources (Hemmenway et al. 1990). In the changing world of health care in which controversy abounds, separating the distress of altruism from that of self-interest can be difficult (Berlin 1969; Zieman 1993), yet mental health professionals must try to detach themselves from decision making based on self-interest.

Communication

Miscommunication lies at the root of some of this controversy. *Psychotherapy* has multiple meanings, and managed care concepts are new and unfamiliar. Moreover, psychotherapy is a diverse field; therapists come from varied training backgrounds, disciplines, theoretical orientations, and cohorts. A psychologist educated in the 1960s by staunch behaviorists may hold very different views from a psychiatrist educated in the 1980s by biological psychopharmacologists or a social worker educated in the 1990s by an ego-analytic supervisor. When there are as many definitions of *psychotherapy* as there are books written about it (Kleinke 1994), the potential for miscommunication grows exponentially.

Clinicians come from diverse therapy orientations, and they vary widely in knowledge of and experience with managed care (Austad et al. 1993). Although the majority of therapists have limited contact with managed care systems, a minority of them are well informed about its general history, structure, and philosophy (Nelson 1987). Some clinicians are attracted to the philosophy of managed care; others are repelled by it. As managed care proliferates, so do new terms, vocabulary, and concepts (e.g., preferred provider organization [PPO], employee assistance program, broker model, Employee Retirement Income Security Act). Mental health professionals are conversing in a rapidly changing health care world without the benefit of a common tradition of shared memories. When the alphabet soup of managed care is coupled with the vagaries of defining psychotherapy, a virtual Tower of Babel is erected.

To illustrate this point, imagine a conversation conducted by the following three therapists. Provider A has dealt with managed care company X, a fly-by-night PPO that closed its doors leaving behind many unpaid providers and patients. Provider B has signed up with a panel of company Y, a large, successful, and financially stable conglomerate whose bureaucracy is inefficient and whose reviewers are inconsistent. Provider C is an employee of company Z, a well-run staff-model health maintenance organization (HMO) with a social mission that reports excellent customer satisfaction. Provider A adheres to a psychodynamic model of therapy, provider B adheres to a family systems model of psychotherapy, and provider C is eclectic. What provider A means by managed care and psychotherapy may not be what provider B or provider C means by managed care and psychotherapy. When speaking to one another, the potential for miscommunication is significant.

To engage in constructive conversation, participants must agree on the meaning of the following key concepts: managed care, psychotherapy, and the parameters of a mental health benefit package. Although other chapters in this book address these issues, in the next part of this chapter I operationally define concepts that are relevant to this discussion so no miscommunication occurs here!

Defining Managed Mental Health Care

Managed care has evolved so swiftly since the 1980s that its definition must remain fluid. Broadly interpreted, the term is applied to many products and services ranging from simple preauthorization of treatment to provider-negotiated delivery systems (Callan and Yeager 1991).

Mental health services can coexist with general managed care health systems or be delivered within them, or they can be carved out of general health care plans and contracted to specialized companies who are responsible for utilization control, provider selection, payment of services, and quality assurance (Boaz 1988; Goran 1992; Levin 1992). The mental health care benefit varies as a function of the type of managed care company and the diverse sets of local and regional requirements and regulatory concerns that center on fiscal soundness, quality assurance standards, and adequacy of provider networks (Davis 1990; Hastings 1990). For the purpose of this chapter, a managed care benefit package is defined as one that is similar to that of a staff-model HMO or a carve-out or PPO model of managed care in that it allows for no fewer than 20 sessions of mental health care including a copayment that does not prohibit patients from using the benefit. Common sense, as well as some data, informs us that the benefit design will have a profound effect on what types or models of psychotherapy will be conducted within managed care settings.

Effects of Benefit Design on Psychotherapy

Essentially, therapists are faced with the choice of selecting models of treatment compatible with the managed care benefit design or not practicing in managed care. What forms of psychotherapy can be used effectively within managed care settings? Long-term models with inflexible parameters (e.g., interminable weekly 50-minute sessions) will not flourish. The "pure gold" of psychoanalysis—long-term psychoanalytically oriented therapies—cannot be included. Like most cosmetic surgery, long-term therapies can rarely be classified as medically necessary and will not be paid for with insurance funds. Long-term treatment will be available, however, to those who pay out-of-pocket or finance a significant percentage of the cost themselves (Austad and Hoyt 1992; Hoyt and Austad 1992; Kisch and Austad 1989).

This still leaves a plethora of treatment models from which a therapist can choose. With the proliferation of psychotherapies in use today, there are many short-term models (Karasu 1992; Kleinke 1994) compatible with managed care benefit packages. Before discussing specific models, in the next section I describe the core features of effective models of psychotherapy in managed care settings.

Principles of Short-Term Psychotherapy

The first five traits described below are characteristic of all forms of short-term therapy, and the remaining are specific to effective short-term therapy in managed care settings (Austad 1993; Austad and Berman 1991; Austad et al. 1989; Bauer and Kobos 1987; Bistline et al. 1991; Boaz 1988).

1. *Focused assessment.* The therapist arrives at a rapid, accurate assessment of what patients need in the here and now to help themselves meet their expectations of treatment. The therapist accepts what patients say at face value and does not interpret meaning at a level that delays taking immediate, helpful action. The clinician is not bogged down in theoretical constructs but must respond to the demands of real people in the real world and evaluate what interventions are "necessary and sufficient" to develop and execute an effective treatment plan.
2. *Pragmatic therapeutic alliance.* Because managed care therapists know that the therapeutic relationship accounts for a significant percentage of change in therapy (Lambert 1991), a strong therapeutic alliance is rapidly established. Both therapist and patient incorporate the reality of limited time and resources into their work together. The nature of the therapeutic relationship is practical and realistic. The therapist encourages autonomy and independence rather than transference and dependence. In this team-like alliance, elements of consumerism are openly acknowledged. Patient satisfaction is considered an important ingredient in the criterion of success.
3. *Active positive therapist.* The role of the therapist is active with an emphasis on fostering positivity and strength within the client. Structuring therapeutic contacts, the therapist recommends alternative interventions for the patient. The therapist involves significant others in the therapy process as needed. The therapist is authoritative, but not authoritarian. His or her role might be described as that of *expert consultant.* The preferred orientation is one in which the therapist's role in the patient's life is demystified.
4. *Clearly defined goals and responsibilities.* The responsibilities of patient and therapist are clearly articulated. A contract for specific, achievable goals is negotiated. The scheduling of sessions and the duration of treatment are agreed on by therapist and patient. The patient's responsibilities include, at minimum, bringing relevant material to the sessions, cooperating in extrasession assignments, and implementing behavioral change outside therapeutic meetings. The therapist clearly defines his or her role in the life of the patient and acts as a mental health consultant and adviser, ready to offer current and empirically based information and treatment.
5. *Rapid response to need or crisis intervention preparedness.* Prompt handling of emergencies is absolutely essential. The therapist knows that early access to psychotherapy can avoid an exacerbation of clinical symptoms and decrease the risk of overintensive therapeutic involvement.

6. *Parsimony and flexible use of intervention.* To be eclectic is to be versatile. The therapist's first interventions are those that are least extensive, least expensive, and least intrusive (Spoerl 1974) unless more aggressive approaches are clinically necessary. All legitimate therapeutic methods are considered. Group therapy, psychoeducation, community resources, family intervention, religious and spiritual counseling, and self-help groups are seen as valued forms of treatment, not just ancillary aids to individual therapy. Alternative treatment approaches and programmatic interventions are also considered. Self-help groups are seen as significant resources. The frequency, length, and timing of treatment are chosen with parsimony in mind.
7. *Life span developmental orientation.* People are seen from a life span development perspective, and the therapist realizes that people are most likely to seek psychotherapy at the time or point in their lives when they face increased levels of stress. Some of these occasions include approaching developmental milestones, situational and "anniversary" crises, and activation of an endogenous mental illness. Once an initial psychotherapeutic relationship is established, if it is of good rapport and high quality, the therapist can act as a guide to help the patient negotiate his or her way through the life span (Cummings 1991).
8. *Psychological family physician or primary care orientation.* The psychotherapeutic dyad is seen as a continuous, intermittent interaction between the therapist and the patient, and it can extend throughout a lifetime. The psychotherapist sees himself or herself in a role similar to that of the psychological family doctor (Cummings 1991). The patient is treated in brief episodes over long periods during the life span through a succession of interrupted, crisis-oriented episodes (Morrill 1983).
9. *Medical or nonmedical collaboration.* The nonmedical mental health provider is able and ready to relate to medical providers. With an increasing need to integrate behavioral and biomedical science, the therapist helps patients comply with medical regimens, adjust to medical conditions, and cope with disability and death through the use of psychological interventions (Belar 1991). Communication with both primary care physicians and psychiatrists is essential to integrate psychopharmacology and psychotherapy. Whether the therapist works in a staff-model setting where it is relatively easy to interact with primary care physicians or in a PPO where contact is less likely and accessible, a relationship with the psychiatrist and the primary care physician improves the quality of treatment by viewing the patient holistically.

10. *Awareness of need for review or information.* The therapist is willing to participate in quality assurance reviews and also initiates his or her own quality assurance system or participates in global management information systems. He or she recognizes the link between quality, cost, and utilization management. Because the therapist is committed to delivering cost-effective therapy, the appropriate use of data and feedback about practice habits are not viewed as a threat and are, in fact, welcomed. The development of adequate management information systems to assess treatment outcomes is considered to be an integral part of practice. Therapists believe that they need to define quality and clinical effectiveness, obtain outcome measurements, and use the data to document their own performance and the appropriateness of their procedures. They are equally aware that measuring outcome accurately in mental health is fraught with difficulties at this time. Their orientation is to support the development of scientifically determined universal standards for outcomes assessment.
11. *Outpatient versus inpatient treatment orientation.* Inpatient treatment is the intervention of *last resort* because it is maximally intrusive, is potentially stigmatizing, fosters dependence, and is expensive. All efforts are made to treat the person in an outpatient setting. There is a strong adherence to the belief that the least restrictive environment is preferable to one that is overintrusive.
12. *Current knowledge about research.* The managed care therapist keeps abreast of research relevant to mental health treatment. Whereas practical considerations limit the amount of available information, the therapist's breadth of knowledge is deep enough to facilitate an informed choice of models. Because so much practice is based on theory and not on research, therapists maximize their ability to select the most effective therapeutic interventions based on empirical research.

Models of Psychotherapy in Managed Care

In this section I describe a sampling of three types of therapy models that incorporate the features—the cornerstones of effective psychotherapy in managed care—outlined above. First, a model that possesses the unique potential to unify many disparate models of psychotherapy (Bennett 1984; Morrill 1983; Spoerl 1974) will be examined. The broad conceptual assumptions of intermittent brief psychotherapy throughout the life cycle (Cummings 1991) can serve as an umbrella under which many less comprehensive models can be organized and integrated. Second, therapy models that provide therapists with a set of assumptions and themes from which to view patient problems will be reviewed (e.g., interpersonal-developmental-existential, problem solving, pathogenic belief). Third, specific models with specific interventions designed for use with specific populations will be briefly described.

Principles of Psychotherapy Throughout the Life Cycle

Cummings' (1991) model of intermittent psychotherapy throughout the life cycle is based on the notion that the role of the therapist is similar to that of the family physician. Psychotherapy consists of brief, intermittent psychotherapeutic encounters to help a patient cope and grow throughout life's inevitable recurring crises and vicissitudes. The patient stops seeing the therapist for regular sessions when sufficient treatment has occurred.

Cummings' model provides a framework for the conduct of "long-term psychotherapy in a short-term setting" and challenges a number of traditional assumptions. Cummings (1991) denies that there is a "right" or "best" model of psychotherapy or that the "ideal therapist" exists, that is, someone who can do all things for all people. The therapist uses a flexible schedule of sessions and does not keep patients in treatment until every conflict in the recess of the unconscious has been analyzed. Termination is not a difficult and painful process; rather, it constitutes a rapprochement that puts the patient on the path of independence.

Cummings' (1991) simple but elegant model is based on a life span view of human development. Life consists of a series of typical and predictable developmental tasks and junctures that can sometimes be difficult to negotiate. Some individuals may undergo excessive stress when encountering developmental milestones such as entering school, beginning adulthood, becoming a parent, divorcing or separating, midlife crises, approaching old age, and ultimately facing death. Depending on a person's early learning history, he or she responds to these crises in a prototypical way. Psychotherapy is indicated if and only if the individual needs help to learn more effective and adaptive ways of dealing with perceived threats. Once the patient achieves mastery, he or she stops coming to therapy and returns only when more help is needed to accommodate to life situations. Therapy is interrupted, not terminated, when the presenting problem is resolved. The notion that psychotherapy *cures* mental health problems is minimized. A patient is not kept in an elongated therapy and attends sessions only to learn how to cope with specific problems as they arise throughout the life cycle. After the initial phase of therapy, each crisis takes fewer sessions to master and resolve. The long-term relationship between the patient and the therapist is of sufficient quality and strength so that the patient sees the therapist as a *psychological family physician* (i.e., a resource to be visited when necessary). Intermittent psychotherapy throughout the life cycle is not only appropriate for individual therapy, but it can also be used in a group therapy format.

Intermittent Group Therapy

Zimet (1979) discussed the developmental task and crisis group therapy model. Based on the same assumptions as the intermittent model of individual therapy, this model extends the tenets of developmental stage theory and crisis intervention to group therapy. A group format allows a number of persons who are struggling with similar life issues to come together and benefit by interacting with one another and a group leader. By focusing on specific developmental tasks while facing the realities of time limits, group members learn to make good use of therapeutic resources. Sharing age-related and stage-related issues with others reduces feelings of isolation. Examples of developmental groups are those that deal with separating from home, midlife transitions, career changes, divorce and separation, bereavement, premarital groups, empty nest syndrome, and retirement. Intermittent therapy throughout the life cycle can help individuals negotiate significant transitions throughout their life span at all stages of development.

The Single-Session Therapy Approach

The briefest of the brief therapies is single-session therapy (Bloom 1992; Talmon 1990). Advocates of brief therapy remind us of the well-established and confirmed statistic that *one* is the most commonly repeated number for psychotherapy because approximately 50% of people leave therapy after a single session (Phillips 1985). Every therapy session should be conducted as if it were the only moment in time that the therapist has to make a lasting impression on the patient. This model does not claim that most problems can be solved completely in a single session, but it reinforces the idea that the first session sets the stage for future therapy. Specific techniques for the therapist to use include 1) identify the focal problem, 2) try to formulate comments in 10 words or less, 3) be prudently active, 4) explore and present interpretations tentatively, 5) encourage the expression of affect, 6) keep track of time, 7) keep factual questions to a minimum, 8) do not be overconcerned about the precipitating event, 9) do not overestimate or underestimate the patient's ability, 10) use education, 11) mobilize social supports, 12) start a problem-solving process, and 13) build in a follow-up plan (Bloom 1992). The therapist chooses the nature of the focus of treatment from among intrapsychic, characterological, interpersonal, or systemic therapy models and then selects appropriate interventions from among educational, behavioral, psychodynamic, systemic, experiential, and medical techniques. A narrow theme rather than a broad theme is used; the patient learns to expect and tolerate change just as the therapist does. Although the necessary therapeutic work is sometimes completed during a single session, other times it is initiated or redirected in more sessions or in life experiences. For example, telling a 25-year-old patient that he has a severe alcohol problem may fall on seemingly deaf ears, but when the patient turns 40 the seeds planted in that single session may finally yield a harvest of recognition—the patient will recognize the nature of his problem. A visit to Alcoholics Anonymous 15 years after the single session may be the fruit of a therapist's earlier work.

Interpersonal-Developmental-Existential Therapy

Developed by Budman and Gurman (1988), the interpersonal-developmental-existential model of psychotherapy provides a systematic framework that allows the therapist to conceptualize the client's problems as *core* issues. There are a number of major themes under which the client's problems can generally be categorized: 1) the loss of significant others or beliefs about oneself or the world; 2) developmental lags or a lack of significance and meaning in life because of not having attained a developmental goal such as an intimate relationship, parenthood, or professional success; 3) specific symptoms that cause discomfort or a desire to deal with a particular habit disorder with no desire to explore overall personality style; 4) interpersonal complaints; and 5) personality disorders. To arrive at an appropriate interpersonal-developmental-existential focus for a particular patient, the therapist obtains the following information: Why is the patient seeking therapy now? At what stage of development is the patient, and what are the pertinent life cycle issues facing him or her? Are any significant anniversaries taking place? What kind of support might the patient have? Are any chemical dependency problems present? Are any outside forces exerting pressure on the individual to come for therapy? What has been the response to prior treatment? Does the patient want limited symptom relief or other types of changes? The therapist uses eclectic techniques to help patients reach their goals, including psychodynamic, behavioral, and hypnotic interventions; individual, group, and marital treatment formats; and between-session homework assignments as needed.

Possibility-Oriented Psychotherapy

In the possibility-oriented model, the therapist invites patients to use their own resources to identify and reach a well-specified goal. According to Friedman and Fangor (1991), the therapist adapts a wellness model and diminishes the role of patient pathology and diagnosis. The therapist applies the following guiding principles within the therapeutic dyad: 1) think small; 2) complicated situations do not always require complicated solutions; 3) consider the client's resources seriously; 4) collaborate to create a context for change; 5) choose small, defined goals; 6) do just one thing differently; 7) the client contains the seeds of the solution; 8) change is inevitable; 9) help to form a supportive network; and 10) maintain an optimistic stance about change. The therapist uses a number of techniques to help patients use their own resources. The therapist tries simple interventions first, focuses on solutions, maintains the therapy focus on the initial request, uses possibility language, focuses on resources and strengths, reframes difficulties in developmental contexts, and maintains and communicates a sense of humor.

Pathogenic Belief Model: Donovan

Donovan (1987) asserted in his pathogenic belief model that a crippling self-belief causes the individual to maintain a neurotic or negative pattern of interpersonal relationships. This conviction represents a childhood attempt to solve unresolvable conflicts. Although the defense was a useful means of survival in childhood, in adulthood it produces bad feelings and is no longer adaptive. The therapist helps the patient identify and reframe the pathogenic belief, resulting in the formation and use of more productive self-constructions.

The three phases of psychotherapy consist of a search for the pathogenic belief, reversal of past trauma, and reframing the pathogenic assumption. This therapy is based on psychodynamic assumptions that were altered to fit the structure of short-term work.

No judgmental or confrontational events occur during this empathy-building process. Reframing the pathogenic belief, the key to successful therapy, is accomplished through a number of techniques, including using the therapist as an alternative object, increased self-awareness on the part of the patient, and support by the nontraumatic selfobject therapist-patient interaction. These ingredients help patients suspend unconscious guilt and leave them freer to conduct the business of life.

Interventions With Specific Populations

Supporters of managed care argue that it is possible to treat a wide variety of patients in a managed care setting if therapists are willing to experiment with creative and innovative models of treatment. In this section I describe a number of treatments designed to help specific populations with specific problems.

Persons With Personality Disorders

Individuals diagnosed with personality disorders are often difficult to treat and are frequently management problems. Although long-term psychotherapy has often been touted as the best method of treatment for these patients, a number of managed care therapists have used group and individual cognitive therapies effectively (Budman and Gurman 1988). Strosahl (1991) described a group cognitive-behavior treatment model used at Group Health Cooperative with concrete, feasible, and practical guidelines. Therapeutic goals were to teach patients skills that helped them identify, challenge, and correct distorted beliefs that resulted in dysfunctional lifestyles. A partial list of what members can learn in the 14-session group therapy includes the following:

- to challenge what causes dysfunctional behavior;
- a basic cognitive model to encourage change;
- to make changes in thinking;
- behavioral skills to increase interpersonal effectiveness and conflict resolution; and
- relapse prevention and change maintenance skills.

Nearly 80% of patients using this method achieved at least one therapeutic objective, such as changing negative beliefs to more positive beliefs, flexing rigid thinking, improving affective regulation, and changing to a more adaptive behavior scheme (e.g., increasing assertiveness, improving conflict resolution skills, improving planning skills, and increasing relaxation and tension-reducing abilities).

Adolescents

The treatment of adolescents entails specific challenges and management problems. Adams (1991) described an adolescent services division within a staff-model managed care setting that offered intervention services for adolescents and their families in the areas of parenting and step-parenting, attention-deficit disorders, teen issues, separation and divorce, integrated medical or psychosocial chronic illness, enuresis, encopresis, and other disorders. Using the Rush Center model, crisis intervention teams worked through windows of opportunity for substantial positive change by addressing current issues. In this model, patients have up to six visits to solve the crisis. Therapy is intended to mobilize a family member's coping responses and encourages him or her to look for social supports to sustain change. Gunstad and Sherman (1991) reported a model of adolescent inpatient care that interfaced with outpatient therapy to increase the continuity of care. Crisis was seen as an agent of change as well as an opportunity to mobilize family resources. Involvement of the family during a child's hospitalization was a way to help parents regain control of the child and to evoke structural family changes.

The Chronically Disabled Patient

Chronic mentally and emotionally disabled patients, many with biologically based disorders, have also been treated effectively in managed care settings. DeStefano and Henault (1991) described creative and flexible methods used at Community Health Care Plan of New Haven, Connecticut. They worked with a number of chronic patients quite effectively (successful outcomes were measured by the ability to keep seriously mentally ill patients from decompensating to the point where they require long-term hospitalization). They attributed success to rapid assessment, installment therapy, pharmacotherapy, and family and social involvement in care. Infrequent individual therapy, supportive group therapy, and collaboration among mental health providers, medical providers, and family and community support systems produced a treatment environment that integrated seriously disturbed individuals into the community.

Persons With Depression and Anxiety

For persons with depression and anxiety disorders, there are a number of specific treatments that have demonstrated therapeutic effectiveness and are easily conducted in the managed care environment. For example, the effectiveness of Beck's cognitive therapy of depression and anxiety and Klerman's interpersonal therapy (IPT) has undeniable empirical support (Bloom 1992). Schulberg and Scott (1991) discussed the high compatibility between the managed care setting and the directed, problem-solving, and present-oriented forms of cognitive therapy. Lasting 16 sessions, IPT can be used alone or with pharmacotherapy. The therapeutic focus is on one of four interpersonal problem areas: 1) grief reactions, 2) role transitions, 3) interpersonal role disputes, and 4) interpersonal deficits. The patient is able to decrease depressive symptoms by resolving interpersonal problems or learning to cope more adaptively with them.

Pediatrics

Herman and Cofresi (1994) described a pediatric mental health consultation model. At the request of the pediatrician, families deemed in need of mental health care who were unwilling to pursue mental health services because of a perceived stigma, inability to afford co-payments, or inability to obtain transportation were offered a consultation with a mental health provider. After dealing with typical presenting problems, the consultant met with the patient and pediatrician and other nonmedical providers. A two-session follow-up was conducted after which the patient was referred for mental health treatment, referred to community services, or told no further intervention was needed. Outcome measures of patient and pediatrician satisfaction demonstrated that satisfaction with this model of mental health intervention was quite high.

Elderly Persons

Robinson (1994) described a program offered at Group Health Cooperative of Puget Sound that integrated the medical and behavioral care of elderly persons. Outcome data from several group programs showed that treatment had successfully facilitated changes in patients in the areas of medical compliance, networking, and subjective distress. Group therapy for elderly depressed women was reported at a New Haven staff-model HMO (Austad and Henault 1989). Meeting every other week, the group served as a source of support for aging women confronted with various diseases and family crises.

Somatizing Persons

Somatizing patients have been treated successfully with short-term, targeted interventions in managed care. Chapter 15, by Cummings, provides an extensive review of how somatization can be reduced through appropriate therapy and how cost savings can be obtained through the *medical cost offset effect.*

Chemically Dependent Persons

Chemical dependency treatment provided within managed care settings may have an advantage over outpatient, nonmanaged care in that there is a greater likelihood that medical and psychological care can be coordinated. Consultation with the patient's physician can increase the likelihood of appropriate detoxification. Numerous programs have been described in many staff, PPO, and network model managed care programs (Gragg 1991).

Behavioral Medicine

Behavioral medicine is an interdisciplinary field that develops and integrates behavioral and medical science techniques and applies this knowledge to prevent, diagnose, treat, and rehabilitate patients with various comorbid conditions (Belar 1991). When a patient experiences medical problems, a variety of accompanying psychological and behavioral components can compound the problem. Some of these problems can be relieved or diminished through the use of behavioral-medicine interventions. Some of the problems that have been treated effectively in managed care settings are chronic pain and other conditions; terminal illness; Alzheimer's disease; headaches; smoking addiction; cardiac disease; and sexual dysfunction. The behavioral-medicine methods that have been used in addition to supportive, verbal, and insight therapies include education, information, biofeedback, skills training, and contingency management.

Example Case Using the Framework of Intermittent Psychotherapy

The case of J. and Dr. S. illustrates how a therapist can use intermittent psychotherapy during the whole life cycle to help patients throughout their lives. When Dr. S. first meets him, J. is an adolescent, brought to therapy by his parents. J. is failing in school and acts like a bully at home. The therapist intervenes, using both individual and family therapy to help J. deal with the stress associated with his parents' pending divorce. J. forms a trusting relationship with Dr. S. and learns to use new coping techniques that help him manage his problems. For 10 weekly individual sessions, Dr. S. chooses to use Donovan's (1987) model of *pathogenic belief*, because J. seems receptive to this kind of therapeutic intervention and it seems that his self-image needs to improve at this early age. Dr. S. refers J. to group psychotherapy with other adolescents who have similar problems. J. attends group therapy weekly for 12 sessions. While J. is in group, individual therapy is conducted once every 3–4 weeks. Dr. S. consults with the group therapy leader to monitor J.'s progress. Within 6 months, J.'s problems are under control. Dr. S. and J. agree that they no longer need to meet in regular sessions. J. is assured that he can return if he feels the need or desire to do so. Until he graduates from high school, J. does reappear every 2 to 3 months to grapple with issues related to pathogenic beliefs.

Six years later, J., married with a child of his own, experiences severe marital discord. He and his spouse consult with Dr. S., who uses cognitive behavior therapy to help the couple improve their communication. Four years later, J. finds himself in a major depression. When he returns to his psychological family physician, Dr. S. intervenes with methods from cognitive therapy and IPT and arranges a psychiatric consultation and monitoring for pharmacotherapy. Five years later, when J. is 33, he returns to his therapist (who is 65) and asks for help to mourn his father's death. Dr. S. uses Budman and Gurman's (1988) interpersonal-developmental-existential model of therapy, focusing on the impact of a significant loss. When his individual grief work is done, J. enters a bereavement support group where he gains even greater understanding. Much improved, J. stops seeing his therapist, adding, "I'll call you if I need to. Thanks, Doc!" The next time J. seeks therapy, he knows where to return and to whom he should report.

By envisioning psychotherapy as occurring intermittently yet throughout life, Dr. S. was free to use any permutation and combination of therapy models he believed to be most helpful to his patient. The therapist was able to give J. necessary and sufficient mental health care at crucial developmental points in his life and at times of increased stress and during crisis. As a therapist in a managed care setting, Dr. S. expresses the opinion that being the psychological family physician is rewarding. Because the therapist-patient relationship is central to positive change in the patient, the therapist's thoughts and feelings about the context in which psychotherapy is conducted are pivotal to success. In the next section, I discuss the attitudes of therapists toward psychotherapy in managed care.

The Therapist's Perspective

Because the quality of the patient-therapist relationship is fundamental to the change process in psychotherapy, it is important to understand the feelings, attitudes, and thoughts of front-line psychotherapists. Catapulted into a world of change, psychotherapists of today are confronted with a challenge to accommodate their practice style or risk a loss of status, income, and feelings of competency and personal satisfaction (Berlin 1969; Hoyt 1991). Only a few studies have addressed this neglected aspect of psychotherapy practice (Kohrman 1986; Lange et al. 1988; Marion-Merril Dow 1989).

In interview and survey studies (Austad 1992; Austad et al. 1992, 1993), several hundred providers working in staff-model managed care settings were asked a series of questions to help clarify how they adapted their practice styles in their new settings. The following changes were typical of a number of traditional therapists who found themselves working in a managed care environment. The culture shock of practicing managed care caused most therapists to evaluate the usefulness of traditional psychotherapy models and training. Belief in, and use of, short-term therapy in lieu of long-term therapy grew. Over time, many of the therapists shed psychodynamic models to don more eclectic models. The percentage of therapists who primarily used the psychodynamic model decreased, and the percentage of therapists who ranked eclectic and "other" as their most frequently used therapy orientation increased. Many therapists reported that their practice style became more focused, goal directed, and short-term, incorporating a view of the therapeutic relationship that emphasized health and independence and de-emphasized pathology and dependence. The majority of therapists thought that the mental health benefit package (20 visits per year) was adequate to treat most patients for their presenting problems. Therapists also believed that the overall quality of care they were giving to patients was high and increased over time.

When clinicians reported feeling "burnt out," they usually attributed the cause of burnout to too large a case load and too little support from administrative, collegial, and staff interactions. On-call responsibilities also contributed to burnout. To prevent burnout, the therapists sought supervision, obtained peer support, took continuing education courses, set limits, and scheduled vacations. Some clinicians endorsed the view that working part-time rather than full-time elongated work-life expectancy. However, they did not discuss the financial implications of their advice.

When asked to describe how they had changed as a person, 98% of therapists named one or more positive changes, for example, they had grown professionally; had become wiser, more mature, and more patient; and had broadened their views and acceptance of life and human nature. Some therapists reported that working in the staff-model setting and sharing in the lives of so many people had made them better clinicians and human beings by becoming more tolerant of others. One or more negative changes such as feeling more cynical, tired, and less caring were described by 28% of the sample.

The majority of study participants emphatically declared that graduate training did not prepare them for practicing in a managed care setting. The most useful skills for managed care work— competence in short-term therapy and crisis management—had been lacking in their formal training.

The recommendations that follow from the results of these studies are that appropriate, relevant training and subsequent support for the mental health providers are important factors that enable a therapist to continue working effectively in the framework of managed care. Supportive interpersonal processes are most helpful in preventing burnout and exhaustion. The results of these studies indicate that traditionally trained mental health providers can adapt their practice styles to the managed care setting and provide what they believe to be high-quality care to their patients.

What the Research Shows

Before an attempt can be made to answer the question of whether psychotherapy can be conducted effectively in managed care settings, it is essential to examine the conclusions from the vast number of psychotherapy studies that have been conducted over time. To summarize the findings of relevance, the effects of psychotherapy are generally positive, exceeding the effects of placebo controls and spontaneous remission. However, psychotherapy can also yield negative effects, leading to patient deterioration (Lambert 1991; Strupp 1986). Although a few therapies have demonstrated unique effectiveness with specific disorders (e.g., behavior therapy for obsessive-compulsive symptoms, systemic therapy for marital conflict, cognitive-interpersonal therapy for depression), equivalence in outcome exists for a large number of therapies, modalities, and temporal arrangements (Garfield and Bergin 1986; Koss and Butcher 1986; Lambert, Shapiro, and Bergin 1986; Lambert and Bergin 1992; Prochaska and Norcross 1994). The overall superiority of any one form of therapy compared with another has never been firmly established.

Research efforts to find the best combination of common and specific factors to help patients and ascertain how to generate optimal matches among therapists, patients, and treatments have not yielded definitive results (Prochaska and Norcross 1994). Searching for the common factors that underscore the success of all forms of therapy leads to the conclusion that the active ingredients that make psychotherapy successful or effective are 1) the therapeutic alliance or the positive emotional bond a client feels toward a therapist, 2) positive expectations that the therapy will help, and 3) a strengthening of the clients' self-efficacy about his or her ability to accomplish various goals. A good patient-therapist relationship is formed rapidly, and the alliance that occurs early in treatment is correlated with success (Lambert et al. 1986; Luborsky 1992). Given these general findings from decades of research, together with the information acquired about psychotherapy models used in a managed care setting and clinician adaptations to that setting, it is now possible to answer the question, "Can psychotherapy be conducted effectively in managed care settings?"

The answer to that question, however, is not a simple matter because it is contingent on a number of factors previously discussed: definitions of managed care, assumptions and techniques related to a specific psychotherapy model, the benefit package under which the therapy is conducted, the quality of the managed care entity, and the type of treatment paired to the type of therapist paired to the specific problem. These elements of psychotherapy in managed care must be considered in conjunction with the following facts:

- The history of psychotherapy research findings shows relative equivalencies of all psychotherapies (including short-term and long-term modalities).
- The important active ingredient of therapy is the relationship between the therapist and the patient and the patient's expectations of therapy,
- intermittent psychotherapy can facilitate a positive and long-term relationship that promotes client self-efficacy.
- A good managed care program supplies a benefit package that enables a therapist to render intermittent therapy throughout the life cycle and use targeted interventions necessary to help a particular patient with a particular problem treated by a particular therapist.

- The therapist finds that it is possible to change personal habits and practice patterns in such a way that adaptation to a managed care environment can be seen as positive.

Conclusion

Given the qualifications described above, it *is* possible to conduct effective psychotherapy in managed care settings provided psychotherapy is conceptualized as an active working relationship between the patient and the therapist whereby the goal of therapy is clearly defined as change rather than cure. Disorders must be perceived not only in terms of pathology but also in terms of developmental stages and life stresses. The therapist acts like a psychological family physician, an eclectic clinician who uses various models of therapy at various stages in the life of the patient to help master psychological trauma and challenges.

It is just as likely, or even more likely, that effective psychotherapy can be conducted in a managed care setting as in any other setting. An effective managed care setting provides a unique opportunity to render high-quality treatment to patients. It also provides a forum to examine some of the basic assumptions that underlie traditional models of psychotherapy and mental health practice. By making psychotherapy accessible to many people, and by making many forms of psychotherapy available, managed care practice can yield positive results for the great majority of individuals who seek the psychotherapist's skill and compassion as a healer.

References

Adams J: Family crisis intervention and psychosocial care for children and adolescents, in Psychotherapy in Managed Health Care: The Optimal Use of Time and Resources. Edited by Austad CS, Berman WH. Washington, DC, American Psychological Association Press, 1991, pp 111–126

Austad CS: Psychotherapists in independent practice and in managed health care settings: a comparison. Psychotherapy in Private Practice 10:1–6, 1992

Austad CS: Health care reform, managed mental health care, and short-term psychotherapy, in Innovations in Clinical Practice. Edited by VandeCreek L, Knapp S, Jackson TL. Sarasota, FL, Professional Resource Press, 1993, pp 241–256

Austad CS, Berman WH: HMO Psychotherapy, in Psychotherapy in Managed Health Care: The Optimal Use of Time and Resources. Edited by Austad CS, Berman WH. Washington, DC, American Psychological Association Press, 1991, pp 5–19

Austad CS, Henault K: Group psychotherapy with elderly women. HMO Practice 3(2):70–71, 1989

Austad CS, Hoyt M: The managed care movement and the future of psychotherapy. Psychotherapy 29:109–118, 1992

Austad CS, Kisch J, DeStefano L: The health maintenance organization–II. Implications for psychotherapy. Psychotherapy 25:449–454, 1989

Austad CS, Sherman WO, Morgan T, et al: The psychotherapist and the managed care setting. Professional Psychology: Research and Practice 23:329–332, 1992

Austad CS, Sherman WO, Holstein L: Psychotherapists in the HMO. HMO Practice 7(3):122–126, 1993

Bauer GP, Kobos JC: Brief Therapy: Short-term Psychodynamic Intervention. Northvale, NJ, Jason Aronson, 1987

Belar C: Behavioral medicine, in Psychotherapy in Managed Health Care: The Optimal Use of Time and Resources. Edited by Austad CS, Berman WH. Washington, DC, American Psychological Association Press, 1991, pp 65–79

Bennett M: Brief psychotherapy and adult development. Psychotherapy 21:171–176, 1984

Bennett M: The greening of the HMO. Am J Psychiatry 145:1544–1549, 1988

Berlin I: Resistance to change in mental health professionals. Am J Orthopsychiatry 39:109–115, 1969

Bistline JL: Sheridan, SM, Winegar M: Five critical skills for mental health counselors in managed health care. Journal of Mental Health Counseling 13:147–152, 1991

Bloom B: Bloom's focused single session therapy, in Planned Short Term Therapy. Edited by Bloom B. Boston, MA, Allyn & Bacon, 1992, pp 97–121

Bloom BL: Managing mental health services: some comments for the overdue debate in psychology. Community Ment Health J 26:107–124, 1990

Boaz JT: Delivering Mental Health Care: A Guide for HMOs. Chicago, IL, Pluribus Press, 1988

Budman SH, Gurman AS: The Theory and Practice of Brief Psychotherapy. New York, Guilford, 1988

Callan MF, Yeager DC: Containing the Health Care Cost Spiral. New York, McGraw Hill, 1991

Carter R: Mental health policy at a crossroads. Behavioral Healthcare Tomorrow 2(1):27–30, 1993

Cummings N: The dismantling of our health system. Am Psychol 41:426–431, 1986

Cummings NA: Brief intermittent therapy throughout the life cycle, in Psychotherapy in Managed Health Care: The Optimal Use of Time and Resources. Edited by Austad CS, Berman WH. Washington, DC, American Psychological Association Press, 1991, pp 35–46

Davis GS: A managed health care primer, in The Insiders Guide to Managed Care. Edited by Hastings DA, Krasner WL, Michael JL, et al. Washington, DC, The National Lawyers Association, 1990, pp 13–35

DeStefano LJ, Henault KH: The treatment of chronically mentally and emotionally disabled patients, in Psychotherapy in Managed Health Care: The Optimal Use of Time and Resources. Edited by Austad CS, Berman WH. Washington, DC, American Psychological Association Press, 191, pp 138–152

Donovan J: Brief dynamic psychotherapy: toward a more comprehensive model. Psychiatry 50:167–183, 1987

Feldman S (ed): Managed Mental Health Services. Springfield, IL, Charles C Thomas, 1992

Flinn DE, McMahon TC, Collings MF: Health maintenance organizations and their implications for psychiatry. Hosp Community Psychiatry 38:255–263, 1987

Friedman S, Fangor MT: Expanding Therapeutic Possibilities: Getting Results in Brief Therapy. Lexington, MA, Lexington Books, 1991

Garfield S, Bergin A: Introduction and historical overview, in Handbook of Psychotherapy and Behavior Change. Edited by Garfield S, Bergen A. New York, Wiley, 1986, pp 3–22

Goran, MJ: Managed mental health and group health insurance, in Managed Mental Health Services. Edited by Feldman S. Springfield, IL, Charles C Thomas, 1992, pp 27–43

Gragg DM: Managed health care systems: chemical dependency treatment, in Psychotherapy in Managed Health Care: The Optimal Use of Time and Resources. Edited by Austad CS, Berman WH. Washington, DC, American Psychological Association Press, 1991, pp 202–219

Gunstad M, Sherman CF: A model of inpatient adolescent treatment, in Psychotherapy in Managed Health Care: The Optimal Use of Time and Resources. Edited by Austad CS, Berman WH. Washington, DC, American Psychological Association Press, 1991, pp 138–152

Hastings DA: Legal and regulatory issues in managed mental health care, in The Insiders Guide to Managed Care. Edited by Hastings DA, Krasner WL, Michael JL, et al. Washington, DC, The National Lawyers Association, 1990, pp 203–240

Hemmenway D, Killen A, Cashman SB, et al: Physicians' responses to financial incentives. N Engl J Med 322:1059–1062, 1990

Herman B, Cofresi A: The pediatric population. Paper presented at Group Health Institute of America, Miami Beach, FL, January 11, 1994

Hoyt M: Teaching and learning short-term psychotherapy, in Psychotherapy in Managed Health Care: The Optimal Use of Time and Resources. Edited by Austad CS, Berman WH. Washington, DC, American Psychological Association Press, 1991, pp 98–107

Hoyt M, Austad CS: Psychotherapy in a staff model health maintenance organization: providing and assuring quality care in the future. Psychotherapy 29:109–118, 1992

Hoyt MF: Therapist resistances to short-term dynamic psychotherapy. J Am Acad Psychoanal 13:93–112, 1985

Karasu TB: The worst of times, the best of times. Journal of Psychotherapy Practice and Research 1:2–15, 1992

Kisch J, Austad CS: The health maintenance organization, I: historical perspective and current status. Psychotherapy 25:441–448, 1989

Kohrman CH: Medical practice where HMOs dominate: the perspective of physicians in Minneapolis–St. Paul. J Med Pract Manage 2(2):81–89, 1986

Kleinke C: Common Principles of Psychotherapy. Pacific Grove, CA, Brooks-Cole, 1994

Koss MP, Butcher JN: Research on brief psychotherapy, in Handbook of Psychotherapy and Behavior Change. Edited by Garfield S, Bergin A. New York, Wiley, 1986, pp 627–670

Lambert M: Introduction to psychotherapy research, in Psychotherapy Research. Edited by Beutler L, Crago M. Washington, DC, American Psychological Association Press, 1991, pp 1–11

Lambert M, Shapiro D, Bergin A: The effectiveness of psychotherapy, in The Handbook of Psychotherapy and Behavior Change. Edited by Garfield S, Bergin A. New York, Wiley, 1986, pp 157–211

Lambert P, Bergin AE: Achievements and limitations of psychotherapy research, in History of Psychotherapy: A History of Change. Edited by Freedheim DK. Washington, DC, American Psychological Association Press, 1992, pp 360–390

Lange Chandler-Guy, Forti R, Foster-Moore C, et al: Providers' views of mental health services. Psychotherapy 25:455–470, 1988

Levin BL: Mental health services within the HMO group. HMO Practice 6(3)16–20, 1992

Luborsky L: The Penn Research Project, in History of Psychotherapy: A History of Change. Edited by Freedheim DK. Washington, DC, American Psychological Association Press, 1992, pp 282–285

Marion-Merrill Dow: Attitudes of physicians with HMO experience toward managed healthcare, in Marion Managed Care Digest. Kansas City, MO, Marion-Merrill Dow, 1989

Morrill J: The future for mental health in primary health care programs. Am J Psychiatry 135:1351–1355, 1983

Nelson J: The history and spirit of the HMO movement. HMO Practice 1(2):75–86, 1987

Pearson J: Managed mental health: the buyer's perspective, in Managed Mental Health Services. Edited by Feldman S. Springfield, IL, Charles C Thomas, 1992, pp 127–143

Phillips EL: A Guide for Therapists and Patients to Short Term Therapy. Springfield, IL, Charles C Thomas, 1985

Prochaska JO, Norcross JC: Systems of Psychotherapy: A Transtheoretical Analysis. Pacific Grove, CA, Brooks-Cole, 1994

Robinson P: The elderly. Paper presented at Group Health Institute of America, Miami Beach, FL, January 11, 1994

Sammons JH: Inside Medical Washington: Standing up for the Doctors Rights in the Nation's Capital. Washington, DC, Whittle Direct Books, 1991

Schulberg HC, Scott CP: Depression in primary care: treating depression with interpersonal psychotherapy, in Psychotherapy in Managed Health Care: The Optimal Use of Time and Resources. Edited by Austad CS, Berman WH. Washington, DC, American Psychological Association Press, 1991, pp 153–171

Sederer LI, St. Clair L: Quality assurance and managed mental health care. Psychiatr Clin North Am 13:89–97, 1990

Spoerl OH: Treatment patterns in prepaid psychiatric care. Am J Psychiatry 131:56–59, 1974

Starr P: The Social Transformation of American Medicine. New York, Basic Books, 1982

Strosahl KD: Cognitive and behavioral treatment of the personality disordered patient, in Psychotherapy in Managed Health Care: The Optimal Use of Time and Resources. Edited by Austad CS, Berman WH. Washington, DC, American Psychological Association Press, 1991, pp 185–202

Strupp H: Psychotherapy research, practice, and public policy: how to avoid a dead end. Am Psychol 41:120–130, 1986

Talmon M: Single Session Therapy. San Francisco, CA, Jossey-Bass, 1990

Truscott AM: Cost and quality—are they compatible? HMO Practice 6(2):3–10, 1992

VandenBos G: Psychotherapy research: a special issue. Am Psychol 41:11–112, 1986

VandenBos G, DeLeon P: The use of psychotherapy to improve physical health. Psychotherapy: Theory, Research, Practice, and Training 25:335–343, 1989

Zieman G: Information systems and capitation contracting: basic specifications for group practices. Behavioral Healthcare Tomorrow 2(1):40–43, 1993

Zimet C: Developmental task and crisis groups: the application of group psychotherapy to maturational processes. Psychotherapy, Research, and Practice 16:2–8, 1979

Zimet CN: The mental health care revolution: will psychology survive? Am Psychol 44:703–708, 1989

Chapter 17

Can Psychiatrists Be Retrained for the Future?

Robert K. Schreter, M.D.
Carol A. Schreter, M.S.W., Ph.D.

In the 1980s, payers of health care began demanding cost containment, accountability, and standardized services. Professional healers began to be seen as part of a giant for-profit industry, labeled by Relman (1980) as the *medical-industrial complex*. The managed care industry emerged as a means to control costs. In response, the entire health care system is changing.

Psychiatry is in the midst of its own industrial revolution. Until recently, psychiatry centered on independent clinicians, solo practitioners with small caseloads providing personalized services to patients. With disdain, critics now dub this a *cottage industry*. Instead, to gain access to third-party payers, mental health professionals are being forced to join cost-conscious groups and to develop alternatives to hospital-based care and the 50-minute hour. "Every psychiatrist over the age of 35 must be retrained," insists Paul Fink (personal communication, 1995), a past president of the American Psychiatric Association (APA).

To compete in this new environment, psychiatrists should refine existing skills, learn new skills, and offer their services in new treatment settings. In this chapter we focus on why psychiatrists must change, what they need to change, and avenues for retraining.

Must We Change?

Many psychiatrists are still struggling to preserve the "good old days." Others are trying to adapt to the relentless economic, political, and social forces transforming health care. As clinicians look to the future, they should anticipate that managed care will not disappear, it will only evolve. The main question is whether it will evolve with or without the cooperation and guidance of psychiatrists. Who will manage the care? Who will make the rules?

As clinicians look to the future, they should anticipate the following trends:

- *Demand for cost controls will continue.*
- *Integrated systems of care will emerge.* Vertical integration occurs when giant insurers purchase hospital chains, utilization review firms, health maintenance organizations (HMOs), and even physician practices. Horizontal integration occurs as corporate entities develop the capacity to provide a wide range of mental health services.
- *Clinicians in integrated systems will be responsible for populations, not individuals.*
- *Control will pass from provider to payer.* When payers sign contracts, they will insist on maintaining control over many aspects of patient care.
- *Costs will continue to affect clinical decisions.* Costs will limit the types of providers, types of reimbursable services, definitions of *medical necessity,* and the size of co-payments by patients.
- *Focus on outcomes will increase.* Clinicians must be prepared to show they are achieving the desired results.
- *Attention will be focused on value.* Exclusive attention to cost is being replaced by the desire to maximize clinical outcome and patient satisfaction for each dollar invested in patient care.
- *A shift from office- and hospital-based interventions to community-based services* (e.g., in schools, workplaces, community residences) will occur.
- *Competition will come from other providers*, including professionals with less training and delivery systems organized by insurance companies.

Obstacles to Change

Managed care has had a devastating impact on the emotional lives of most psychiatrists. Many interpret the conflicts with managed care as personal assaults on their identity and income. Many psychiatrists have been unwilling or unable to respond to the trends in mental health care (Schreter 1993), placing their careers in jeopardy. To adapt, the critical first step is to recognize and overcome obstacles to change. Psychiatrists, who devote their lives to promoting change in their patients, are now being asked to change themselves.

The Mourning Process

Understanding facilitates change. It may help to think of psychiatry's resistance to managed care in the framework of grief over a great loss. The normal mourning process, as described by Elizabeth Kübler-Ross (1969) in her book *On Death and Dying*, involves five stages:

1. *Denial.* At first, psychiatrists seemed to ignore managed care. They denied its potential impact and refused to join managed care networks as long as private patients were still available. They resented the idea of submitting treatment plans for review and complying with limitations on authorized visits. As evidence of this denial, APA members seemed not to notice that their professional organization developed a utilization review program where the APA, in collaboration with industry, served as a care manager. This program operated for 5 years before members took notice and objected vigorously. As a result, the APA lost its major contract in 1989, and the program ended.
2. *Anger.* In 1990 the APA created a managed care hot line to collect complaints about managed care practices. Psychiatrists talked of jointly financing class action suits against the industry. Personal attacks on managed care executives were not uncommon.
3. *Bargaining.* When psychiatrists grudgingly joined managed care systems, they would bargain on behalf of their patients, arguing for more inpatient days or outpatient sessions. Such arguments, equally distasteful to clinicians and reviewers, highlighted the need for medical necessity criteria and standardized treatment guidelines that would objectify and detoxify the process.
4. *Depression.* Clinicians felt hopeless and helpless as they struggled to accept a loss of control, autonomy, and income. As in the classic mourning process described by Bibring (1953), they felt overwhelmed, gave up, and were unable to change.
5. *Acceptance.* By 1993 it seemed that some clinicians were working through their anger and sadness. Contributors to our first book, *Allies and Adversaries: The Impact of Managed Care on Mental Health Services* (Schreter et al. 1994), voiced a surprising level of willingness to begin cooperating with managed care, so as to manage care, not just dollars. In 1995 the APA managed care hot line, a depository for complaints, was expanded to include a managed care help line—offering advice on how to cooperate with managed care.

Character Traits as an Obstacle to Change

Most mature physicians do not want to be managed. Gabbard (1992) suggested that the following characteristics are frequently found in people who choose medicine as a career: perfectionism, chronic self-doubt, guilt feelings and a tyrannical conscience, an exaggerated sense of responsibility, conflicts about overt expressions of anger, and conflicts about dependency. These traits make physicians vulnerable to distress and demoralization when confronted with the scrutiny, demands for compromise, and implied criticism that are part of the managed care era.

Conflicting Values and Beliefs

Most established psychiatrists were trained in hospital-based programs in which long-term treatment organized around the 50-minute hour was the intervention of choice. The dyadic physician-patient relationship was considered to be the instrument of therapeutic change. To these psychiatrists, the Hippocratic oath is an obligation to do the utmost for each individual patient, without regard to cost. These fundamental beliefs are scorned by managed care.

Managed care prefers to finance short-term therapies, in episodes. The value system of short-term therapists, as described by Budman and Gurman (1988), meshes better with managed care. Short-term therapists value parsimony and small change as more important than cure. They view patients from an adult developmental perspective rather then seeing development as static. Short-term clinicians focus on patient strengths and resources instead of pathology. They see change as occurring largely outside the office, between treatment sessions.

The Eclipse of Confidentiality

Routine managed care procedures threaten the long-standing practice of patient confidentiality. To access insurance benefits for psychiatric care, the patient's story is passed to strangers on paper, by phone and computer, and passed to reviewers who authorize treatments, piece by piece. To date, this issue has escaped public attention and debate. Clinicians need to work with insurers to develop safeguards, so that patients are not discouraged from seeking mental health care.

Reluctance to Retrain

Another obstacle to participating in managed care is the clinician's reluctance to pay the double costs of retraining, paying tuition fees while incurring a loss of practice income. Perhaps more important, mature psychiatrists see themselves as teachers, not learners.

This reluctance to retrain may be short-sighted. After World War II, Japanese industry revitalized with the help of W. Edwards Deming (1986), an American management consultant. From him the Japanese learned the importance of research and development, training and retraining workers, and continuous quality improvement. Psychiatry, now at a crossroads, may need such an overhaul.

What Needs To Be Changed?

Retraining in psychiatry will involve adopting new attitudes, learning new roles and skills, and identifying new treatment settings.

New Attitudes and Beliefs

Managed medical care is a rather new concept, an experiment. Cooperating clinicians must be flexible and convinced that quality patient care is possible in a cost-conscious environment. At the least, they must recognize and accept two fundamental principles that underlie all of managed care practice: 1) the *population-based perspective* and 2) the *principle of parsimony.*

The population-based perspective encourages clinicians to look beyond the needs and optimal treatment of an individual patient and to consider instead the health of society—with attention to preventing illness and treating as yet unidentified patients. Thus managed care is the allocation of limited resources to achieve maximum utility, not simply to contain cost (Sabin 1993). This perspective is not foreign to clinicians with public health and public sector experience.

The principle of parsimony is a second bulwark of managed care. This principle implies that clinicians use the least intensive, least expensive of the suitable interventions, unless there is strong evidence that another treatment will produce a superior outcome.

New Clinical Roles

Psychiatrists, best trained in one-to-one communications, are now filling an array of more public roles. These include the following:

- *Provider.* Psychiatrists will continue to be highly valued for their special skills in valuation, diagnosis, and treatment planning. Their therapeutic arsenal must be flexible, expanded to include time-limited and supportive psychotherapies for individuals, couples, and families, as well as group treatments. The recent approval of naltrexone for alcoholism invites developments in treating substance abuse disorders.
- *Emergency service clinician.* The demand for hospital diversion will produce mobile crisis teams, home-based mental health care, and the subspecialty of emergency psychiatry.
- *Triage clinicians.* Given an array of services of different intensities at different settings, sometimes called the *continuum,* someone must decide

where to assign new patients. Psychiatrists should be directly involved in this process or be available as back-up to those who make these decisions.

- *Team member.* Systems of care create the need for teams of multi-specialty clinicians who collaborate to optimize patient outcome.
- *Team leader.* As predicted in the report by the Group for the Advancement of Psychiatry (1992), mental health care is becoming increasingly demedicalized. Clinicians with a wide range of preparation and experience are providing service at every level of care. Psychiatrists will continue to assume leadership and supervisory roles.
- *Consultation-liaison clinician.* Many patients have concurrent medical and psychiatric disorders and physical conditions affected by psychological factors. In cost-conscious systems, psychiatrists will earn new respect for providing anxiety and substance abuse treatments that help patients avoid costly medical and surgical services.
- *Clinical manager.* Within the managed care administrative structure, clinicians now play a role in the management of provider networks and in the design of medical necessity criteria, practice guidelines, quality assurance, and outcome data systems.
- *Psychiatrist-administrator.* Although psychiatrists, by personality and skills, are often poorly suited to the business world, it will be important to have administrators with a mental health perspective contributing to corporate strategy and operations.
- *Psychiatrist-owner.* Psychiatrists as owners of managed care organizations are still relatively rare. We should, however, anticipate a significant increase in their number as groups of clinicians unite to form behavioral group practices (Schreter 1994) and as physician-owned multispecialty medical groups take on capitated populations or joint ventures with managed care organizations.

New Skills

To fill these roles, psychiatrists will need to develop new skills. Sabin (1991) described six core skills essential for today's high-volume, high-turnover practice: designing treatment interventions and programs to address the needs of populations, applying an adult developmental model within an expanded array of treatment methodologies, and directly addressing the ethical and advocacy dilemmas that confront clinicians in managed care settings. Others have suggested additional necessary skills (Bennett 1992; Blackwell and Schmidt 1992; Sabin and Boris 1992; Schneider-Braus 1987).

Perhaps the most important skill within the managed care arena is comfort with short-term therapies. Research indicates that outpatient treatments have always been brief, averaging six or fewer sessions. Until recently, that occurred by default, not by design. The pioneers in short-term treatments were long-term therapists, including psychoanalysts (Beck 1976; Davanaloo 1978; Malan 1976; Mann 1973; Sifneos 1979). Spurred by managed care, other short-term strategies are being developed (Budman et al. 1980; De Shazar 1988).

The short-term therapist will develop a practice typical of the medical internist. Treatments of a high level of intensity will address acute issues in episodes over a long-term relationship, if the managed care contract permits. Patients with major psychiatric disorders superimposed on character pathology, as well as child and adolescent patients, will do least well with that mode of treatment.

New Treatment Settings

Psychiatric treatment is rapidly moving out of the hospital and into the community. A continuum is developing (i.e., an array of treatment options between 24-hour inpatient care and weekly outpatient sessions). These were initially valued for their cost savings but will probably proliferate because they have proven to have special clinical advantages. Options along this continuum include observation and respite beds, partial hospitals, therapeutic group homes for adults, residential treatment centers and foster placement for children, mobile crisis teams, and home-based services. (Schreter et al., in press). In the future, care is likely to move into the workplace and schools. This expansion of treatment settings will hasten the demedicalization of mental health services. Few of the workers in facilities at lower levels of care will be physicians.

Avenues for Retraining

When Fink warned that every psychiatrist over age 35 must be retrained, he was not suggesting additional education in psychopharmacology. Instead, he was encouraging clinicians to be creative in preparing for the future.

There are existing avenues for retraining, and others could be developed. To be most effective, trainers should include people from managed care companies. Some companies already play a role in the initial training of residents. They should be encouraged to participate in retraining established clinicians.

Note, however, that retraining will be viewed with skepticism until managed care and academic centers can prove the value of short-term, episodic therapies, new treatment guidelines, and quality assurance standards.

Avenues for retraining include the following:

- *Continuing education workshops.* Budman and Armstrong (1993) described three principles of adult education that should guide retraining efforts:

1. Adults have a wealth of experience to draw on when faced with new ideas.
2. Adults decide what they want to learn and when.
3. Adults apply their new learning immediately.

Bennett (1993) expanded on these principles for continuing education:

1. Teach in small groups to emphasize active as opposed to passive learning.
2. Draw on trainees' clinical experience.
3. Provide ample opportunity for feedback and processing.
4. Use intermittent reinforcement.
5. Be sure teaching is relevant to what learners need to know.
6. Ensure that teachers are creditable clinicians.
7. Keep the didactic portion brief.

Thus, continuing education workshops seem advisable. They should be practical and patient focused, with time for discussion. Participants' actual conflicts with utilization reviewers and material from the APA managed care hot line could be used to discuss inpatient care. Videotaped patient encounters and participants' experiences could provide a platform for discussing outpatient care, including treatment focus, frequency, and choice of modality.

- *Continuous case conferences.* Psychotherapy has been taught via individual supervision and group continuous case conferences. These valuable arenas should now focus on short-term interventions and case management skills. At case conferences adapted to the managed care environment, clinicians could follow one provider's entire panel of patients in treatment and case management. Or a group of providers could follow selected patients over time during their course of treatments at various settings.
- *Managed care networks.* These networks differ considerably. Become familiar with a range of managed care organizations before joining one. Choose the one whose treatment philosophy seems most congruent with your own. A good working alliance with a managed care case manager can be an instructive experience for both parties.
- *Group practice.* Membership in behavioral group practices and multispecialty mental health groups will provide access to a large number of patients, management information systems, and outcomes data. The group of providers then grapples with the allocation of resources and learns together.
- *Reorganization of individual practice.* Reorganizing your practice is a form of self-instruction. Experimenting with time slots and treatment settings causes changes in the treatment approach. Typical managed

care innovations include sessions of varying lengths and frequency, never giving a patient a "regular hour," and favoring couples and group sessions over individual work. Start delivering care in the home, school, or workplace. Experiment with the use of physician extenders such as nurses, physicians' assistants, and social workers.

- *Risk-sharing group practice.* Membership in a risk-sharing group contract offers the best training ground for modern psychiatric practice. A single fee, referred to as capitation, prospectively covers payment for a large population. The Advisory Board Company (1994), a strategic research firm, reported that medical groups taking on such contracts decreased the use of many medical services by an astounding 15%–60%. These groups commonly developed alternative treatment approaches. Be careful to build in safeguards to protect the group from serious financial loss. Be alert to the danger that just as fee for service encourages overutilization, capitation is an incentive for underutilization, for refusing to provide needed care.
- *Peer study and support groups.* Hospital administrators have discovered that published quarterly reports comparing physician-prescribing practices alter physician behavior. By comparing their practice patterns, psychiatrists could learn from others who are effectively adapting to diminishing financial resources. Organized psychiatry could devote district branch meetings and academic medical center rounds to information sharing by clinicians and groups who describe how resource allocation decisions are made and how this has changed over time.
- *Managed care consultation programs.* Invite managed care consultation to your community. APA is developing a managed care consultation program to help independent clinicians, groups, and academic medical centers. A planned five-volume interactive textbook and experiential workshop sessions will help those who are new to managed care. For groups more sophisticated with managed care, consultants will include APA members, nationally recognized accountants, actuaries, business managers, and legal advisors.
- *Degrees in related fields.* For those interested in becoming clinician–administrators in managed care, a degree in business or public health will be useful (Lazarus 1995).

Conclusion

This is a period of painful disruption, but stress enhances the possibility for change. Some psychiatrists will not be willing to change. Others will be unable to make the necessary adjustments, but of necessity, most psychiatrists who wish to practice their art into the 21st century will change. For them, retraining must be part of the process.

References

Advisory Board Company: Capitation I: The New American Medicine. Washington, DC, Advisory Board Company, 1994

Beck AT: Cognitive Therapy and the Emotional Disorders. New York, International University Press, 1976

Bennett MJ: The managed care setting as a framework for clinical practice, in Managed Mental Health Care: Administrative and Clinical Issues. Edited by Feldman J, Fitzpatrick R. Washington, DC, American Psychiatric Press, 1992, pp 203–219

Bennett MJ: The importance in teaching the principles of managed care. Behavioral Healthcare Tomorrow 2(3):28–32, 1993

Bibring E: The mechanism of depression, in Affective Disorders: Psychoanalytic Contribution to Their Study. Edited by Greenacre P. New York, International University Press, 1953, pp 13–48

Blackwell B, Schmidt GL: The educational implications of managed mental health care. Hosp Community Psychiatry 43:962–964, 1992

Budman SH, Armstrong E: Training for managed care settings: how to make it happen. Psychotherapy 29:416–421, 1993

Budman SH, Gurman AS: Theory and Practice of Brief Psychotherapy. New York, Guilford, 1988

Budman SH, Bennett JM, Wisneski MJ: Short term group psychotherapy: an adult developmental model. Int J Group Psychother 30:63–76, 1980

Davanaloo H (ed): Basic Principles and Techniques in Short Term Dynamic Psychotherapy. New York, Spectrum, 1978

Deming WE: Out of Crisis. Cambridge, MA, MIT Center for Advanced Engineering Studies, 1986

De Shazer S: Keys to Solutions in Brief Therapy. New York, Norton, 1988

Gabbard GO: The big chill: the transition from residency to managed care nightmare. Academic Psychiatry 16:119–126, 1992

Group for the Advancement of Psychiatry: Psychotherapy in the Future (GAP Report No 133). Washington, DC, American Psychiatric Press, 1992

Kübler-Ross E: On Death and Dying. New York, Macmillan, 1969

Lazarus A: From spreadsheet to stethoscope: the physician with an M.B.A. The Pharos 58(2): 20–23, 1995

Malan DH: The Frontiers of Brief Psychotherapy. New York, Plenum, 1976

Mann J: Time Limited Psychotherapy. Cambridge, MA, Harvard University Press, 1973

Relman A: The new medical industrial complex. N Engl J Med 303:963–970, 1980

Sabin JE: Clinical skills for the 1990s: six lessons from HMO practice. Hosp Community Psychiatry 42:605–608, 1991

Sabin JE: The moral myopia of academic psychiatry. Academic Psychiatry 17:175–179, 1993

Sabin JE, Boris JF: Mental health teaching and research, in Managed Mental Health Care: Administrative and Clinical Issues. Edited by Feldman J, Fitzpatrick R. Washington, DC, American Psychiatric Press, 1992, pp 185–199

Schneider-Braus K: A practical guide to HMO psychiatry. Hosp Community Psychiatry 38:876–879, 1987

Schreter RK: Ten trends in managed care and their impact on the biopsychosocial model. Hosp Community Psychiatry 44:325–327, 1993

Schreter RK: Outpatient services: the clinician's view, in Allies and Adversaries: The Impact of Managed Care on Mental Health Services. Edited by Schreter RK, Sharfstein SS, Schreter CA. Washington, DC, American Psychiatric Press, 1994, pp 60–68

Schreter RK, Sharfstein SS, Schreter CA (eds): Allies and Adversaries: The Impact of Managed Care on Mental Health Services. Washington DC, American Psychiatric Press, 1994

Schreter RK, Sharfstein SS, Schreter CA (eds): Managing Care, Not Dollars: The Continuum of Mental Health Services. Washington, DC, American Psychiatric Press (in press)

Sifneos P: Short Term Psychotherapy and Emotional Crises. Cambridge, MA, Harvard University Press, 1979

Section V

Administration and Management

Chapter 18

What Factors Should Managed Behavioral Health Programs Consider When Designing Their Operations?

Monica E. Oss, M.A.
Mark Tidgewell, C.P.A.

As policymakers, payers, managed care organizations, and provider-sponsored integrated delivery systems consider designing managed behavioral health programs, there are a number of issues to examine. Unfortunately, there is no single program design or structure that is "best" because the objectives of the health plan and the characteristics of the beneficiaries have a dramatic effect on the design elements adopted.

Generally, the issues under consideration in the design of a managed behavioral health program fall into six categories: 1) benefit parity or limitations, 2) beneficiary options in provider selection, 3) program access design, 4) carve-out or primary care integration, 5) contractual payment arrangements, and 6) information systems and claims payment.

Behavioral Health Benefit Parity or Benefit Limitations

One of the first decisions to be made in the design of a managed behavioral health program is what mental health and chemical dependency treatment services are to be paid and at what level. There are basically two schools of thought with regard to behavioral health benefit levels. One belief is that with a managed care program in place, payers can safely offer behavioral health benefits at the same level, or at parity, with other health care services. In this case the plan limitations in terms of dollars, days, and so on would be equal to those imposed on all health care services. However, for many payers, decision makers are unwilling to extend parity in coverage to mental health and chemical dependency benefits.

The Debated Costs of Parity

Discriminatory behavioral health benefits are an antiquated artifact from an earlier era in medicine when little was known about the etiology of behavioral health problems and their relationship to physical health. Mental health benefits are prime candidates for benefit redesign, restructuring, and restriction to correct the disparity between coverage of behavioral health problems and coverage of all other health problems. Considerable progress has been made nationally to destigmatize mental illness. Along with destigmatization there has been an increased awareness of the dysfunction related to mental disorders and the increasing cost of treatment in both the public and private sectors. Awareness of the cost issue has in turn increased concerns that mental health services are unaffordable, require management and containment, and are often of questionable value. Despite this view, many now agree that it is unethical to subject a small group of Americans to a lesser quality of life and possible financial ruin because they or a member of their family suffers from a chronic condition.

Nondiscriminatory coverage for treatment of mental health and chemical dependency problems is presently the exception, rather than the rule, in most public and private sector health benefit plans. As the United States moves forward toward reform of its health care system, there is an opportunity to gain equal coverage for treatment of behavioral health problems and a first-class system for this care. Limiting behavioral health coverage in a national health care plan forces the continuation of a backup second-class system of care through a hodgepodge of federal block grants, state programs, state hospitals, and private fee for service. Without a basic entitlement to care, persons with mental illness will continue to face the problem of assembling the necessary health care services in a fractured system—a system that national health care policy is supposedly dedicated to eradicating. Without a unified system of care, mentally ill and chemically dependent Americans will continue to be forced to seek care from charitable institutions, in homeless shelters, and through prisons or court-ordered treatment programs.

The moral and ethical issues are being debated at the state level as well. Proposals for limited parity for serious mental illness to full parity are being discussed and enacted. States such as Virginia have mandated unlimited nondiscriminatory benefits for medication evaluation and medication maintenance visits. Maryland recently passed a mental health insurance parity bill. The new law greatly expands mandated mental health and substance abuse benefits, including the elimination of separate lifetime maximums and aggregate limits. The law does allow for separate co-payments for outpatient services. Full parity in all other respects is effective July 1, 1995.

The current practice of allowing discriminatory benefits promotes cost shifting. State hospitals, the community mental health system, and community resources serve as the ultimate stop-loss arrangement for indemnity plans, managed care plans, and Medicare. As long as limitations other than medical necessity are placed on behavioral health benefits, there will be a requirement for a public system to serve those needs.

Several studies assessing the cost of serious mental illness have been conducted over the past few years as legislatures have considered limited parity. Generally, the serious mental health diagnoses account for < 20% of the inpatient admissions in a commercial managed care plan. A 1992 study (Krizay and Oss 1992) showed that parity for serious mental illness would increase the cost in Maryland by $0.89 per employee per month. Furthermore, it was found that full parity for health maintenance organizations (HMOs) would raise rates $1.29 per employee per month. The authors went on to state, "If the Maryland insurance parity bill reduces the state's hospital census by only 3.5% as a result of the shift back to private insurance, it will cover the entire increase in the state's employees' health benefit" (p. 10).

Actual payment experience for the military's Civilian Health and Medical Program of the Uniformed Services (CHAMPUS) health plan (which provided virtually unlimited behavioral health coverage) provides a good basis for analyzing behavioral health costs. Data adjusted for age distribution suggest that full coverage for behavioral health can be provided for less than $200 per person per year. Only about one-third of this behavioral health cost is attributable to *severely mentally ill* persons (defined as those with a primary diagnosis in *International Classification of Diseases, 10th Edition* [ICD-10], categories F20 through F25).

Another study, *Psychiatric Benefits In Employer-Provided Health Care Plans: 1992 Report* (Hustead 1992), also found that nondiscriminatory coverage of mental health and chemical dependency benefits can be provided with relatively little additional cost if the behavioral health benefit plan design covers the entire continuum of care. To equalize behavioral health benefits with physical health benefits, the study found health plans would pay between $0 and $11 more per person per month, depending on their current behavioral health coverage and their current physical health coverage.

Typical Behavioral Health Plan Limitations

In an effort to cap spending on behavioral health benefits—either with or without the use of managed care—many types of specific limitations can be found in a review of health plans:

- *Annual and lifetime maximum dollar limits.* Some health plans have limits on the reimbursable spending for behavioral health benefits that is permissible in a year or a lifetime. Some plans have limitations as low as $10,000 in a patient's lifetime.
- *Inpatient or residential day limits.* Plans range in reimbursable inpatient and residential days from as few as 3 to as many as 365 per year.
- *Nonresidential acute care service limitations.* Some health plans specify the amount of services and types of alternatives to traditional residential service that are reimbursable. These limitations can be a dollar amount, a visit limit, or a reimbursement limit with a preestablished fee schedule.
- *Outpatient treatment limitations.* Many traditional indemnity plans have very specific limitations on outpatient mental health treatment. Some very regressive plans have limitations of as little as $500 per year for all outpatient services. Other plans limit psychotherapy but have unrestricted reimbursement for medication management. Other plans limit specific forms of outpatient services such as group therapy or home visits.
- *Limitations by type of provider.* Health plans can often limit providers who are eligible to provide services by licensure category (limited only to psychiatrists and psychologists, for example) or by accreditation category (Joint Commission on Accreditation of Healthcare Organizations or Commission of Accreditation of Rehabilitation Facilities, for example).
- *Specific exclusions in behavioral health plans.* Many health plans have specific limitations on reimbursement by type of mental health or chemical dependency problem. A survey of a number of public and private health plans found the following specific exclusions: court-ordered treatment, psychological testing, inpatient treatment for adolescent conduct disorders, AIDS dementia, organic brain syndrome or Alzheimer's disease, smoking cessation, gambling addiction, marriage and family therapy, and developmental disabilities.

Again, the debate in the next several years will be whether these specific limitations and exclusions are necessary in managed behavioral health plans.

Beneficiary Options in Provider Selection

A fundamental issue in the design of a managed behavioral health plan is how much flexibility the beneficiary should have in provider selection. The most cost-effective plans limit beneficiary selection to a limited panel of behavioral health professionals and treatment programs. This cost-effectiveness is a result of the ability of managed behavioral health programs to select participating providers for consumer satisfaction and cost-effective treatment patterns.

Plans that reimburse for behavioral health services outside the established provider network are more costly to payers (and to consumers, if they share in premium payments) but are generally more desirable to consumers. If the plan is going to allow out-of-network benefit payments, the level of required co-payments and allowable reimbursement levels should be a part of the health plan.

Program Access Design

How beneficiaries access the mental health and chemical dependency treatment services is also a fundamental design issue in managed behavioral health programs. Options available in program design include the following:

- Mandatory toll-free telephone access that can either direct the patient to a specific clinical evaluator or to providers in the network at large.
- Mandatory access through specific clinical evaluation centers or through specific employee assistance professionals.
- Access through primary care physician referrals.
- Open access to any participant in the behavioral health provider network.

Carve-Out Models Versus Primary Care Integration

For most payers, the issue is whether to finance behavioral health benefits with primary medical care benefits or through a separate financing structure—often referred to as a *carve-out*. There are three basic options with regard to this decision:

1. *Primary care model.* Pool behavioral health benefit dollars with medical plan dollars into a single financing pool, with a single administrative plan.
2. *Total carve-out.* Carve out all behavioral health benefit dollars from general medical dollars into two separate financing pools with two separate administrative plans.
3. *Indemnity carve-out.* Carve out behavioral health benefit dollars from the general medical funding in the indemnity-style health plans, leaving the primary care model financing of behavioral health benefits in HMO plans.

In the mid-1980s, managed behavioral health carve-out programs emerged as a solution to the cost management issue. Two designs were dominant, specialized utilization management and the full-risk carve-out. Both designs recognized three factors that affect utilization:

1. A relatively small minority of persons generate the great majority of demand for mental health services.
2. Most of the variation of intensity in mental health services provided is variably but positively correlated to patients' severity of illness, the desire to seek treatment, and local practice patterns.
3. The degree of utilization management in the setting in which mental health service is rendered will affect the continuing utilization frequency per user but not necessarily the number of individuals seeking services.

Managed behavioral health programs that concentrated on specialized utilization management were sold directly to large employers with self-funded plans or to health plans that in turn offered minimum premium and administrative services only (ASO) financing vehicles to their accounts. ASO financing arrangements were initially developed in response to market demands for full experience rating. Faced with escalating health care expenses, large accounts were unwilling to pay premiums based on the experience of a pool. Traditional insurance products had become too inefficient in managing risk. Specialized behavioral health care companies provided immediate relief by introducing sophisticated utilization review and case management processes. These companies effectively used these tools to develop more predictable results by intervening in the delivery process with precertification and concurrent review. The companies employed specialty personnel and provided an intensive focus to processes that were not well understood by health plans.

Other strategies were developed by the managed behavioral health care companies involving specialty networks, credentialing processes, discounts, and administrative processes. Early networks emphasized size, geographic coverage, and access. The common perception seemed to be that more providers led to improved access. These large networks are typically accompanied by a credentialing process, provider profiling, negotiation of discounts, and strict administrative protocols for certification of inpatient and outpatient care. Outpatient management has emerged as the most difficult area to manage. Unlike inpatient care, outpatient treatment in a broad network is difficult to manage. There is a high volume of low-dollar transactions, lack of direct involvement in the treatment process by the managed care company, and payment to providers based on a discounted fee-for-service model.

The success these programs have enjoyed has been a result of their ability to influence the decisions of patients and providers that affect demand for service. Generally, these plans have shown significant decreases in use of inpatient services with limited increases in outpatient care.

Full-risk carve-out programs were first offered as a solution for the utilization management of HMOs in the late 1970s and early 1980s. HMOs by design held the full risk and had developed risk transfer arrangements through specialty pools, provider withholds, independent practice association contracting, and a variety of other mechanisms. The emergence of specialty managed behavioral health care programs that would accept full risk for mental health and chemical dependency care was seen as simply another step in the process of managing risk through transfer.

The programs that accepted full risk on a carve-out basis were faced with a more difficult task than the companies that specialized in utilization management. Survival of these programs depended on their ability to manage both inpatient and outpatient care within the projections used in establishing the capitation paid by the HMO. Early versions of these programs tended to be staff models in which all outpatient care was rendered by employed or contracted clinicians. This model evolved into a network by the mid 1980s. However, the successful networks were tightly managed and tended to be smaller than the broad networks offered by the utilization management programs.

Beneficiary reaction to these programs was not always positive. The intensity of management required to achieve the cost management goals positioned these programs to be portrayed as insensitive to the pressures of the provider community and employee relations issues.

For any payer evaluating carve-out financing mechanisms for behavioral health, there are distinct advantages and disadvantages to both approaches. Advantages include the following:

- Specialized approach to managing behavioral health treatment services—clinical criteria, case managers, provider network, and so on.
- Separate and customized benefit plan design for managing behavioral health benefits.
- Assurance that an adequate proportion of health benefit dollars will be allocated for mental health and chemical dependency treatment services.
- Referrals for service exclusive of the primary care network.

The following are some of the disadvantages to payers:

- Duplicate administrative systems for primary medical and behavioral health services, with resulting additional operational administrative costs and contract administration costs.

- Confusion of two delivery systems for beneficiaries.
- Lack of coordination of behavioral health benefits with the primary care system.
- Lack of ability to capture *offset* effects of behavioral health treatment services in the reduction of primary care dollars.

Contractual Payment Arrangements

The final, but critical, issue for payers to consider in the design of a managed behavioral health plan is the type of contractual arrangement between the payer and the behavioral health plan. Payers basically have five options, in increasing order of risk assumption:

1. *Standard ASO arrangement.* Under these arrangements the fee to the managed behavioral health program is a fixed amount for the management of the program, although the payer pays the actual amount required to reimburse providers.
2. *Performance-based ASO arrangement.* In this variation of the standard ASO arrangement, payment to the managed behavioral health program is increased or decreased based on its actual performance on administrative, clinical, or financial parameters. Under these arrangements, bonuses or penalties to manage behavioral health programs can range from 5% to 25% of administrative fees.
3. *Risk-limitation arrangements.* Under these arrangements, the managed behavioral health program administers the behavioral health benefit under a typical ASO arrangement but guarantees the payer that total behavioral health benefit costs will not total more than a fixed amount. In this case, the managed behavioral health program not only administers the plan for a fee, but also provides the payer with the equivalent of aggregate stop-loss insurance.
4. *Risk corridor arrangement.* Risk corridor arrangements most closely resemble full-risk capitation without having the managed behavioral health plan assume complete fiscal risk for the provision of behavioral health benefits. In these arrangements, the managed behavioral health plan is paid on an ASO arrangement for managing behavioral health benefits. However, the contractual relationship between the payer and the managed behavioral health program stipulates ranges of behavioral health benefit costs in which penalties will be paid by the managed behavioral health program if costs exceed certain targeted amounts or bonuses will be paid by the payer if costs are below certain targeted amounts.
5. Full-risk capitation arrangements. In these arrangements, the payer gives the managed behavioral health program a fixed fee, or premium,

for both the administration and the provision of mental health and chemical dependency benefits.

Information Systems and Claims Payment

The behavioral health industry's demand for precise, integrated data on the cost, quality, and utilization patterns of mental health and chemical dependency treatment is being met by an evolving technology of sophisticated management information systems (MISs). Payers want to know three simple things: 1) Does treatment work? 2) How often is treatment required? 3) How much will it cost?

When choosing a MIS, managed behavioral health programs should carefully consider their individual needs. Large provider groups with several capitated contracts will need to process and maintain information that differs from that of a community mental health organization that primarily is reimbursed through publicly funded fee-for-service contracts. The basic information required by all managed behavioral health programs includes client demographic information, client payer information, client treatment information, and provider performance information.

A MIS for each provider must support access to the information listed above. It is not absolutely necessary for a MIS to be fully automated, but the larger the provider organization, the greater the need for computer hardware and software tools to support this effort. It is important not to confuse the computer hardware and software tools with the MIS. The computer hardware and software are simply *tools.* The MIS is an organizational system that is supported by people and an assortment of information collection, processing, and reporting software tools. It is advisable to seek consultative assistance in choosing a MIS. A mistake can be extremely costly.

There are a wide variety of MIS systems. Most large, multifaceted systems offer a full spectrum of services, and most are sold with the software necessary to maintain an integrated battery of information programs. The MIS should support subsystems that supply and integrate many types of data, including but not limited to membership enrollment, financial information, benefits management, and utilization and quality improvement data. In choosing a MIS system, personnel issues must be addressed. These issues generally relate to implementation and use of the system. Because MIS technology changes so quickly, managers must make decisions with implications that extend beyond the first or second year of utilization. Important issues to consider include the initial configuration and installation of the system, its integration with existing systems, and training clinicians and personnel to use it. A MIS interface is an ongoing commitment.

Implementation and utilization decisions have to made with an eye toward the future.

Conclusion

There are many considerations in the structure and organization of any managed behavioral health program. Decisions about the extent of benefits, consumer access, integration with general medicine, and financing arrangements depend on both the goals of the payer and the needs of the beneficiary population. Government policymakers and health plan executives need a comprehensive understanding of these issues—and the effects of managed behavioral health program structure on both quality and cost—to optimize monies available for mental health and chemical dependency treatment.

References

Hustead EC: Psychiatric Benefits in Employer-Provider Health Care Plans: 1992 Report. Washington, DC, Hay/Huggins Company, 1992

Krizay J, Oss ME: Equal coverage costs estimated at $2.32 monthly in Maryland. Open Minds 4(10):10, 1992

World Health Organization: The ICD-10 Classification of Mental and Behavioral Disorders. Geneva, World Health Organization, 1992

Chapter 19

How Should the Profit Motive Be Used in Managed Care?

Christine S. Spencer, Sc.D.
Richard G. Frank, Ph.D.
Thomas G. McGuire, Ph.D.

An alarming rate of increase in expenditures on mental health care threatens employer willingness to provide mental health insurance benefits (Frank et al. 1992). These cost increases have often been blamed on the fee-for-service (FFS) payment system, which rewards providers for increased utilization, and on insurance, which encourages consumers to demand more medical care. Insurance is designed to protect consumers from financial risks associated with treating illness. However, in providing this protection, insurance also provides consumers with incentives to demand an increased amount of medical care. (Manning et al. 1984). Furthermore, FFS reimbursement methods provide no incentives to providers to limit supply (McFarland 1993). Although consumer and provider behavior is linked through the insurance system, the risk protection component for the consumer can be preserved and separated from the reimbursement component for the provider. Managed care organizations provide an alternative way to structure provider reimbursement while continuing to provide financial protection.

The term *managed care* can refer to organizations that are essentially administrative shells that process claims and administer certain programs such as second opinion and utilization review. In this chapter, we refer to managed care organizations (MCOs) as entities that assume some direct financial risk for the costs of care supplied.

MCOs have arisen in part as a response to the worrisome features of the FFS system. MCOs often operate on a prospective fixed or per capita budget so that incentives to providers act as a check on utilization of services. However, the use of such payment mechanisms has generated a new set of concerns. When MCOs assume some financial risk for the cost of providing services, this risk creates financial incentives for MCOs to be more efficient but also to engage in practices that may be undesirable from a social point of view (Mechanic and Aiken 1989). For example, putting providers at risk for costs creates strong incentives for health plans to pursue a favorable risk selection of enrollees from the general population. The MCO may achieve this favorable selection of enrollees through underwriting practices or through the design and administration of benefits. Underwriting practices such as preexisting condition exclusions can be used to discourage the enrollment of high-cost individuals (Starr 1992). If underwriting practices fail to keep high-cost enrollees from enrolling in the MCO, plans may encourage disenrollment of enrollees that are high cost and difficult to treat through the design and administration of benefits. Some plans deny coverage to enrollees who develop a severe and persistent mental illness (e.g., schizophrenia) while enrolled, charge higher co-payments for mental health visits, and limit the annual inpatient mental health care and outpatient mental health visits (Peterson et al. 1992). Insurance plans may be able to rationalize underservice to individuals with serious mental health conditions if a public system serves as a backup (Jellinek and Nurcombe 1993).

Unlike the cost-based reimbursement mechanism that is intended to insulate providers from the pursuit of profits, the managed care framework more explicitly employs profit incentives to motivate provider behavior. In this chapter we explore the role of profits in developing reimbursement methods that encourage desirable provider behavior. We pay special attention to the related problems of paying organizations according to the financial risks they bear while attenuating incentives to undertreat. The chapter is organized into five sections. The second section addresses the incentives within a managed care setting, the third section discusses managed care and special issues in treating mentally ill persons, the fourth section illustrates a design for reimbursement that would provide appropriate incentives for managed care providers, and the last section provides some conclusions about use of profit as an incentive in the managed care setting.

Incentives Within Managed Care Organizations

MCOs have evolved over the past 15 years to include a spectrum of organizational forms. The most well-known organizational form is the health maintenance organization (HMO), but preferred provider organizations and point-of-service plans are also included. Although these organizations vary along several dimensions, they all are designed to manage utilization and quality of care through explicit use of financial incentives. Techniques that managed care organizations use to control utilization and quality of care include utilization review, mandatory second opinion, primary care physician gatekeepers, and nonphysician case managers (Smith 1993). MCOs are freer than FFS insurance plans to use a broader array of services that may lead to the use of less costly treatment settings. MCOs may also use prior authorization, concurrent review, and improved information systems to increase efficiency and lower costs (Frank et al. 1992; Jellinek and Nurcombe 1993).

MCOs are most often financed through a prospective budget, either fixed or per capita (Smith 1993). The fixed-budget approach sets an overall dollar amount to finance all covered services for a given population. If the number of individuals is known, then this amounts to a capitation plan. However, in many public plans, such as community mental health centers, the number of service users in a population is not known in advance (Paulson 1988). Under the fixed-budget approach, MCOs have incentives to fill available "slots" with less costly users that satisfy the eligibility criteria (McFarland 1994). Because it is often difficult to identify the target population, payers may not be able to easily (or at low cost) determine whether the appropriate individuals are being served or if they are receiving appropriate services. If the amount of the fixed budget is not tied to the number of individuals enrolled, the MCO may also have an incentive to enroll fewer individuals. Under capitation, an MCO receives a fixed fee per individual enrolled. When the amount of capitation does not vary by risk group, the MCO has an incentive to attempt to engage in practices that lead to favorable risk selection.

Whether MCOs are financed through a fixed budget or capitation, revenues per person are fixed and therefore net revenues (profits) decrease as costs increase with service utilization. In Figure 19–1, MCO net revenues (profits) are graphed against the costs, where on the vertical axis amounts greater than zero represent profits and amounts less than zero represent losses. The diagonal line shows how net revenues fall with cost increases. The intersection of these two lines represents a zero-profit point for the MCO. In other

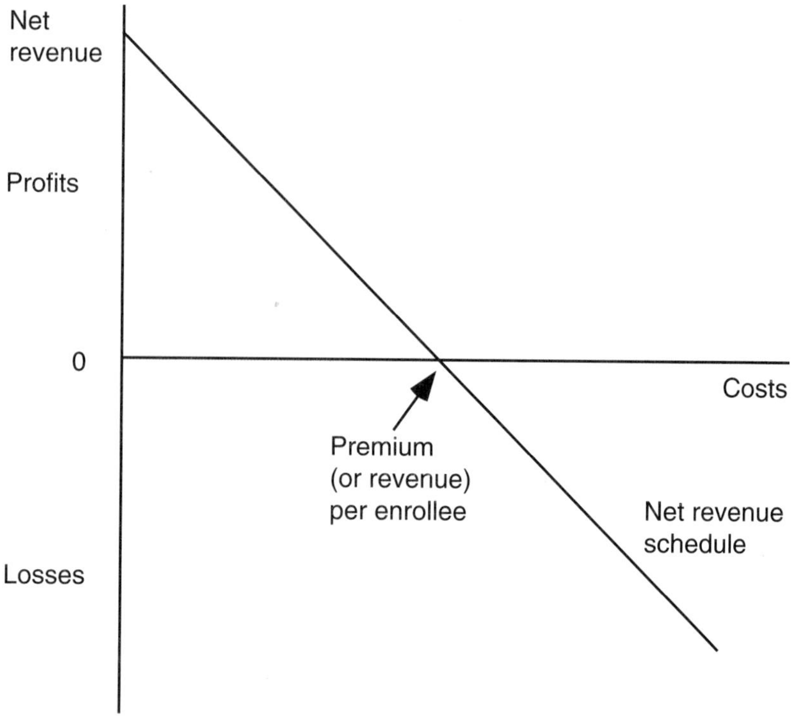

Figure 19–1. Net revenue and costs per enrollee in managed care. See text for explanation.

words, points on the line to the left of the zero-profit point represent net revenue, or profit, received by the MCO but not used on services for enrollees. The points on the net revenue line to the right of the zero-profit point represent losses when costs exceed net revenue. This diagram illustrates that to the right of the zero-profit point, every dollar of service use represents a dollar of loss, whereas to the left of the zero-profit point, every dollar of service use not spent represents a dollar of profit. This profit and loss diagram characterizes the strong incentives at work in the capitated framework.

Ideally, putting MCOs at risk for costs furnishes an incentive to improve efficiency in the provision of services and thus lowers costs. The hope is that MCOs will use mechanisms such as case management, utilization controls, and a broader array of service settings to improve efficiency while maintaining an appropriate level and quality of care.

Managed Care and Mental Health Services

In principle, medical care quality is maintained within the managed care framework through consumer choice of provider and plan. If a consumer is dissatisfied with any dimension of service, such as appointment time or in-office waiting time, type of care provided, or location of ancillary services, that consumer may switch to a new provider or managed care plan at the time of contract renewal (usually once a year). The ability of the consumers to change plans guarantees that the plan has an incentive to remain responsive to consumer demands. In the case of mental health services, these constraints on provider behavior are often not operative because of the very nature of mental illness. Individuals with mental illnesses may be less capable of understanding the benefits of their health insurance policy. In this way, they may function poorly in the consumer role (Arons et al. 1994). Severely mentally ill persons are an especially vulnerable population who may not be able to assess the relevant dimensions of service.

Not only are individuals with severe mental illnesses not likely to function well as consumers, they also can be very susceptible to negative incentives within a payment system. For example, inpatient psychiatric care has been shown to be very responsive to prospective payment systems (Harrow and Ellis 1992). In general, the response of psychiatric inpatient length of stay to per case prospective payment is roughly twice as large as that found in general medical inpatients (Frank et al. 1987; Freiman et al. 1989; Harrow and Ellis 1992).

When the provider is at risk for cost there are three types of behavior that are potential causes of concern. MCOs may 1) select patients who are healthier at the outset and require less care, 2) transfer costly patients to the public sector, or 3) provide an inappropriately low quantity of services (Ellis and McGuire 1993). Government regulation can attempt to correct certain manifestations of the problem by requiring minimum benefit packages and open enrollment and by prohibiting exclusions based on preexisting conditions. However, when there are strong financial incentives, it is difficult to impede the creativity that plans may exhibit in determining methods to discourage enrollment of those with high expected costs.

Prepaid mental health care offers a relevant example. Many HMOs are required to cover 20 outpatient mental health visits and offer annual open-enrollment periods. In most HMO services, however, to access the mental health benefit the patient must first see a primary care provider and receive approval for specialty treatment. A good deal of evidence suggests that non-financial mechanisms to allocate mental health care are employed by prepaid group plans. In the RAND Corporation Health Insurance Experiment, for example, participants in the prepaid group practice arm of the study used only 25% of the visits consumed by those in the free-care, fee-for-service plan, despite similar demand characteristics. For non-mental health visits, HMO enrollees used 50% of the available services compared with

FFS plan users. Mental health services were rationed more closely by the HMO than were other medical visits. Many HMOs control mental health care costs simply by limiting the available number of mental health professionals (Christianson et al. 1992).

Providing services for individuals with mental illness in a risk-bearing situation may be even more problematic and financially risky for MCOs than providing general medical services for the following three reasons. First, mental illness is expensive to treat. The average case of schizophrenia covered by insurance plans of large firms in the United States required mental health payments of $5,600 in 1988. For individuals with schizophrenia using hospital care, the average payment was $25,000. Nearly 10% of individuals hospitalized for mental health reasons in 1988 had hospital payments of more than $30,000 for their treatment. Second, mental illness tends to be persistent. Although for 50% of the people with an episode of major depression the first episode will be their last, once someone has experienced a second episode, the probability of another within several years reaches 89% (Kupfer 1991). Roughly 24% of individuals hospitalized for depression and schizophrenia are rehospitalized within 2 years. Of those rehospitalized once, 35% have a third hospital episode, and 42% of those are hospitalized a fourth time (R. G. Frank and R. Brookmeyer, Cost sharing, managed care and inpatient psychiatric utilization in private insurance, unpublished manuscript, 1993). Finally, patients with mental illness have higher expected costs for treatment of other (nonmental) conditions (Shatkin 1990).

Although managed care plans create an incentive to reduce treatment or to avoid high-cost patients, appropriate financing arrangements can create incentives to provide suitable treatment while not avoiding certain high-cost patients. In the mental health area, these high-cost patients are often chronically mentally ill. MCOs have incentives to shift these patients to publicly financed systems of care such as community mental health centers and state psychiatric hospitals. Economizing on these patients may be accomplished through a variety of internal mechanisms designed to limit access to care for these patients. For example, in addition to the use of copayments and additional payments to provide mental health benefits, MCOs may impose lifetime limits on hospital utilization, have lengthy waiting lists, or provide mental health services at an inconvenient location (Shadle and Christianson 1988).

Design of a Supply-Side Cost-Sharing Payment System

In this section we discuss methods for using profit incentives as a tool to encourage MCOs to enroll patients, including those likely to be high cost, while maintaining an incentive to provide efficient care. Two basic methods have been proposed to pay MCOs fairly: a classification system that uses risk adjusters to differentiate high- from low-risk groups and a payment system that uses risk sharing between the purchaser and the managed care plan. The risk-adjustment approach merely regulates the level of payment, leaving the capitation incentives intact. The risk-sharing mechanism actually changes the profit incentives of the MCO, thus offering an additional tool to create appropriate incentives for MCOs.

The first method is a risk-adjustment system in which insurance premiums vary according to risk-group identifiers such as age or other family characteristics. Classification systems such as the Ambulatory Care Groups (Weiner et al. 1991), the Diagnostic Cost Groups (Ash et al. 1989), and the Payment Amount for Capitated Systems (Anderson et al. 1990) have been shown in research studies to improve the prediction of expenditure levels for the Medicare population compared with what is possible using only demographic predictors. Each of these classification systems makes some use of past mental health utilization for purposes of prediction.

However, current risk-adjustment methodologies have been criticized by a number of researchers as inadequate to prevent risk selection (Newhouse 1994). Existing risk-rating systems in the mental health area are not well developed enough to be able to capture enough of the variance in expected future use to forestall large gains from a selective enrollment policy.

The second method uses risk sharing between the purchaser and the MCO to provide appropriate incentives to the MCO. In fact, in the private sector, sophisticated contracts between purchasers and MCOs are increasingly being used to minimize negative incentives while maintaining the beneficial features of managed care. Private contracts do not generally use a classification system, but base payment between the purchaser and the risk management company on past and current utilization by the group in question. Past utilization can be used to project utilization targets for the MCO while the risk of financing current utilization costs that diverge from the targets can be shared by the purchaser and the MCO.

In terms of ability to bear risk, it is not at all obvious that purchasers are less able to bear claims cost risk than are MCOs, who tend to be small in terms of total revenue in relation to the purchasers for whom they work. The risk-sharing nature of the contracts may have more to do with incentives purchasers wish to give to MCOs to control costs than with the need for purchasers to shed simple risk. In this section of the chapter, we explore what such a contract might look like and the way in which profits can be used to alter incentives.

Contracts between purchasers and MCOs are composed primarily of three dimensions: 1) target cost of services per enrollee, 2) an administrative fee, and 3) the amount of risk sharing between the MCO and the purchaser. Current private sector contracts typically base the payment target between the purchaser and the MCO on past and current utilization by the group in question. Although the risk in the contract is sometimes assumed totally by the MCO, most often it is shared between the MCO and the purchaser. The MCO will have different incentives to reduce utilization, according to the amount of risk it bears. When total payment by the purchaser is independent of the actual utilization in the current period (a *pure-premium* contract), the financial risk for current utilization is assumed completely by the MCO and maximizes the incentives to the MCO to reduce cost. When the MCO is at no risk for the cost of current utilization, the incentives of the MCO to reduce cost are minimized.

In the competition for contracts, MCOs evaluate the previous 1 or 2 years of the claims experience of employees and project future health care costs based on that experience and the MCO management process. The MCOs then present bids to the purchaser. The bids usually consist of a claims target and an administrative fee. The purchaser then chooses an MCO to provide managed care services to the employee group.

The various risk-sharing mechanisms within the contract influence the strength of the incentives to the MCO to provide appropriate services to the enrollees. For example, when the MCO assumes complete risk, it receives the target amount specified in the contract per person and the administrative fee, or a pure premium. If utilization exceeds that target, then the MCO bears the full loss. If utilization is less than the projected target, the MCO reaps the entire financial gain. The financial arrangement provides strong incentives for the MCO to reduce utilization and potentially shift costly patients into the public system.

An alternative to the pure premium approach illustrated in Figure 19–1 is to structure a contract that contains a risk-reward feature. A contract specified in this way reduces the actual risk to the MCO of excessive claims and lessens the potential for windfall profits. For example, if the claims target is $100 per enrollee and the administrative fee is $20, when use is just at the target, the total payment by the purchaser to the MCO is $100 plus $20 per person. The MCO receives $20 per person after payment of the $100 claim. If actual use deviates from the $100 target, the risk-reward feature would regulate losses and gains of the MCO. For example, the risk feature might be such that if costs are between 100% and 120% of the target, the MCO loses 5% of its fee for each 1% that the costs exceed the target, up to a 50% loss. Then, for example, if costs are at 120% of the target or above, the MCO would only receive 50% of its negotiated fee. The reward feature may work on a similar basis so that when costs are < 90% of the target, the MCO may keep the surplus up to some specified maximum amount.

Figure 19–2 shows a risk-reward contract versus a pure-premium approach to risk sharing. The kinked line reflects the profits to the MCO under the risk-reward contract design, and the diagonal line shows the profits or losses to the MCO under the pure-premium payment method. In the risk-reward contract design, if costs are kept between 0 and point A, then MCO profits are capped at a predetermined level. Between points A and B profits fall as utilization increases. This provides the MCO with an incentive to contain costs but only to point B. Between points B and C, profits remain stable for the MCO at the level defined by the administrative fee. Between points C and D, the increased costs lower the amount of the administrative fee received by the MCO, which provides a strong incentive for utilization control. Beyond point D, losses are capped as well. This last feature prevents financial risk from catastrophic loss caused by caring for an unexpectedly high-cost population.

Under the pure-premium contract, all of the risk is assumed by the MCO when costs diverge from the target. Profits or losses move directly with the discrepancy between the actual and target amounts, dollar for dollar. The risk-reward contracts offer the MCO much less exposure to losses and much

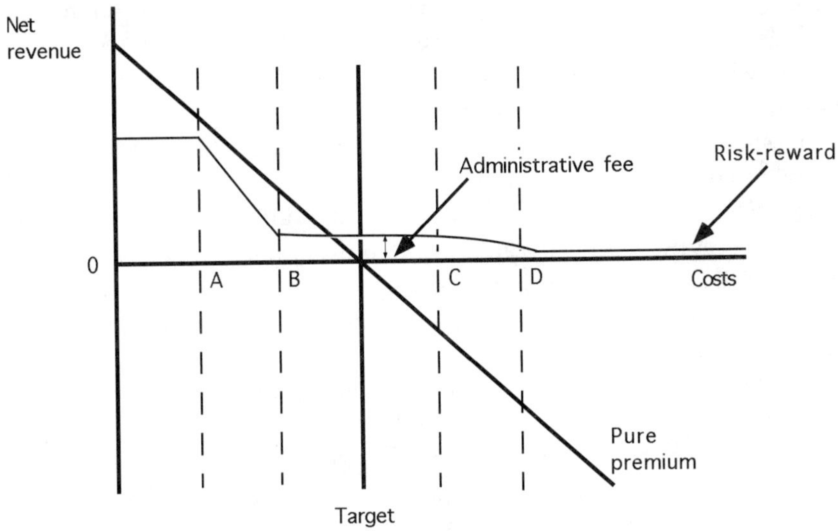

Figure 19–2. Net revenue in "pure premium" versus "risk-reward" managed care contracts. See text for explanation. *Note.* Assumes pure-premium contract sets premium at target amount.

less opportunity for profits. These "flattened" profit opportunities as shown in Figure 19–2 provide incentives to control utilization by the plan enrollees while protecting MCOs from extreme losses if utilization is higher than expected. Under these circumstances, MCOs have less incentive to risk-select because obtaining a bad risk from the population will not mean the financial ruin of the company.

Furthermore, because these need not be single-year contracts, other influences may minimize the effect of negative incentives on MCO performance. The multiyear nature of many contracts will mean that deviation from the target expenditure in a given year can be used to adjust the target in the following year. MCO behavior will affect future opportunities of business with that purchaser and, through reputation, with other purchasers. Satisfaction of the covered population may influence the purchaser's likelihood of renewing a contract with an MCO.

Conclusion

There are two main financing concerns related to paying MCOs for providing mental health services: paying plans fairly and maintaining incentives to be efficient. First, MCOs must be paid fairly. To ensure that this is done, MCOs must not be faced with excessive financial risk in providing care for mentally ill individuals. Most risk-adjustment systems do not adequately account for differences in costs between individuals and groups, thereby encouraging practices that result in biased selection of patients into health plans. Furthermore, current risk-adjustment technology in MCOs is so primitive that MCOs may avoid high-cost patients, not necessarily to pursue profits but to protect themselves against financial loss.

Second, incentives to maintain efficiency must be present. Mental health care is responsive to the financial incentives contained in various types of prospective payment systems. The responses are sufficiently strong so as to raise concerns about undertreatment and shifting responsibility of care for difficult-to-manage patients to the public sector.

However, within the private managed care sectors, contracts with purchasers are becoming increasingly sophisticated. These contracts use profits to counteract negative incentives inherent in a capitated or fixed-budget managed care system. Profits can be used in these contracts to provide positive risk-reward features. A more complex contract than a pure-premium design can be developed so that large swings in profits and losses are not possible. With the potential for losses from unpredictable, high-cost patients eliminated and the potential for windfall profits through selective enrollment forestalled, an MCO will have no economic incentive to avoid a group of potential enrollees, either by direct discrimination or by reducing services used by the group. Profits are an important tool that can be used to achieve socially desired outcomes in the managed care arena.

References

Anderson GF, Steinberg EP, Powe NR, et al: Setting payment rates for capitated systems: a comparison of various alternatives. Inquiry 27:225–233, 1990

Arons BS, Frank RG, Goldman HH, et al: Mental health and substance abuse coverage under health reform. Health Aff 13(1):192–205, 1994

Ash A, Porell F, Gruenberg L, et al: Adjusting Medicare capitation payments using prior hospitalization data. Health Care Financ Rev 10:17–30, 1989

Christianson JP, Lurie N, Finch M, et al: Use of community-based mental health programs for HMOs: evidence from a Medicaid demonstration. Am J Public Health 82:790–796, 1992

Ellis RP, McGuire TG: Supply-side and demand-side cost sharing in healthcare. J Econ Perspect 7:135–151, 1993

Frank RG, Lave JR, Taube C, et al: The impact of Medicare's prospective payment system on psychiatric patients treated in scatterbeds, in Advances in Health Economics and Health Services Research, Vol 8. Edited by Scheffler RM, McGuire TG. Greenwich, CT, JAI Press, 1987, pp 1–21

Frank RG, Goldman HH, McGuire TG: A model mental health benefit in private insurance. Health Aff 11(3):98–117, 1992

Freiman MP, Ellis RP, McGuire TG: Provider response to Medicare's PPS: reductions in LOS for patients treated in scatterbeds. Inquiry 26:24–34, 1989

Harrow B, Ellis RP: Mental health providers response to the reimbursement system, in Economics and Mental Health. Edited by Frank RG, Manning W. Baltimore, MD, Johns Hopkins University Press, 1992, pp 19–39

Jellinek MS, Nurcombe B: Two wrongs don't make a right: managed care, mental health, and the marketplace. JAMA 270:1737–1739, 1993

Kupfer D: Long term treatment of depression. J Clin Psychiatry 52:28–34, 1991

Manning WG, Leibowitz A, Goldberg GA, et al: A controlled trial of the effect of a prepaid group practice on use of services. N Engl J Med 310:1505–1510, 1984

McFarland B: Capitation and mental health, in Focus on Mental Health Services Research. Washington, DC, Foundation for Health Services Research, 6(1): 1–8, June 1993

McFarland B: Health maintenance organizations and persons with severe mental illness. Community Ment Health J 30:221–241, 1994

Mechanic D, Aiken LH: Capitation in mental health: potentials and cautions, in Paying for Services: Promises and Pitfalls of Capitation. Edited by Mechanic D, Aiken LH. San Francisco, CA, Jossey-Bass 1989, pp 5–18

Newhouse JP: Patients at risk: health reform and risk adjustment. Health Aff 13:32–146, 1994

Paulson RI: People and garbage are not the same: issues in contracting for mental health services. Community Ment Health J 24:91–102, 1988

Peterson MS, Christianson JB, Wholey D: National Survey of Mental Health, Alcohol, and Drug Abuse Treatment in HMOs: 1989 Chartbook. Excelsior, MN, Interstudy Center for Managed Care Research, 1992

Shadle M, Christianson JB: Mental health care for children and adolescents in health maintenance organizations, in The Financing of Mental Health Services for Children and Adolescents. Washington, DC, National Center for Education in Maternal and Child Health, 1988, pp 29–44

Shatkin B: Health care utilization of children of alcoholics (doctoral dissertation). Boston, MA, Brandeis University, 1990

Smith GR: Managed care, managed competition, and mental health, in Focus on Mental Health Services Research. Washington, DC, Foundation for Health Services Research, 1993 vol 6(1):1–8, June 1993

Starr P: The Logic of Health-Care Reform. Knoxville, TN, Grand Rounds Press, 1992

Weiner JP, Starfield BH, Steinwachs DM, et al: Development and application of a population-oriented measure of ambulatory case-mix. Med Care 29:452–472, 1991

Chapter 20

Can Providers and Payers Collaborate?

William R. Dubin, M.D.

Perhaps no other issue has polarized psychiatry like that of managed care. There are psychiatrists who believe that their livelihood as well as the future of psychiatry is threatened by managed care. There are other psychiatrists, some who work for managed care companies, who view managed care as an opportunity to provide cost-effective treatment and improve the current mental health care delivery system. At times the intensity of the debate between these groups has become so acrimonious and affect laden that rational discourse has become difficult, if not impossible.

In this chapter I review the negative and positive impact of managed care on psychiatric providers, cite examples of how psychiatric organizations collaborate and negotiate with managed care companies, and describe a unique experience in Philadelphia. Psychiatrists from managed care companies and members of the Philadelphia Psychiatric Society met for nearly 2 years to develop a consensus on clinical criteria that would be suitable for reimbursement purposes.

Negative Impact of Managed Care

There are numerous articles citing the negative impact of managed care on psychiatry. Gabbard (1992) elegantly described the effect of managed care on the morale of psychiatrists. He asserted that the conflict physicians have with the concept of managed care stems from certain psychological characteristics of physicians. These traits include perfectionism, chronic self-doubt, guilt feelings, an exaggerated sense of responsibility, conflicts about expressing anger, and conflicts about dependency. Gabbard (1992) also described how psychiatrists can withdraw into sullen anger, apathy, and depression when confronting the realities of working in a managed care environment.

Fink (1993) described feelings of ambiguity that psychiatrists experience when working in managed care settings. Managed care companies may limit the roles of psychiatrists to evaluating patients, prescribing medication, and providing supportive psychotherapy. Fink (1993) raised the possibility that psychiatrists' roles may be trivialized or eliminated altogether by managed care. He noted that the treatment team, under the supervision of a case manager, often takes responsibility for the patient. Occasionally the patient may be assigned to a nonphysician therapist for the bulk of care.

Some psychiatrists have been excluded from networks developed by managed care companies and pitted against psychiatrists who have not been excluded. Similarly, adversarial relations have been created by peer review in which values, background, and training shared by reviewing and attending psychiatrists have been ignored. Fink (1993) noted that managed care companies want to recruit psychiatrists who understand managed care. Yet the distinction between the provision of psychiatric care and the provision of managed care is unclear, although it "obviously exists in the minds of some people" (p. 724).

Gabbard and associates (1991) described the impact of managed care and utilization review on inpatient psychiatry. They noted that the time formerly devoted to treatment has been appropriated by extensive requirements for documentation, weekly or even daily phone calls with reviewers, and letters to justify continued hospitalization. Gabbard et al. (1991) further described how concurrent review may promote "splitting" in treatment, impede a patient's ability to separate from the hospital, and paradoxically reinforce a patient's illness.

Borenstein (1990) observed that concurrent utilization review disrupts the therapeutic relationship between the physician and the patient. Review organizations seldom employ reviewers who are not cost-effective. Knowing that their jobs may depend on decreasing expenditures for psychiatric treatment, reviewers must find ways to cut costs. Borenstein (1990) concluded that such pressure makes it highly unlikely that reviewers can objectively evaluate another physician's treatment. Moreover, certain types of treatment may be reviewed intensively in an effort to terminate care or change treatment so that it becomes less costly. Attending psychiatrists may be asked to write detailed progress reports and call reviewers with the results of their evaluation. Borenstein (1990) believed that managed care and utilization review clearly led to rationing psychiatric treatment. Likewise, Jellinek and Nurcombe (1993) noted that "there is little to check profiteering from under-utilization" (p. 1738).

Dr. Paul J. Fink and I described an experience with a health maintenance organization (HMO) in which our hospital suffered financial losses because of major philosophical differences over the delivery of treatment (Fink and Dubin 1991). Our hospital, Belmont Center for Comprehensive Treatment, became a subcontractor of a managed care subcontractor for an HMO to provide only inpatient care. Belmont had no control over outpatient treatment, and an overwhelming number of patients were referred for evaluation by inexperienced outpatient therapists who were unable to tolerate or manage any level of acute illness. Many patients were hospitalized, costing the hospital more than the capitation fee. It became apparent that an emergency service with a holding area would be necessary to divert admissions from the hospital (Gillig et al. 1989). However, the capitation fee was so low that such a service could not be implemented. The result was that the contract was canceled.

From this experience, our hospital administration concluded that for a capitated system to be successful, the entire spectrum of care should be delivered by one entity. We also noted the gross disparity between the benefits described by the HMO and the dollars available to provide them. Finally, we noted that such organizations rarely talk about the profit motive and the need to satisfy shareholders, which, in reality, is the underlying goal of many of these organizations. In summary, we concluded that there is "no free lunch" for psychiatric hospitals who do not control all aspects of treatment and who contract with managed care companies that underutilize psychiatrists in their outpatient provider networks.

Westermeyer (1991) described seven patients who received less than adequate psychiatric treatment because their care was not managed by a psychiatrist. Five patients committed suicide, one patient became psychotic, and one patient became permanently physically disabled. When psychiatric consultation was sought, psychiatrists were used primarily as psychopharmacological consultants. In three cases, the psychiatrists' recommendations were not followed or were poorly implemented. In six cases, mismanagement of psychotropic medications by a nonpsychiatrist was a factor in the negative outcome.

Despite these reports, there are a number of articles that have described positive experiences providing managed care, have reported successful treatment based on the concepts of managed care, and have pointed out that bad outcomes are not unique to managed care settings (Lazarus 1995).

Positive Impact of Managed Care

Patterson (1990) argued that cost-effective mental health care using the principles of managed care is possible. His model includes the following: assignment of clinical functioning by level of expertise, epidemiological accountability, fiscal responsibility, direct patient access, incentives for prevention, alliances between management and providers, choice of services, outcomes assessment, and collaboration between public and private providers. Patterson (1990) believed there was a way to link private practice with managed care so that a rational treatment delivery system could be forged.

Sabin (1991) observed that clinical practice in many HMOs during the past 25 years essentially serves as a model of good managed care. HMO practice involves population-oriented practice management, population-oriented program development, an ability to apply an adult developmental model to understanding psychopathology, command of a broad repertoire of treatment methodologies, and ethical analysis and advocacy. Many experienced HMO clinicians possess and use these skills daily. The HMO style of practice reaches a larger percentage of patients than does a fee-for-service practice, yet it provides relatively less treatment time per patient.

Several inpatient programs have negotiated successfully with managed care companies to develop programming consistent with the principles of managed care. Consequently, costs have been reduced, inpatient length of stay has decreased, and use of partial hospital services has increased (Baker and Giese 1992; Olden and Johnson 1993). Furthermore, there has been no increase in recidivism as a result of these changes.

Moore and associates (1992) evaluated treatment satisfaction among patients and clinicians in an HMO based at a private psychiatric hospital. They concluded that treatment outcome was satisfactory or very satisfactory in more than 80% of cases. In more than 60% of cases there was no perceived interference from the managed care component. The authors concluded that managed care is workable if benefits are not severely limited, authorization review puts patients' needs first, providers understand managed care concepts and are willing to conform their practice to certain restrictions, a strong management information system is in place, and providers and management know each other and trust each other.

Carson (1993) described the changes that took place at Timberlawn Psychiatric Hospital in Dallas, Texas, after the hospital administration decided to move into the managed care arena. The results have been gratifying, and most patients have done well with shorter hospital stays. Many patients have avoided hospitalization by utilizing intensive outpatient services. Unfortunately, the residency training program was forced to close because of financial stresses created by the hospital's contracts with managed care plans.

Pomerantz and colleagues (1994) described a unique model for delivering managed psychiatric care in HMOs. In their model, discussed in Chapter 2, local psychiatrists supervised the treatment of a network of interdisciplinary mental health providers. Fifteen *outpatient professional affiliation groups* were organized. Each group consisted of a psychiatrist and three to six nonmedical therapists who were linked by geographic preference, specific request, or special expertise. With an emphasis on outpatient treatment and diversionary programs, rather than inpatient treatment, this model achieved a 10% reduction in costs and a 94% patient satisfaction level.

Dr. Bruce J. Berg and I described the successful operation of an outpatient substance abuse program as an alternative to a traditional 28-day inpatient program (Berg and Dubin 1990). This program was developed in response to a request for proposals from a local HMO. In a 2-year period, 680 patients were treated in our outpatient department and an additional 197 patients were initially hospitalized because they met the criteria for inpatient detoxification. The average length of stay for this group was 4.9 days, followed by referral to the outpatient program. Of the 680 outpatients, 466 were detoxified from alcohol or a combination of alcohol and other drugs. We felt that this program demonstrated the effectiveness of outpatient treatment for substance abuse disorders and that inpatient treatment should be reserved for the most severely ill patients.

Lazarus (1994) described ways in which practicing psychiatrists, primary care physicians, nonmedical therapists, and managed care administrators effectively collaborate to enhance patient care. He noted the complexities involved in "sharing" patients among caregivers and discussed the type of interactions between caregivers and third and fourth parties that lead to expeditious treatment. Lazarus (1994) suggested that collaboration, rather than competition, best served the needs of patients, practitioners, and administrators in managed care settings. A similar model of care, based on the premise of *shared accountability*, was proposed by Bennett (1994).

An article in *Psychiatric Times* (1993) reported a study conducted by the National Association of Psychiatric Health Systems. The study indicated that the relationship between psychiatric health care facilities and managed care firms was improving. In 1992, 36% of facilities reported that relationships with managed care had improved, whereas in 1993, 78% felt that relationships had improved. Better relations were attributed to increased use of clinicians to conduct utilization review and a greater willingness of managed care firms to disclose review criteria. This study was conducted by survey and focused on relationships between member hospitals of the association and managed care companies rather than individual physicians and managed care companies.

Organized Psychiatry and Managed Care

Debate over the merits of managed care will probably continue for some time as the literature presents both "good" and "bad" forms of managed care. While this controversy has persisted, there have been efforts by psychiatric organizations to meet with managed care companies to try to resolve some of the issues that have led to negative perceptions about managed care.

Sederer and St. Clair (1989) described several attempts by psychiatric societies to collaborate with managed care organizations. The Philadelphia Psychiatric Alliance was an organization established in Philadelphia in response to Independence Blue Cross and Pennsylvania Blue Shield after the insurance companies established a preferred provider organization with limited psychiatric benefits and low reimbursement fees. The Philadelphia chapter of the American Psychiatric Association district branch, Psychiatric Physicians of Pennsylvania, created the Philadelphia Psychiatric Alliance as a separate organization because of concerns about restraint of trade. A $50 enrollment fee asked of the 500 psychiatrists who joined was used to create the alliance, establish a board, and hire staff. The alliance had some success in bargaining with "the Blues" for enhanced, clinically flexible benefits, and it identified questionable managed care systems, first by word of mouth and then by publication. The alliance was also active in discouraging hospitals and psychiatrists from contracting with insurers who were perceived as problematic.

Similar to the Philadelphia Psychiatric Alliance, the Physicians' Association of New Haven County was formed and funded by the Connecticut Medical Society. The Physicians' Association was established separate from the Medical Society to analyze managed care contracts for prospective physician providers. The Connecticut Medical Society added $100 per year to the dues of its members to help pay for the association. A newsletter *Informed Consent*—was published monthly or bimonthly and distributed to all members of the Connecticut Medical Society. The newsletter contained information about managed care systems in the area and described what it was like to contract with them.

The Task Force on Managed Care of the Massachusetts Psychiatric Society, also described by Sederer and St. Clair (1989), developed standards for certifying managed mental health plans and standards for certifying and monitoring utilization review organizations. A second-opinion service was also developed.

In 1988 the American Psychiatric Association sponsored a 3-day invitational symposium titled Psychiatry and Managed Care Systems: A Resource Symposium (Sederer and St. Clair 1989). Psychiatrists, management consultants, business executives, government representatives, and attorneys attended. Subjects included an overview of mental health services in managed care, the practitioner in managed care systems, issues related to practice, perspectives of various mental health care constituents, quality of care, and initiatives of the medical community. Following the symposium, the American Psychiatric Association established a Committee on Managed Care. This committee, which is still active, was given several important tasks, including determination of how managed care affects psychiatrists and psychiatric practice, trying to facilitate positive relationships between managed care companies and psychiatrists, investigating complaints from the American Psychiatric Association managed care hot line and reviewing these complaints with managed care companies, and representing members of the American Psychiatric Association in negotiations with managed care companies.

The Philadelphia Criteria

In 1988 I was elected president of the Philadelphia Psychiatric Society (PPS). The PPS represented 1,200 psychiatrists in the Philadelphia area. Between 1986 and 1988 managed care companies were moving into the Philadelphia area and having an impact on psychiatric treatment. They were insisting on preadmission certification, shorter hospital stays, and treatments other than inpatient hospitalization. Previously, these companies had dramatically altered the nature of substance abuse treatment by insisting that most treatment occur in an outpatient setting. Now the focus was clearly on inpatient mental health treatment.

As managed care grew, disputes over the locus of treatment occurred more frequently. There was increasing anxiety, anger, and feelings of helplessness among local psychiatrists. Although most managed care organizations had level-of-care criteria on which to base their certification decisions, the criteria were considered proprietary and were not shared with the psychiatric community. I decided during my year as president of the society that I would develop criteria from a consensus of the Philadelphia psychiatric community. Four committees were established: adult, child and adolescent, substance abuse, and outpatient. Each of these committees was given the task of developing criteria for inpatient, partial hospital, residential, and outpatient treatment. In addition to individuals I appointed, each committee invited psychiatrists from appropriate specialty societies.

For example, psychiatrists from the American Academy of Psychiatry in Alcoholism and Addictions served on the substance abuse committee. The child and adolescent committee had many members from the Regional Academy of Child and Adolescent Psychiatry. Society members who had an interest in any of these areas were also invited to serve on committees of their choice. For 16 months, committees of approximately 10–15 members met monthly to work on the criteria.

After the criteria were developed, a town meeting was held and more than 100 psychiatrists attended. The criteria were presented to the attendees and Dr. Steven Sharfstein was invited to comment on them. After the criteria were approved, they were distributed to the executive council members of the Psychiatric Physicians of Pennsylvania and to presidents of the Pennsylvania District Branch chapters. Their comments were reviewed and the criteria underwent further revision. The final version was approved both by the executive council of the PPS and the executive council of the Psychiatric Physicians of Pennsylvania. Although these criteria represented the consensus of Pennsylvania psychiatry, they were referred to as the *Philadelphia criteria* because of their place of origin.

Following the publication of the criteria, the executive committee of the PPS established a managed care committee. The committee decided to approach the managed care companies in the Philadelphia area and meet with their medical directors to develop further consensus regarding the Philadelphia criteria. This idea was greeted enthusiastically both by members of the psychiatric community and by the medical directors of the managed care companies.

The committee met with medical directors or other physician representatives from six managed care companies for 18 months. Because of the size of the group (12–15 participants) and scheduling difficulties, meetings were held approximately every 8–10 weeks. Throughout the time the committee met, an open and honest dialogue prevailed.

The first criteria discussed were the adult level-of-care criteria. A consensus was reached, although it took 14 months. The committee then began to focus on the adolescent criteria. However, at about this time, significant changes occurred in the managed care market in Philadelphia that altered the course of the committee. Managed care companies had generally become more acceptable. They had shifted their attention to outcomes measurement and quality in contrast to focusing on utilization management. The committee felt that the continuing focus on level-of-care review criteria was less relevant in view of the changing focus of the managed care companies. In addition, the entry of several new managed care companies diluted the autonomy of the committee because representatives of these companies lived in other parts of the United States. Continued collaboration between local managed care companies and the PPS would have excluded many companies from doing business in the Philadelphia area.

One factor that had facilitated the original work of the committee was the preexisting relationships between many representatives of the managed care companies and the committee members. The Philadelphia psychiatric community is large but close-knit, and most of the medical directors of local managed care companies had trained and practiced in Philadelphia. The preexisting relationships thus contributed to the collegiality and success of this endeavor.

The Philadelphia Managed Care Committee provided the managed care medical directors with a close view of the issues confronting front-line psychiatrists who were trying to adjust to the challenges of managed care. Similarly, practicing psychiatrists became more cognizant of the concerns of the managed care companies. By the end of this 16-month process, each member of the committee had gained insight and had become sensitive to pressing issues confronting all psychiatrists.

Conclusion

Initially, I was heartened by my experience in the Philadelphia Managed Care Committee. I thought both sides could develop common goals and shape the delivery of care in a way that was best for patients. However, the succeeding years have diminished my enthusiasm as additional barriers have been erected between psychiatrists and managed care companies.

A major problem has been the expansion of managed care organizations to provide direct treatment. Managed care companies have leased beds in local hospitals (Lazarus, in press) and developed their own outpatient clinics to compete directly with established psychiatrists. Furthermore, many of the policies in these organizations appear to have been made by individuals other than psychiatrists. The new managed care organizations that have entered Philadelphia have depersonalized many treatment procedures. When the Managed Care Committee met, there were only five or six major companies in the area. The number of new companies has skyrocketed, and there are currently more than 50 organizations in business in the Philadelphia area. Many of these companies are distant from Philadelphia and have preempted the warm relationships that once existed between attending psychiatrists and reviewing psychiatrists. Philadelphia psychiatrists, like most other psychiatrists, are now dealing with anonymous reviewers who do not live in the community.

Another contentious issue is the policy of companies to develop discrete provider panels that exclude psychiatrists in a given geographic area. This practice has had significant economic implications for psychiatrists who have been excluded from the network and have lost a significant portion of their practice and income. Patients are also affected by this change because in many instances psychiatrists have had long-standing relationships with them. Sadly, it has become common to hear a patient say, "I used to see Dr. Dubin and I liked him very much, but my insurance company told me that I have to see someone else now."

Nonetheless, psychiatrists will continue to interact with managed care companies in provider panels, networks, and a variety of other clinical affiliations. I do not think this interaction will be marked by the openness that existed during the life of the Managed Care Committee in Philadelphia. Instead, relationships will be more reserved and tense because psychiatrists will be in a subordinate position and will have little negotiating power. As long as managed care companies can wield economic power over psychiatrists it will be difficult to re-create the ambience that characterized the Managed Care Committee. Alternatively, if managed care companies dedicated themselves to building partnerships of service with providers, and providers share some of the economic risks with managed care organizations, a rewarding collaboration may be possible.

References

Baker NJ, Giese AA: Reorganization of a private psychiatric unit to promote collaboration with managed care. Hosp Community Psychiatry 43:1126–1129, 1992

Bennett MJ: Are competing psychotherapists manageable? Manag Care Q 2(2):36–42,1994

Berg BJ, Dubin WR: Why 28 days? An alternative approach to alcoholism treatment. Hosp Community Psychiatry 41:1175–1178, 1990

Borenstein DB: Managed care: a means of rationing psychiatric treatment. Hosp Community Psychiatry 41:1095–1098, 1990

Carson D: Managed care: a provider perspective, in Managed Mental Health Care. Edited by Goldman W, Feldman S. San Francisco, CA, Jossey-Bass, 1993, pp 81–87

Fink PJ: Psychiatrists' roles in managed care programs. Hosp Community Psychiatry 44:723–724, 1993

Fink PJ, Dubin WR: No free lunch: limitations on psychiatric care in HMOs. Hosp Community Psychiatry 42:363–365, 1991

Gabbard GO: The big chill: the transition from residency to managed care nightmare. Academic Psychiatry 16:119–126, 1992

Gabbard GO, Takahashi T, Davidson J, et al: A psychodynamic perspective on the clinical impact of insurance review. Am J Psychiatry 148:318–323, 1991

Gillig PM, Hillard JR, Bell J, et al: The psychiatric emergency service holding area: effect on utilization of inpatient resources. Am J Psychiatry 146:369–372, 1989

Jellinek MS, Nurcombe B: Two wrongs don't make a right: managed care, mental health, and the marketplace. JAMA 270:1737–1739, 1993

Lazarus A: A proposal for psychiatric collaboration in managed care. Am J Psychotherapy 48:600–609, 1994

Lazarus A: Managed care practice and psychiatric deaths: must we assign blame? Administration and Policy in Mental Health, 22(4):457–461, 1995

Lazarus A: Leased psychiatric beds. Psychiatr Serv, in press

Moore RA, Moore C, Lindley C: Hospital-based HMO: an outpatient study. Psychiatr Hosp 23:79–82, 1992

Olden KW, Johnson MP: A "facilitated" model of inpatient psychiatric care. Hosp Community Psychiatry 44:879–882, 1993

Patterson DY: Managed care: an approach to rational psychiatric treatment. Hosp Community Psychiatry 41:1092–1095, 1990

Pomerantz JM, Liptzin B, Carter AH, et al: The professional affiliation group: a new model for managed mental health care. Hosp Community Psychiatry 45:308–310, 1994

Psychiatric Times: Study says relationship with managed care firms improving. Psychiatric Times 10:36, 1993

Sabin JE: Clinical skills for the 1990s: six lessons from HMO practice. Hosp Community Psychiatry 42:605–608, 1991

Sederer LI, St. Clair RL: Managed health care and the Massachusetts experience. Am J Psychiatry 146:1142–1148, 1989

Westermeyer J: Problems with managed psychiatric care without a psychiatrist-manager. Hosp Community Psychiatry 42:1221–1224, 1991

Chapter 21

Do Employers Want Mental Health and Substance Abuse Benefits for Their Employees?

Dorothy E. Dugger, M.D.
Paul R. McCarthy, Ph.D.
John C. Burroughs, M.S.S., M.B.A.

Employers and other payers have increasingly come under fire from patient groups, professional associations, and government officials involved in health care reform. These groups have criticized payers (employers) for their apparent unwillingness to assume an increasing amount of the health care funding burden, especially in the area of mental health and substance abuse treatment. Some politicians have even tried to paint a caricature of employers as "the bad guys," rolling in excessive corporate profits and concerned only with profits at the expense of their employees' welfare. In fact, much of the current cost of health care is borne by employers. Employer funding decisions are therefore of prime importance. In this chapter, we explore a number of the variables affecting employers' decisions and attitudes regarding mental health and substance abuse treatment in the group health, disability, and workers' compensation arenas.

Group Health

A senior consultant with a large employee benefits consulting firm paraphrased her experience with the attitude of a number of employers toward mental health and substance abuse (MH/SA) coverage as nothing works, and nobody needs it anyway. This assessment of employer attitudes—and it is hoped the attitudes are only those of a small minority— does not take into account the wide range and complexity of factors facing employers in evaluating benefits design for employee MH/SA coverage.

Before the 1950s, MH/SA coverage was not included routinely in most insurance plans (Glaser 1991). Since then, there has been a trend toward progressive inclusion of these benefits in the health plans purchased or funded by many employers. However, traditional coverage for MH/SA has been and continues to be significantly more limited in terms of the number of inpatient days or the total dollars of coverage than the medical and surgical benefits within the same company. It is common that some companies have a very generous medical-surgical benefit (e.g., 1 million dollars or unlimited lifetime benefit), yet MH/SA benefits may be covered at a lifetime maximum of $10,000–$50,000 with annual day limits and a 20% co-payment for inpatient care, as well as limited outpatient visits, often with a higher co-payment of 50%. The "dental or mental" choice between coverages offered by some employers in a cafeteria-style or flexible benefits plan has been interpreted as implying that MH/SA care is less relevant than medical-surgical care.

It is important to identify the primary factors that may drive employers' benefits-design decisions, resulting in unequal coverage for MH/SA care. These factors include economic concerns, the employer's attitude toward employees, the employer's understanding of mental illness, and the differences between current MH/SA and medical-surgical delivery systems.

The importance of economic factors cannot be underestimated in the employer's decision-making process for all health care benefits. Health care spending in the United States has been rising dramatically. Indeed, in a recent survey conducted by Foster Higgins (a large benefits consulting firm) it was the consensus of large managed care organizations that their customers (i.e., employers) considered the price of benefits coverage over specific quality-of-care measures in guiding their purchasing decisions for health care coverage (Foster Higgins 1995).

In 1991, the Department of Health and Human Services estimated that health care spending was $738 billion, or 13.1% of gross national product (GNP), and predicted it would reach $1.61 trillion, or 16.4% of the GNP, by the year 2000 if it continued at the same rate of inflation. Despite multiple cost containment strategies, health care spending was estimated at 14.1% of the GNP in 1992 by the Congressional Budget Office. A more recent estimate predicts 1.68 trillion—18% of the GNP—will go toward health care by 2000 (Barge and Carlson 1993).

What has focused attention on MH/SA benefits coverage in particular is the fact that the rate of inflation for these benefits has been significantly greater than the double-digit rate of inflation for medical-surgical benefits. MH/SA benefit costs per employee increased 27% in 1987 and 18% in 1989. Nationally, MH/SA costs accounted on average for 10%–15% of total benefit costs. However, in some companies MH/SA costs represented between 25% and 35% of the total benefit costs. These numbers are rather astounding in view of reports placing the incidence of mental illness near 20% with approximately 3%–7% of this population in treatment at any given time. It is not surprising that employers would focus on an area where 7% of their employee population accounted for 33% of total benefit dollars. Further analysis of the costs and lengths of stay for inpatient treatment indicated that in 1985–1986, adolescent admissions accounted for 25% of inpatient admissions, 40% of inpatient days, and up to 40% of inpatient costs (Medical Care 1988). Equally disturbing to employers was evidence that 63% of adolescent admissions were for nonserious problems (The Center for the Study of Youth Policy).

There were many reasons for the increased utilization and costs in the 1970s and 1980s. The supply of MH/SA services grew, and there was a diagnosis-related group exemption for psychiatry. There was increased awareness of the need for substance abuse treatment, and specialized adolescent services were developed. A number of social factors were also active in this situation, including the proliferation of illegal drugs, the destabilization of the nuclear family caused by a high divorce rate, and the decreased stigma associated with seeking treatment. Aggressive marketing became a major force in increasing the utilization of MH/SA services, with scare tactics in public advertising for both print and broadcast media (e.g., act now or the consequences could be dire!). Some providers even paid for a prospective patient's cross-country airfare after a telephone screening interview by nonmedical personnel.

Not surprisingly, all payers, including both insurers and employers, became concerned about both the costs and the value of the services they were purchasing. The inherent value of MH/SA treatment services was not always apparent. For example, some employers found that they were paying for multiple 28-day substance abuse admissions with no observable improvement in their employee. Employers have demanded accountability for treatment, adding impetus to the quality assessment and outcomes movements.

However, their concerns also have been reflected in a tendency to restrict MH/SA benefits. This tactic met with apparent short-term success, because identified expenditures for MH/SA were more limited. Some employers attempted to manage these costs through the use of utilization review, case management, discounted provider networks, and modified benefits plans.

Another economic driver of health benefits decisions has been the ability of American industry to be competitive in the national and international marketplace. With rising health care costs, many companies found their profits eroding. A survey of *Fortune* 500 companies and 250 large nonindustrial companies indicated that between 1981 and 1983 total health care costs accounted for 24% of after-tax corporate profits (Butler and Haiselmaier 1989). Concurrently, the ability of companies to reinvest in their business has been reduced substantially, as well as the ability to develop and bring new products to market. Some small companies in highly competitive markets could not afford to offer health insurance because they would have to price their products out of the market to do so. In 1989, 26% of corporate net earnings went to cover health care costs. This figure accelerated to 45% in 1990 (Barge and Carlson 1993). Employee health care costs more than doubled between 1984 and 1991, fueled by annual increases in the double-digit range. Accordingly, health care costs in the United States represent a far more significant percentage of the GNP than in any other major industrialized country (Schieber et al. 1991).

International competition and the recession of the late 1980s and early 1990s focused the attention of employers on expense management. Limiting benefits was one of many initiatives; other cost-cutting initiatives included downsizing, doing more with less, outsourcing, and eliminating many nonessential and unprofitable activities. Although the United States ranks first in health care spending, it ranks with third-world countries and developing countries in terms of population indicators of health such as the infant mortality rate. Furthermore, consumer ratings of satisfaction with the health care system place the United States last out of 10 major democratic nations (Blendon et al. 1990).

An employer's attitude toward employees can span a continuum from highly paternalistic to complete disregard for employees and their well-being. Many rich MH/SA plans still exist with paternalistic employers, but it is with million-dollar and unlimited plans that extraordinarily high utilization and lengths of stay frequently are found. For example, one plan with unlimited benefits experienced more than 1,000 outpatient visits per 1,000 employees, and on the inpatient side, nearly 400 bed days per 1,000 employees. This further fuels employers' existing fears of expanding the demand for services by offering high-dollar coverage with low co-payments and deductibles. This fear may be well founded as it has been observed that there is unlimited demand for free services. This applies equally to MH/SA and to medical-surgical services.

An employer's understanding of mental illness may also influence coverage decisions. The views of employers reflect societal views of mental illness. Some consider MH/SA disorders to be real, viewing their treatment as equally important as the treatment of more clearly defined physical illnesses. Others regard MH/SA disorders to be character flaws or to be volitional in nature. That view has been especially prevalent in regard to substance abuse disorders. For a number of employers, mental illness is seen as a black box, totally mysterious in nature. The latter conceptualization is unfortunately reinforced by the excessive use of technical jargon in the mental health field as well as structural differences between the current MH/SA and medical-surgical delivery systems.

The MH/SA delivery system is substantially different from the medical-surgical delivery system in several key ways. These differences only reinforce employers' concerns regarding the value of treatment services. There is no natural triage point, such as the family physician in medical-surgical services, who ideally determines the diagnosis and the need for specialty treatment. Numerous studies indicate that primary care medical physicians are not effective for MH/SA assessment and triage. Generally, they tend to misdiagnose and undertreat mental illness (see Chapter 3). Clearly, if misdiagnosed, these disorders cannot be effectively treated. More often, however, patients are self-diagnosed and self-referred, frequently on the basis of the "mental illness of the week" showcased on daytime TV talk shows. Aggressive advertisements and toll-free telephone screening lines are other common sources of patient self-diagnosis and referral.

Another difference between MH/SA and medical-surgical services is that MH/SA diagnoses often do not indicate the appropriate treatment or provider. Psychosocial factors may significantly shape the course of the illness, and many competing philosophies of treatment claim equal effectiveness despite the lack of outcome data or data to the contrary.

The mental health treatment system is complex, with numerous treatment levels on the continuum of care. Many patients need assistance in negotiating the system to receive necessary and appropriate care. Additionally, there is substantial variation in cost within and among types of providers and across types of treatment.

One factor frequently cited as a cause of rising cost and inpatient utilization has been the poor design of the benefit plan itself. With relatively rich inpatient benefits with a low co-payment, limited outpatient benefits with a high co-payment, and inadequate coverage for intermediate levels of treatment, the plan itself was set up to provide incentives toward the overuse of the most intensive level of care. However, this traditional MH/SA benefits plan reflected a different assumption about the nature and purpose of health insurance. Originally, health insurance, unlike other forms of insurance, was designed to provide steady cash flow to hospitals in the Great Depression. The acute-care front-end coverage was never meant to protect patients from catastrophic illness and financial loss. Subsequently, health insurance evolved into a vehicle to cover routine care. By comparison, Americans do not expect their auto insurance to pay for fuel and regular upkeep and repairs. As a result of heavy subsidization of health care costs by employers and state governments, Americans are largely unaware of the cost of medical care. Consequently, they have come to believe they are entitled to receive the best care, regardless of cost or efficacy, and they have the expectation that it should cost them nothing. Again, there is endless demand for free services.

As indicated earlier, restricting benefits met with apparent success. The problems incumbent on excessive restriction of MH/SA benefits are significant but largely invisible to the employer. The invisible costs include a shifting of costs from MH/SA providers to the medical-surgical arena, where MH/SA problems are often misdiagnosed and inappropriately treated, thereby significantly increasing total health care costs. There is also lost productivity, absenteeism, higher cost, longer duration, and increased frequency of short- and long-term disability claims, as well as cost shifting to the workers' compensation system.

Many employers, however, have tried to address the issues of early detection of mental illness and intervention. This effort is reflected in the increased use of employee assistance programs (EAP) and the expansion of their role from the evaluation and treatment of only substance abuse problems to now include mental health problems, with some offering financial and legal counseling as well. There is a strong movement among employers to use EAPs as gatekeepers. However, although EAPs often do utilization review, the employer's primary motive is not cost containment. Rather, the employer views the benefit of using an EAP to be early diagnosis and referral to treatment, the underlying assumption being that this will avoid more costly medical problems in the future. In fact, employers with EAPs reported significantly higher medical costs ($272 versus $200 per employee) according to a 1994 Foster Higgins survey (Foster Higgins 1995). However, it appears EAPs may have been effective in lowering average per-employee cost increases.

Workers' Compensation and Disability

In the workers' compensation and disability arena, the question of what MH/SA coverage employers would like is moot. Employers rarely have control over the care and treatment of their injured employees, because workers' compensation benefits are state mandated and vary from state to state. There are also differences between the workers' compensation and the health care benefits systems in objectives, goals, and administration, as well as economic and social differences. Although integrating the two systems may be desirable, there are many challenges to combining them (Meszaros 1994). However, employers and their carriers are increasingly turning to managed care techniques used in the group health industry and applying those tools to the workers' compensation arena (Reagan 1994). Assuming such tools can be used under state law, managed care organizations must adapt to the unique employer incentives present in the workers' compensation system.

Traditional wisdom in the business, insurance, and employer communities holds that MH/SA is generally insignificant in workers' compensation and disability because stress claims account for only 2% of these costs. Although it is recognized that stress claims pose a significant problem in states such as California, Pennsylvania, and Florida, the nonpsychiatric community has not recognized the tremendous role of psychosocial factors in workers' compensation claims.

Workers' compensation costs have been spiraling out of control. Overall costs in workers' compensation increased from $34.8 billion in 1986 to $47.1 billion in 1988, a 35% increase in a 2-year period. In 1990, job-related injuries cost approximately $60 billion in direct workers' compensation expenses. Notably, that represents a doubling in the past 5 years, and estimates are that costs may double again by 1995 to more than $100 billion, according to a 1990 study (Tillinghast 1991). In contrast to group health costs, for every dollar spent in direct cost (e.g., medical treatment) there are two dollars spent in indirect costs for workers' compensation claims. Part of the indirect cost is attributable to lost productivity and part is the indemnity, or wage replacement, cost. According to a Gallup survey sponsored by the New York Business Group on Health (Allen 1990; Mangan 1991; McDonald 1990), approximately 25% of workers in the United States suffer some kind of health problem related to stress at an estimated annual cost of $150 billion. It is estimated that if workers' stress claims continue to grow at the current rates through the 1990s they will lead all other claims. For many employers, indeed, stress claims are considered to be among the top 10 work-related problems, given that they are roughly twice as expensive as the average industrial injury claim.

Stress Claims

Stress claims fall under the occupational disease category. Occupational disease is defined by the lack of any kind of single, identifiable, traumatic onset and includes cumulative trauma (e.g., carpal tunnel syndrome) and mental illness. There are three classifications of stress injuries.

1. Physical-mental claims: an initial physical injury with subsequent psychological sequelae.
2. Mental-physical claims: a physical disease ostensibly resulting from stress (e.g., cardiac disease, hypertension, and ulcers).
3. Mental-mental claim: purely mental illness or injury caused by emotional or psychological factors. These mental-mental injuries sometimes are referred to as *nonscheduled disabilities* simply because they are based on subjective complaints, often without a clearly defined accidental onset.

It is interesting to note that the number of nonspecific complaints increases as the average age of the workforce increases. For each 10-year increase in age of the workforce, nonspecific complaints increase by 15%.

There are generally two types of compensable mental injury. One is the single traumatic event in which there is a specific job-related event that ostensibly causes the stress. This event can include something as minor as being reprimanded by a supervisor or narrowly missing getting into an accident if one is driving as part of one's duties. These are less frequent than the gradual job stress category claims, in which the psychological injury has developed over time as a result of general employment conditions. These mental-mental claims have really only become significant in the workers' compensation market in the past 15 years since they have become eligible for compensation. For example, there was a 700% increase in stress claims between 1979 and 1988 in California because of enabling legislation. Currently, only 10 states require a physical injury as a prerequisite for claiming any occupational mental injury. Legislation clearly influences the prevalence and incidence of stress claims in any particular state. California, Pennsylvania, and Florida have traditionally been particularly open to considering any type of stress claim. California's law is so permissive that the employee's general level of emotional health or disease is irrelevant, the fact that another person was not upset by the same traumatic event is irrelevant, and in the gradual stress category it is not relevant that there may have been emotional stressors outside the job such as marital difficulty, substance abuse, or financial problems that may have contributed to the illness.

Many of the data on stress claims come from California because California was the forerunner in this type of legislation and has had the most experience. Overall, workers' compensation costs in California in 1989 accounted for $5.3 billion in disability payments, 10% higher than they were in 1988. Stress claims accounted for $389 million, which was paid to employees and unemployed workers for various stress complaints ranging from headache to insomnia to depression. California has the second highest insurance rate in the nation, second only to Montana, which has a large high-risk segment that includes industries such as mining and timber. Adding to the cost of stress claims in California is the high litigation rate (98%). This rate is greater than twice the rate of other injury claims, and 90% of those cases actually receive some kind of compensation payment, with the average cost being $13,002. One example of the extent to which stress claims can influence a business is that of Security Metal Corporation, which, like other companies, had to lay off employees in the past few years because of the poor economy. Of those laid-off employees, 30% claimed mental stress caused by the layoff and filed for claims for up to $25,000 each. The insurance company settled the claims for up to $10,000 each. Consequently, the company moved out of California because it could no longer sustain those costs. Other examples of frivolous claims include the woman who was traumatized and on disability for 2 years as a result of the stress of hearing a sexist remark while on the planning committee for the company picnic (a fellow employee jokingly suggested having a wet T-shirt contest) (Katz 1990). In another example, a bank guard accidentally shot and killed a bank patron. He was so distressed, he immediately shot and killed himself. The family filed a stress claim, contending he would not have committed suicide were it not for the job stress (Nordstrom 1990).

There are a number of reasons why workers' compensation stress claims and costs have increased so rapidly. There is cost shifting from group health, where there are many cost controls, to workers' compensation. Mental illnesses do not go away because benefits have been curtailed. People with mental health problems may go to their family physician with physical or psychological complaints. Mental illnesses are often underdiagnosed or inappropriately treated in this setting. Alternatively, there is an incentive to attribute problems to work because workers' compensation is the last blank check with first-dollar coverage (no deductibles), no co-payments, no preexisting condition exclusion, and no waiting period. Many states have limited the extent to which managed care techniques can be applied to workers' compensation, so this arena may provide greater freedom of choice as well as more generous benefits for the treatment of mental illness. In addition, provider income limitation resulting from cost-containment measures and federal government initiatives, such as the resource-based relative-value scale and diagnosis-related groups, may result in some providers cost shifting to workers' compensation insurance coverage in an effort to maintain income.

The nature of our economy is changing. The growth area is service rather than manufacturing, and it is in service industries that stress claims are most likely to occur. More younger women are in the workforce and tend to be employed in white-collar positions in the service industry. Not by coincidence, this is also the group most likely to file a workers' compensation stress claim.

The United States economy has been in a recession/depression over the past several years. In American culture, workers are considered dispensable and often laid off, although they may be rehired when the economy improves. Given that the current economic climate is one characterized by reorganizations, downsizing, and layoffs, it is not surprising that people are stressed by changes in the workplace, especially by anything that seems to threaten their job security. For some employees, the workers' compensation system offers a way to maintain income with dignity in the event that job loss is imminent. Workers' compensation is being used, in effect, as an economic safety net.

Litigation is also an important contributor to the increase in workers' compensation costs, particularly stress claims. As mentioned previously, there is a great deal of litigation in the area of stress claims, much more than for other occupational diseases or industrial injuries. Litigation does tend to prolong a case. The relationship of a psychiatric illness to the job may also be somewhat more subjective and harder to quantify than physical illness, and that fact contributes to the increased litigation and higher costs. A number of companies settle because they do not want to get involved in costly litigation with an uncertain outcome, a circumstance that also inadvertently encourages fraud and abuse in this area.

Malingering, fraud, and abuse have contributed to rising costs in workers' compensation and disability. Malingering in this context refers to the exaggeration of a disability for the purpose of prolonging benefits. Taricco distinguished between fraud and abuse. He defined *abuse* as "an exaggerated statement, willfully made, for material gain, with the intent to confuse." *Fraud* is defined as "a false statement, willfully made, for material gain, with the intent to deceive" (Greenwood and Taricco 1992, p. 27). In both cases, the intent is to access benefits that would not otherwise be available.

Thomas Jacob and Associates (Chelius et al. 1992) has estimated that the large employers pay at least $1 million annually in unnecessary disability, with fraud being a key contributor to this problem. Notably 20% of claims account for 80% of the total of disability benefits. Examples were plentiful in a feature aired on *World News Tonight* (July 3, 1991). The topic was California "stress claims mills," which is a less than complimentary description of medical clinics and legal offices that specialize in recruiting claimants and filing stress claims. In one example, 40 of 90 employees of the same company filed stress claims on the same day through the same legal office with nearly identical symptoms. At the time, California law required only 10% of the illness to be work related.

The problem of fraud had become so rampant in California that there was an antifraud law (SB1218) enacted that made it a felony to be involved in any kind of fraudulent workers' compensation claim. It penalized physicians and lawyers who employ case finders to identify clients and recruit them to file workers' compensation claims. If convicted, they could be sentenced to 5 years in jail and fined $50,000 or double the amount of the fraud. The law made it easier to disbar lawyers and revoke the licenses of physicians involved in fraud, and it penalized physicians who publish misleading ads about compensable injuries. This antifraud law assesses employers and insurers about $3 million annually for the purpose of fraud investigation and prosecution. California had also enacted workers' compensation reform (AB971), which bars stress claims in the first 6 months on the job.

The best management of stress claims is prevention, and this is most effective at the employer level. Attitude and employee satisfaction are major determinants of whether an employee will bring a workers' compensation stress claim. Most workers' compensation stress claims are filed by employees who are dissatisfied with the way the company or people in the company have treated them and handled their claims.

In a 1990 study (Tillinghast 1991), it was noted that 87% of employers who use integrated group health, disability, and workers' compensation benefits and data systems find them to be effective, although only 17% of employers used them. A study by Federal Express, which used integrated data capabilities to track employees' benefit usage, was informative. In tracking mental health claims for 4 years, the company found that 89% of employees used no mental health benefits, but 88% of mental health claims expenditures in accident and health insurance coverage were attributable to 2.3% of its employees. Of those employees in the high-utilization group, two-thirds of them had filed more than two workers' compensation stress claims. Federal Express targeted these high users for interventions in terms of education and health promotion and approached them from the perspective of helping them to protect themselves as valuable human capital. Notably, Federal Express's interventions focused on the employees' attitude toward themselves as valuable resources as well as specific medical educational intervention.

Purely Physical or Mental-Physical?

What do MH/SA issues have to do with physical claims? Ostensibly, nothing, or so says the traditional view of physical injury and disability. However, although safety and prevention programs (including ergonomic improvements) have contributed significantly to the physical safety of our working environment, each year there are more workplace injuries and illnesses at greater cost. More than 9 million people annually suffer work-related illness and injury, with workers' compensation claims costs increasing an average of 14% per year since 1976. These claims costs now account for more than 20% of payroll expenses in most industries. Disability, both job related and non–job related, is a growing concern in our workforce as more working-age people become disabled. Although the working-age population grew 38% between 1959 and 1984, the number of people in this working-age category with severe disabilities grew 158%. If the workplace is physically safer, why do we have such an alarming increase in illness and claims, whether they are workers' compensation or disability? The missing variables that account for this discrepancy may be biopsychosocial in nature.

The effects of mental illness and substance abuse on physical injury and recovery are not unknown in the MH/SA community; the literature is filled with theorists. Weiss and English (1949) defined the area of psychosomatic medicine, and Hans Selye elaborated on it in *The Stress of Life* in 1956. Subsequently, in 1967 Holmes and Rahe developed the Social Readjustment Rating Scale to quantify the stressors of life and predict the likelihood of developing a physical illness. In 1977, George Engle coined the term *biopsychosocial* to describe an approach to understanding the sick person; this term became more popular under the concept of holistic health. With this concept came the recognition that stress and coping style influenced the etiology and onset of disease, the course and outcome of illness, the utilization of medical care, and a patient's compliance with treatment and response to treatment. As Richardson (1945) wrote, "Disease is no longer an entity limited to one person . . . and transmissible; rather, disease is an integral part of the continuous process of living" (p. 76). Subsequently, we have seen the emergence of the field of psychoneuroimmunology. For example, various forms of positive imaging in cancer patients have been effectively employed as adjunctive therapy (Ader 1988; Barber 1982).

The concepts of behavioral medicine have to some extent permeated the business community and the workers' compensation and disability systems, as reflected in the mental-physical category, which includes cardiac disease, hypertension, and stress ulcers. However, the significant role that psychosocial factors play in supposedly purely physical injuries such as back pain has not been widely addressed. Emotional factors can affect this purely physical system in several ways. Parallel to Weiss and English's (1949) classifications, depression and anxiety can be a normal reaction to physical illness, and physical injury can exacerbate a current emotional problem or reactivate a past one, which then makes recovery more difficult.

Numerous studies have been done linking behavioral and psychological factors, including stress, anxiety, fatigue, and drug and alcohol use, to performance decrements and a subsequent increase in the risk of accidents. According to Jones (1984), on the basis of an analysis by National Institute of Occupational Safety and Health, the National Safety Council, and the College of Insurance, in 1982 work-related accidents cost $32 billion, and in 80% of the accidents an inability to cope with stress played a significant role. In addition, psychosomatic problems are estimated to contribute to more than 60% of long-term employee disability cases (Shapiro 1985).

Dr. Alexander Hirschfield studied hundreds of workers injured in industrial accidents while investigating the stress-accident connection. He found that many were emotionally stressed before the injury and postulated that stress predisposes one to accidents through fatigue and impaired physical coordination and mental abilities (e.g., poor judgment, inattention, distraction, distorted perception). He also highlighted the adaptive aspect of injury in that the accident may decrease stress by focusing attention on physical symptoms rather than emotional symptoms (Mikkelson 1977).

The notion that symptoms attributed to the workplace really originated elsewhere is supported by Nelson and Sutton's (1990) work, in which distress symptoms reported before beginning a job account for most of the variance in distress symptoms on the job 9 months later. Bacharach et al. (1991) noted that the perception of work role conflict was antecedent to work-home conflict and subsequent job dissatisfaction, suggesting work and home factors are not independent.

Many patients with work-related injuries have a major depression. The failure to diagnose depression in these patients results in long and costly diagnostic and therapeutic procedures that can also cause iatrogenic harm. Hypochondriac patterns are reinforced, and subsequently secondary gain (such as disability payments, dependence on the health care system for social support, and manipulation of social relationships) only serves to maintain physical disability and dysfunction.

Notably, somatization in the United States is correlated with lower socioeconomic status, blue-collar workers, rural living, social isolation, lower educational levels, and affiliation with traditional ethnic groups that discourage expression of emotion (Katon et al. 1992). Many of these variables describe the population that is likely to submit physical injury workers' compensation claims. Physical complaints have social efficacy in that they provide socially legitimate ways to receive and accept nurturance, especially in families or cultural groups that do not encourage the expression of emotional distress. Somatization frequently represents a combination of psychological, societal, and economic concerns. This becomes a problem when these concerns become identified as purely physical in nature. It is clear that the workers' compensation system partially functions to address social and emotional problems that are not primarily a function of employment. As such, managed care mechanisms can and should be made part of this system.

Conclusion

Employers' attitudes regarding the funding of treatment in the MH/SA area are varied and may differ among the medical delivery and payment systems of group health, disability, and workers' compensation. Employers' economic concerns about health care, and especially MH/SA treatment, are noteworthy because these costs may be determinants of the employers' ability to remain in business. Wariness on the part of the employer about the cost and value of MH/SA treatment is understandable, given the blatant examples of fraud and abuse in group health, disability, and workers' compensation. The workers' compensation health care system is, in fact, the last remaining blank check health care system in the United States.

Increasingly, employers have been asked to take responsibility for virtually complete funding of a health care system characterized by perverse financial incentives for overdelivery of high-cost, high-intensity care and with expectations by users for extensive treatment, regardless of the cost or efficacy of treatment. The question, "Do employers want mental health and substance abuse benefits for their employees?" may be more appropriately subsumed under the issues of who should fund health care and how should the limited financial and medical resources in our society be allocated. Until these issues are settled, employers will continue to look to managed care organizations for substantial relief.

References

A. Foster Higgins: 1994 National Survey of Employer-Sponsored Health Plans. New York, NY, A. Foster Higgins and Company, April 1995

Ader R: The placebo effect as a conditioned response, in Experimental Foundations of Behavioral Medicine: Conditioning Approaches. Edited by Ader R, Weiner H, Baum A. Hillsdale, NJ, Lawrence, Erlbaum Associates, 1988, pp 47–66

Allen DS: Less Stress, Less Litigation. personnel. January 1990, pp 32–35

Bacharach SB, Bamberger P, Conley S: Work–home conflict among nurses and engineers: mediating the impact of role stress on burnout and satisfaction at work. Journal of Organizational Behavior 12:39–53, 1991

Barber TX: Hypnosuggestive procedures for the treatment of clinical pain, in Handbook of Clinical Health Psychology. Edited by Millon T, Green C, Meagher R. New York, Plenum, 1982, pp 521–560

Barge BN, Carlson JG: The Executive's Guide to Controlling Health Care and Disability Costs. New York, Wiley, 1993

Blendon R, Leitman R, Morrison I, et al: Satisfaction with health systems in ten nations. Health Aff 11:185–192, 1990

Butler S, Haiselmaier E: Critical Issues: A National Health System for America. Washington, DC, Heritage Foundation, 1989

Chelius J, Galvin D, Owens P: Disability: It's more expensive than you think. Business and Health, March 1992, pp 78–84

Engle GL: The need for a new medical model: a challenge for biomedicine. Science 196:129–136, 1977

Glaser WA: Health Insurance in Practice. San Francisco, CA, Jossey-Bass, 1991

Greenwood J, Taricco A: Workers' Compensation Health Care Cost Containment. Horsham, PA, LRP Publication, 1992

Holmes TH, Rahe RH: The social readjustment rating scale. J Psychosom Res 11:213–218, 1967

Jones JW: Managing Stress to prevent worker accidents. National Underwriter, August 3, 1984, pp 18–19

Katon W, Kleinman A, Rosen G: Depression and somatization: a review. Am J Med 72:127–135, 1992

Katz DM: Workers comp sex cases help to fuel frequency rise, lawyer says. National Underwriter: Property & Casualty/Risk & Benefits Management 26:2, 1990

Mangan JF: Stress related claims: Causes and Controls. Best's Review, March 1991, pp 68, 70, 99, 100

McDonald M: You can control your disability costs, Business and Health, May 1990, pp 21–36

Medical Care: August 26, 1988, p. 8

Meszaros EC: Fixing the leaks. Managed Healthcare 4(8):12–16, 1994

Mikkelson EJ: The psychology of disability. Psychiatric Annals 7:74–95, 1977

Nelson D, Sutton C: Chronic work stress and coping: a longitudinal study and suggested new directions. Acad Manage J 33:859, 1990

Nordstrom RR: Suicide as a compensable injury under workers' comp statutes: a review of judicial decisions. Employee Relat Law J 16(1):37–55, 1990

Reagan ME: Managed workers' comp is final frontier. Managed Healthcare 4(8):26–27, 1994

Richardson HB: Patients Have Families. New York, Commonwealth Fund, 1945

Schieber GJ, Poullier JP, Greenwald LM: Health care systems in twenty-four countries. Health Aff 12:45–55, 1991

Selye H: The Stress of Life, revised edition. New York, McGraw-Hill, 1978

Shapiro E: Stress: The New Disability Claim. Minneapolis-St. Paul Business 3(1): Section 1, p. 1, April 24, 1985

Tillinghast (Towers Perrin) Survey Report. Responding to the workers' compensation crisis: can employers manage and control costs? St. Louis, MO, Tillinghast, January 1991, pp 2–21

Weiss E, English OS: Psychosomatic Medicine. Philadelphia, PA, WB Saunders, 1949

The Center for the Study of Youth Policy: Youth Services Study. Ann Arbor, MI, University of Michigan Press, 1989

Chapter 22

Can Psychiatrists Become Efficient Managers?

Arthur Lazarus, M.D.

Most of the methods suggested for reforming health care in the United States have been based on the principles of managed care. Because of the dangers inherent in managed care practice, many of those proposals have met with skepticism. This skepticism is particularly evident in regard to the mental health field, where managed care has been criticized for disrupting the therapeutic relationship, restricting access to treatment, lowering quality of care, and excluding seriously mentally ill persons from treatment.

Rarely has managed care been presented in a positive light that emphasizes the opportunities created by this new practice—innovative patient care, outcome-driven treatment, and strategic management of resources. If the Eastern philosophers are correct in their belief that a crisis represents both danger and opportunity, then the role of psychiatrists in managed care organizations will be critical in determining which of those two extremes prevails throughout the period of health care reform and in subsequent years.

Psychiatrists have been underused in many managed care programs (Fink and Dubin 1991; Westermeyer 1991), prompting a few managed care firms

---

Reprinted, in part, from Lazarus A: "Opportunities for Psychiatrists in Managed Care Organizations." *Hospital and Community Psychiatry* 45:1206–1210, 1994. Used with permission.

to "elevate" the role of psychiatrists. In organizations that have recognized the value of psychiatrists, psychiatrists have been given greater supervisory responsibilities, more time to see patients, and an expanded role in conducting psychotherapy, not simply prescribing medication.

However, apart from rendering direct patient care for managed care organizations, psychiatrists' potential to contribute in mental health administration remains largely untapped. Mental health management promises to be an area of growth and opportunity for psychiatrists, and they may wish to explore this area further by working for managed care organizations. This topic was discussed briefly in Chapter 1 and merits further consideration now.

Are Physician-Managers Necessary?

One of the great ironies of the American health care crisis is that, in anticipation of the passage of definitive legislation prior to 1995, widespread changes occurred in medical delivery systems even though legislation was not enacted. These changes included mainstreaming Americans into managed care plans, consolidating health care organizations, and requiring health maintenance organizations (HMOs) and health providers to measure treatment outcomes and other quality-related activities. Although the final chapter on health reform has yet to be written, one thing seems certain: the new health care system will most likely be highly regulated, and oversight will be provided by administrators with variable or no clinical experience. In such a highly regulated society, the need for effective physician-managers should be obvious.

The potential domination of health care by business practices has led many physicians to protest health reform proposals fashioned by bureaucrats. Noted medical authority Arnold Relman, M.D., (1993) stated, "Physicians should be preparing now for a new health care system . . . . They should also tell their congressional representatives that the new legislation must pay careful attention to the role of physicians in the health plans" (p. 1,576).

The public appears to be equally concerned about the role of physicians in managed care plans. O'Rourke (1993) commented, "The President has put a lawyer in charge of making doctors cheaper. Next he'll be trying to get our grass mowed for less by calling the plumber to come have a word with the boy who does the lawn" (p. 20). Brookhiser (1994) was equally sarcastic and wrote, "The American health system is the best in the world. It has saved the life of people I know, more and more of them as I grow older. I'm not going to dilute it to please some power-tripping bureaucrat who got his law degree when Abbey Road was released" (p. 64).

The diluted system that Mr. Brookhiser refers to contains an insufficient number of physicians in key management positions. The American Medical Association (AMA) estimates that only about 2% of physicians in the United

States devote most of their time to management (Roback et al. 1994). In a 1986 survey (Schenke 1986) of 848 physicians identified as administrators, fewer than 14% had a degree other than an M.D., and only 1% had a master's in business administration (M.B.A.). A more recent survey (Lloyd and Lyons 1995), however, showed that the number of physicians pursuing an M.B.A. degree has increased. The 1990s may indeed become the decade of the physician-manager (Lazarus 1995).

However, there are several reasons why recruiting physicians into management may be difficult. The reasons include a shortage of physician-executive role models for medical students, a fear of leaving practice, a lack of administrative skills, and uncertainty about how to interface with nonphysician managers. Some of these factors may also explain why the development of management skills in psychiatrists has lagged behind the acquisition of clinical skills in general (Silver and Marcos 1989).

Physician-Manager Role Models

Role models in medicine may significantly influence career choices of medical students (Kassebaum and Szenas 1994). Medical students are rarely exposed, however, to physician leaders in their formative years of medical school. Their contact with physicians during the first 2 years is limited primarily to physicians engaged in research and teaching. In the remaining 2 years, although medical students gain wide exposure to clinical faculty and various specialists, the teaching emphasis is on individual patient care rather than the management of patient populations and medical systems. Furthermore, what little opportunity medical students do have to interact with physician-managers (for example, deans and department chairpersons) is often viewed as irrelevant or is unappreciated.

Because the primary goal of medical school is to teach students factual information and how to integrate that information into clinical practice, management theory and office practice skills are not given a high priority. Even medical schools that offer a combined M.D.–D.O./M.B.A. degree generally contract the M.B.A. teaching component to a graduate school of business. Medical students who pursue a combined degree typically find the curriculum demanding and a deterrent to their clinical training.

Also, the value of a business education early in one's career may be questioned. As medical schools gear their curricula toward educating primary care physicians, they may be less likely to offer important instruction in office and practice management. Perhaps the best a medical student can hope for early in his or her career is to be fortunate to have a clinical preceptor with business savvy who imparts administrative know-how and management skills. For most students, the initial experience in administration will not come until residency, and then only if they become chief resident.

Medicine as a Career

It seems incredible that a college student seeking advice about a career in medicine would alternatively consider a career in business, but this is precisely what happened when surgeon James M. McGreevy (1994) was approached by a college student and was asked whether the student should pursue an M.B.A. degree or an M.D. degree. Dr. McGreevy said, "As a result of this interaction, I became more acutely aware of the public opinion change that is driving students away from medical careers" (p. 32). Increasingly, it seems, physicians are having difficulty mustering enthusiasm about their profession, especially when it involves recommending medicine as a career to their own children (Wehbé 1994).

A fall from the proverbial pedestal (Siegler 1993) appears to be only one of many factors that have discouraged college students from pursuing medical careers. In fact, many of the concerns voiced by college students about practicing medicine, such as threats of malpractice litigation and loss of autonomy as a result of managed care, persist into practice and are magnified by other worries such as increasing third-party interference, competition from other physicians, and personal problems. More than ever, the choice of a specialty appears to be determined by lifestyles and economic considerations (Rosenthal et al. 1994). Furthermore, once established in practice, all physicians are susceptible to burnout and disillusionment with medicine.

Leaving Practice

The decision to leave clinical practice for a career in management must be considered carefully. Common reasons for pursuing nonclinical careers include boredom and disillusionment; increasing interference from third parties; increased threats of malpractice; and personal and financial considerations such as competition from other physicians, erratic work hours, health problems, and aging and retirement (Crane 1988). However, many physician-managers maintain a small private practice, if only to maintain credibility among their peers.

One psychiatrist, a regional medical director of a large managed care organization, coined the term "recovering" clinician (Bennett 1993, p. 45). Another psychiatrist nearly went into management because she was exhausted from dealing with hospital politics, cost-containment edicts, and turf battles. She commented that "my work is challenging, but I feel agitated most of the time" (Crane 1988, p. 133).

The AMA (1993) published a guide for physicians contemplating leaving practice. The AMA and physician search firms have been flooded with inquiries from disenchanted physicians interested in management careers. Practicing physicians who feel pulled toward the challenges of leadership, as opposed to those who feel pushed into management, usually experience less stress and anxiety when making the transition. Physicians who have "outgrown" their specialty or even medicine as a career may find medical management a rewarding alternative to practice.

Perhaps the most difficult part of leaving practice is finding the courage to change and explaining one's motives to friends, family, and colleagues. However, internal and external resistances to change can be overcome. It is not uncommon for physicians considering leaving practice to seek guidance from career counselors, support groups for career changers, and psychotherapists. Others may benefit from courses in conflict resolution and negotiation. According to the AMA (1993), the pressure to not change—to stay in medicine at all cost—may be more unbearable than the pressure for the alternative, switching careers.

Profile of a Physician-Manager

Despite differences that mark medical professionals, there are commonalities among physicians who choose careers in medical management (Hodge and Grebenschikoff 1988). They tend to have a genuine interest in management and are drawn to administrative responsibilities. Although most physician-managers are initially attracted to the practice of medicine, they eventually feel a need to move beyond one-on-one patient care. One administrator, formerly a family practitioner, commented, "I started to realize that I was becoming a much more process-oriented, rather than individual-oriented, person. I wanted to have an impact on the entire system, as opposed to individual care" (Breisch 1994, p. 17).

Many physician-managers are portrayed as incompetent medical rejects when the reality is that they are high achievers. Another physician-executive gave this account: "The reason for my involvement in medical management is not, as some disparagingly suggest, either incapacity to remember medication doses, an inability to build and maintain a practice, or the results of ostracism from the ranks of real doctors. The reason is the maddeningly seductive belief that I would be able to 'straighten things out' if only I were at the administrative helm. This is not a fantasy unique to me. I perceive it to be the major come-on that has ensnared most of the top physician managers . . ." (Sams 1988, p. 54).

Physicians who enter the management field tend to be flexible and open to change. That is why physicians who are truly motivated to manage often have less difficulty leaving practice than those who feel pressured to leave. As creative individuals, physician-managers have a tendency to look for new challenges. They must act decisively when new opportunities are available and be able to adapt to organizational changes. Moreover, the families of physician-executives must be prepared to absorb these changes and make certain lifestyle adjustments.

Administrative physicians usually enjoy working with nonphysicians. Because physician-managers interact with many different people, good interpersonal skills are a prerequisite. The ability to negotiate deals and influence authority figures is important. Introverted physicians and those accustomed to an autonomous practice may have the greatest difficulty making the transition into medical management. Physicians who are part of a group practice or work in a multidisciplinary setting may be able to make the transition with relative ease.

Acquiring Management Skills

Trends indicate that the demand for trained physician executives, and psychiatrists in particular, will continue to increase as mental health becomes more managed and integrated into larger health care delivery systems. Psychiatrist-executives will be challenged to master the necessary managerial skills and to stay abreast of issues affecting today's competitive and changing health care environment.

Psychiatrists have the potential to make excellent managers because of their diverse clinical experience and training (Marcos and Silver 1988). Penzer (1989) noted that psychotherapists possess many of the same attributes as good administrators; for example, they tolerate ambiguity and make difficult decisions, use appropriate judgment to solve complex problems, minister to individuals who are upset and angry, and overcome individuals' resistance to change. Because of their background in mental health, psychotherapists are ideally positioned to move into administrative positions, whereas nonclinicians may lack certain interpersonal skills necessary to be effective managers.

Regrettably, business organizations tend to discriminate against psychiatrists (Lyons and Cejka 1994). This bias is most unfortunate because psychiatric training often provides a strong base in organizational theory and dynamics.

Because the road to medical management has been traveled primarily by first-generation physician-managers who accepted leadership roles that their colleagues were not interested in or were not capable of assuming, many physicians have moved into executive positions without adequate planning. For many first-generation managers, the timing and circumstances were just right for exploring new and interesting alternatives to medical practice, even if they assumed the position by default.

However, a haphazard approach to a career in medical management is not desirable. The field is becoming increasingly competitive and warrants strategic planning that includes course work and other activities to build and demonstrate management skills. On-the-job training may have been common 10 or 20 years ago, but experience alone is inadequate to progress through the ranks of management.

Some psychiatrists working in managed care organizations have pursued formal training in graduate schools of business, public health, and public administration. The M.B.A. degree is arguably the most recognized and desirable of graduate degrees aimed at educating present and future managers (Vavala 1994). The components of a typical business curriculum include marketing, finance, accounting, statistics, economics, strategic planning, human resource administration, and business law and ethics. Differences between health- and business-oriented master's programs are slight because the core requirements are nearly identical.

Executive M.B.A. programs, in which the M.B.A. degree can be achieved through an intensive 2-year course of study, are quite popular. More than 100 executive M.B.A. programs are available in the United States. These programs offer several advantages over traditional programs leading to the M.B.A. degree: there are no prerequisite "foundation" courses; they do not interrupt one's career because classes are usually given on Fridays and Saturdays; and many programs offer seminar-style classes in intimate settings conducive to learning. Most students are in their 30s and 40s and have had at least 10 years of work experience.

Executive M.B.A. students are frequently sponsored by their companies, which help pay tuition and allow time from work to attend classes. Nearly one-half of the schools offer study tours abroad. Although as many as one-fourth of the participants in executive M.B.A. programs may have a background in health care, only a few programs provide electives or specialization in health care management. Tuition for executive M.B.A. programs ranges from less than $20,000 to more than $60,000 for both years.

Physicians with management degrees earn about 7% more than those without them (Mangan 1993). A business degree, in general, can be expected to yield a greater financial return on the educational investment than a medical degree (Weeks et al. 1994). Early in the careers of physician-executives, however, compensation may not match the earnings possible in a strong clinical practice. Supplementing physicians' administrative salary with clinical practice revenue may lower the cost of placing a physician in an administrative position.

Training in management does not necessarily require an advanced degree. Educational needs may be met through selective courses, workshops, and management training seminars. Many universities offer these types of programs; those at Tulane University and the University of Wisconsin–Madison are especially noteworthy. Additional training may also be obtained through seminars offered by various professional organizations, such as the American Psychiatric Association, the American College of Physician Executives, the American Managed Care and Review Association, and the Institute for Behavioral Healthcare, to name a few.

The Transition From Medicine to Management

Changing careers may be intellectually stimulating and genuinely invigorating, but it entails many risks (Lawson 1994). For example, to progress in management, frequent job changes may be necessary, unlike private practice, where stability is the norm. Also, the corporate culture may be ruthless. Job security may be threatened by downsizing, layoffs, and changes in management and organization. The possibility of mergers, acquisitions, spinoffs, and other paradigm shifts also creates instability. Finally, with few exceptions, psychiatrists employed by managed care organizations ultimately report to nonphysician managers. This situation not only can cause tension but also can make mistakes by physicians more visible in light of their being outnumbered by other managerial staff.

Psychiatrists who have become demoralized as managed care has eroded their autonomy may be no more autonomous working for a managed care organization. Also, those who have decried the intrusion of third-party payers may unconsciously experience working for them as "identification with the aggressor." Other realities that confront physician executives are described in Table 22–1.

The most serious challenge awaiting physician-managers is not mastery of the job; rather, it is the ability to develop fruitful and collegial relationships with nonphysician managers (see Chapter 26). There are several reasons for differences between physicians and managers. First and most important is that physicians receive their training in medical school and residency, whereas managers are trained primarily in graduate schools of business. Second, physicians and managers tend to have different value systems. Physicians are more sympathetic to patients and have a lifetime obligation to uphold the Hippocratic oath. Managers are more likely to be interested in financial matters and protecting the company from adverse economic forces. Third, physicians and managers generally have different psychological dispositions. Physicians tend to be introverted, feeling, and perceiving, whereas administrators tend to be extroverted, thinking,

Table 22–1. Realities confronting psychiatrists as managers

The business world is significantly different from the clinical practice world.
Management does not recognize physician entitlement.
Geographical moves may be necessary for career advancement.
Compensation may be less than earnings from clinical practice.
Psychiatrist-executives must continually sell themselves.
A graduate degree other than a medical degree may be necessary for some positions.
Business organizations tend to discriminate against psychiatrists.
Job security is never guaranteed.
Psychiatrist-executives may feel as if they're teaming with the "enemy."
Psychiatrist-executives often report to nonphysician clinicians or to nonmedical personnel.
The desire to see patients may continue to exist and even create administrative conflicts.

Source. Lyons MF, Cejka S: "Getting a firm grip on the realities for physician executives." *Physician Executive* 20(6):8–12, 1994. Adapted with permission.

and judging (O'Connor and Shewchuk 1993). Appreciation of these differences, however, may lead to effective collaboration between physicians and managers.

Psychiatrists working in managed care organizations may benefit from studying relationships between physicians and administrators in other health care systems. The two most widely studied systems are large corporations (Walsh 1987) and hospitals (Shortell 1991), especially emerging physician-hospital organizations. Financial conflicts of interest appear to be inherent in both systems, and organizational demands often intrude on physicians' obligations to individual employees and patients. For example, corporate medical directors are often faced with the dilemma of diagnosing work-related illness in employees, knowing that their company is likely to resist this interpretation. Similarly, physicians employed by managed care organizations must deal with thorny utilization issues that dramatically affect the company's profits (Boren 1994).

Indeed, disputes over payment for hospital services under mental health carve-out programs have been described in the literature (Lazarus 1993). One skeptic asked, "To what extent does 'managed care' mean managed billing that raises costs as it lowers payments for medical services?" (Light 1994, p. 498). The answer to that question may depend in part on whether physicians in managed care organizations are co-opted by fiscal concerns. The black box of medical decision making must be replaced by explicit utilization criteria, and biased decisions must be eliminated in favor of decisions based on reasoned fairness.

Hospital-physician relationships have been fraught with conflict for most of this century. The advent of managed care appears to have exacerbated traditional hospital-physician conflicts, particularly among younger physicians (Burns et al. 1993). The new competitive environment has reduced physician control over medical care decisions, pressured physicians to transfer patients or discharge them prematurely, and second-guessed physicians' use of certain tests and ancillary services. As managed care organizations become entwined with physician-hospital organizations, as is likely to happen under current health reform proposals, the quality of physician leadership will assume great importance. Unless managed care organizations seek out skilled medical leaders, progress in health reform may be slower than anticipated.

Responsibilities of Psychiatrists in Managed Care Organizations

Psychiatrists may be employed by managed care organizations in various capacities, from utilization reviewer to medical director to chief executive and owner of a managed care company. Employment may be part time or full time, depending on the preference of the psychiatrist and the needs of the company. The American Psychiatric Association (1989) recommended that psychiatric medical directors of staff-model HMOs spend 4 hours per week of administrative time per 10,000 covered lives. However, unlike psychiatrists in HMOs, those in other types of managed care firms are likely to find themselves at a disadvantage in competing for an adequate voice in their organizations. Nonetheless, the following areas appear to be fertile ground for psychiatrists who wish to do administrative work.

Utilization Management

The primary objective of psychiatrist reviewers is to ensure proper use of resources, which entails guarding against both under- and overutilization, ensuring timely and appropriate access to treatment, and promoting a continuum-of-care model of service delivery. Various methods may be used to facilitate proper utilization, including serving as a physician adviser to case managers, speaking directly with the attending psychiatrist and members of the treatment team by telephone or on site, and reviewing medical records.

Psychiatrists, whether engaged in utilization review or in having their treatment reviewed, often view utilization management with disdain. Clearly, injustices have been perpetrated both by psychiatrists who conduct utilization review and by psychiatrists who are reviewed (see Chapter 8). Still, negative interactions must be avoided as firm limits are set on utilization (Green 1989). Peer reviewers must try to develop a working relationship with the attending psychiatrist and demonstrate competence without sounding condescending or demeaning. The attending psychiatrist should try to perceive the review as an opportunity to explain the treatment plan and not become overdefensive or uncivil. In situations where there appears to be an impasse, independent adjudication by an appeals panel of psychiatrists could be helpful (Lazarus 1994). Psychiatrists who work for managed care organizations are often instrumental in convening such panels (American Academy of Child and Adolescent Psychiatry 1993).

Quality Management

The concept of total quality improvement is somewhat new in medicine and psychiatry, although quality assurance initiatives have been mandated for federal- and state-supported programs for many years (Wells and Brook 1988). Managed care has been praised for focusing clinicians' attention on quality improvement activities designed to monitor performance, measure outcome, and assess compliance with practice guidelines (Shore 1993).

To ensure quality, psychiatrists in managed care organizations will most likely be asked to conduct focused audits and participate in the development of audits and information systems. Managed care psychiatrists will need to become familiar with computer technology and research-based decision support tools to help organizations achieve a proper balance between quality and cost containment (Gray and Glazer 1994).

Network Development

The creation of select networks of mental health providers is occurring in parallel with consolidation in the health care industry. In fact, the shift to networks is occurring rapidly throughout the United States (see Chapter 25). Because of the sheer number and heterogeneity of mental health providers, some providers will probably be prevented from seeing patients who are enrolled in managed care plans. Thus, the "profiling" of individual providers to show their success in treatment will become extremely important in the formation of mental health networks. Psychiatrists in managed care organizations will be called on to assess the potential of clinicians to be good service providers and to help develop local and national networks. Psychiatrists must become familiar with the attributes and qualifications of potential providers and understand market dynamics in those areas targeted for development.

Credentialing

Once providers are chosen for a network, they will have to be credentialed by the managed care organization. Credentialing is a fundamental risk-management activity; an ill-conceived credentialing process can create enormous liability for the company. As the *ostensible agent* of treatment, managed care companies have an obligation to thoroughly screen all candidates in their network.

Credentialing activities have become more sophisticated in the past few years. Economic credentialing, which incorporates measures of treatment and resource utilization and basic elements related to education and licensing, will serve to bond clinicians more closely to managed care organizations. Psychiatrists who participate in credentials committees for managed care organizations will be asked to evaluate clinicians in depth. In addition, psychiatrists may be asked to render an opinion about specialty capabilities of clinicians. This evaluation has become increasingly difficult given the numerous specialty areas of mental health practice without corresponding certification or qualification by subspecialty boards.

Ombudsman

Managed care psychiatrists often represent their firm to professional societies, businesses, employee assistance programs, and state and national organizations. They serve as liaisons between the managed care organization and the provider community to educate providers in managed care concepts and ensure the delivery of effective clinical services. Complaints must be investigated and occasionally discussed with senior management to achieve an equitable resolution.

When mental health services are provided through carve-out programs, the medical director of the managed mental health care company providing the services is expected to develop a relationship with his or her counterpart in the health plan that contracted for the services. Furthermore, the psychiatrist may be asked to participate in the health plan's quality management committee and help mediate conflict between the managed care organization and the health plan. The interface between the managed care organization and the health plan must be maintained with the medical community at all times.

Internal Support

Psychiatrists in managed care organizations frequently act as supervisors and consultants for internal operations. Claims processing, member services, and corporate affairs are just a few departments that may require additional support. Psychiatrists may find themselves acting as "superego" for managed care organizations and overseeing their medical policies. Effective managed care physicians resist deliberately choosing profit over health. At the same time, they must be keenly aware of these issues and advocate for their companies in appropriate situations.

Conclusion

The field of medical management is certainly not for everyone. Just as our patients may experience a flight into health in the face of a catastrophic illness, so too can physicians spring to new life in management only to find temporary relief from what is really a deep-seated problem. Clearly, the medical management field is not a panacea for unhappy physicians trying to escape the regulation of practice by government and insurance companies. On the other hand, a career in administration deserves serious consideration because health reform will most likely be fashioned by principles based on management and competition.

Many psychiatrists have enjoyed rich and rewarding careers in medical management. Managed care organizations, however, have used psychiatrists primarily for patient care skills rather than administrative skills. The era of managed care provides psychiatrists an opportunity to extend their clinical and leadership qualities in the service of health care reform. Although formal training beyond medical school and residency is not required for psychiatrists to become effective managers, various educational programs are available and are highly recommended.

Having recently celebrated its sesquicentennial anniversary, the American Psychiatric Association should keep alive its commitment to health care administration. Psychiatric managers face daunting challenges ahead. They need the support of their colleagues and managed care organizations. This expanding cadre of talent is an ideal resource for the ranks of major corporations seeking expert medical opinion in "real time." Psychiatrist-executives are infinitely better at making clinical decisions than medically untrained individuals sitting before a computer with a bottom-line–oriented algorithm.

References

American Academy of Child and Adolescent Psychiatry: How to Communicate Effectively With Managed Care Companies When Appealing Noncertification Decisions. Washington, DC, American Academy of Child and Adolescent Psychiatry, 1993

American Medical Association: Leaving the Bedside: The Search for a Nonclinical Medical Career. Chicago, IL, American Medical Association, 1993

American Psychiatric Association: Guidelines for Psychiatric Practice in Staff Model Health Maintenance Organizations. Washington, DC, American Psychiatric Association, 1989

Bennett MJ: View from the fridge: reflections of a recovering staff model HMO psychiatrist. Psychiatr Q 64:45–75, 1993

Boren SD: I had a tough day today, Hillary. N Engl J Med 330:500–502, 1994
Brookhiser R: Barefoot doctors vs. Scroogecare. Time, January 10, 1994, p 64
Breisch SL: Changing course. American Medical News, March 28, 1994, pp 17–18
Burns LR, Anderson RM, Shortell SM: Trends in hospital/physician relationships. Health Aff 12(3):213–223, 1993
Crane M: Thinking about leaving practice? Read this first. Medical Economics, August 15, 1988, pp 132–136
Fink PJ, Dubin WR: No free lunch: limitations on psychiatric care in HMOs. Hosp Community Psychiatry 42:363–365, 1991
Gray GV, Glazer WM: Psychiatric decision making in the 90's: the coming era of decision support. Behavioral Healthcare Tomorrow 3(1):47–54, 1994
Green SA: The process of reviewing peers. Gen Hosp Psychiatry 11:264–267, 1989
Hodge RH Jr, Grebenschikoff J: Medical management: portrait of a profession, in Roads to Medical Management: Physician Executives' Career Decisions. Edited by Curry W. Tampa, FL, American Academy of Medical Directors, 1988, pp 1–5
Kassebaum DG, Szenas PL: Factors influencing the specialty choices of 1993 medical school graduates. Acad Med 69:164–168, 1994
Lawson JS: Difficulties in the transition from clinician to manager. Physician Exec 20(7):19–21, 1994
Lazarus A: Disputes over payment for hospitalization under mental health "carve-out" programs. Hosp Community Psychiatry 44:1134–1136, 1993
Lazarus A: Using an appeals panel to mediate mental health care UR. Medical Interface 7(8):56–58, 76, 1994
Lazarus A: The psychiatrist–executive: new role, new economics. Psychiatric Annals, 25:494–499, 1995
Light DW: Life, death, and the insurance companies. N Engl J Med 330:498–499, 1994
Lloyd JS, Lyons MF: The physician executive "arrives"—a new generation prepares for the future. Physician Exec 20(7):31–36, 1994
Lyons MF, Cejka S: Getting a firm grip on the realities for physician executives. Physician Exec 20(6):8–12, 1994
Mangan D: Lured by the promise of a new career? Read this first. Medical Economics, November 22, 1993, pp 159–169
Marcos LR, Silvery MA: Psychiatrist–executive styles: nature or nurture? Am J Psychiatry 145:103–106, 1988

McGeevy JM: Advice to a college student considering medicine as a career. The Pharos 57(1):32–34, 1994

O'Connor SJ, Shewchuk RM: Enhancing administrator–clinician relationships: the role of psychological type. Health Care Manage Rev 18(2):57–65, 1993

O'Rourke PJ: Mr. Clinton has put a lawyer in charge of doctors. Cortlandt Forum, October 1993, pp 17–20

Penzer WN: Clinician turned administrator: drawing upon clinical experience for managerial expertise. Administration and Policy in Mental Health 17:105–109, 1989

Relman AS: Medical practice under the Clinton reforms—avoiding domination by business. N Engl J Med 329:1574–1576, 1993

Roback G, Randolph L, Seidman B, et al: Physician Characteristics and Distribution in the U.S. Chicago, IL, American Medical Association, 1994

Rosenthal MP, Diamond JJ, Rabinowitz HK, et al: Influence of income, hours worked, and loan repayment on medical students' decision to pursue a primary care career. JAMA 271:914–917, 1994

Sams BJ: Managed care: the need to "straighten things out," in Roads to Medical Management: Physician Executives' Career Decisions. Edited by Curry W. Tampa, FL, American Academy of Medical Directors, 1988, pp 54–62

Schenke RS: Administration. New Physician 35:44–45, 1986

Shore MF: One tentative cheer for managed care. Harvard Review of Psychiatry 1:123–124, 1993

Shortell SM: Effective Hospital–Physician Relationships. Ann Arbor, MI, Health Administration Press, 1991

Siegler M: Falling off the pedestal: what is happening to the traditional doctor–patient relationship? Mayo Clin Proc 68:461–467, 1993

Silver MA, Marcos LR: The making of the psychiatrist-executive. Am J Psychiatry 146:29–34, 1989

Vavala D: A matter of degree: the trend toward physician executives' pursuing master's degrees. Physician Exec 20(7):31–36, 1994

Walsh DC: Corporate Physicians: Between Medicine and Management. New Haven, CT, Yale University Press, 1987

Weeks WB, Wallace AE, Wallace MM, et al: A comparison of the educational costs and incomes of physicians and other professionals. N Engl J Med 330:1280–1286, 1994

Wehbé MA: A father's advice: don't become a physician, my son. American Medical News, April 25, 1994, p 24

Wells KB, Brook RH: Historical trends in quality assurance for mental health services, in Handbook of Quality Assurance in Mental Health. Edited by Stricker G, Rodriquez AR. New York, Plenum, 1988, pp 39–63

Westermeyer J: Problems with managed psychiatric care without a psychiatrist-manager. Hosp Community Psychiatry 42:1221–1224, 1991

Section VI

Health Reform

Chapter 23

Can Managed Competition Reform Mental Health Care?

T. Scott Stroup, M.D., M.P.H.
Robert A. Dorwart, M.D., M.P.H.

Managed care, with its goals of controlling costs and increasing accountability while maintaining quality throughout the health care industry, is fundamentally altering the rules and assumptions of mental health care delivery. Although previous chapters of this book have focused on issues specific to managed care, in this chapter we place managed mental health care in the larger context of health care reform, which is now proceeding incrementally through state and private initiatives.

As we began to write this chapter we expected to concentrate on *managed competition*, the foundation of several comprehensive health care reform bills proposed to the 103rd Congress. As publication nears, there is a Republican-dominated Congress that appears interested in health care reform only as a mechanism to control government expenditures. It is unlikely that the current federal legislature will adequately address the many issues, beyond cost, that were raised during the extensive recent discussion of health care reform. Nevertheless, increased competition and more managed care are expected to be the foundations of continued efforts to improve efficiency in the health sector. Therefore, it is useful to discuss what the reformers hoped to achieve and to describe their efforts.

Health care reform in the United States most often refers to reform of the financing and the delivery of health care, not to reform of the nature of the care itself (Reinhardt 1993). Consistent with this is the belief by many that a reliance on competitive forces is the most effective and efficient means of reforming the American health care system. Managed competition refers to a specific design for market-oriented health care reform promoted by Stanford economist Alain Enthoven and the Jackson Hole Group, which we describe in detail below. It is one strategy to achieve some of the goals of health care reformers through financial reorganization. The term *managed competition* is also used generically to describe health care services organized on principles of management and competition.

The Clinton administration's Health Security Act sought to control costs and maintain health care quality by adapting some of Enthoven's ideas. The approach was market oriented in that it was expected to result in regulated competition among health maintenance organization (HMO)–like health plans, which would have competed for consumers by offering low-cost plans promising high quality (Relman 1993).

To achieve cost control and maintain quality health care services, health reform plans based on managed competition relied heavily on managed care. Several of the difficulties posed by managed care, such as the risk that consumers would receive a minimum amount of care and that choice of physicians would be restricted, would exist under a health care system billed as managed competition. Some difficult issues, such as whether appropriate patient care could be given by physicians who worked for competitive corporations, were not addressed.

The use of market forces to reform clinical practice implicitly transforms health care into a business and medical services into commodities. This scenario is often seen by clinicians as conflicting with their goal of providing care to individuals in need of medical services. Market-oriented reform using managed care techniques raises fundamental ethical issues. Potential conflicts exist between clinicians' loyalties to patients, to managed care companies that employ them, and to the larger community. Research has shown that competition can distort institutional behavior as well as individual physician judgment (Dorwart and Epstein 1993). Managed competition, as it is developing, is likely to have serious ramifications for the organization and delivery of mental health services. In this chapter we focus on how managed competition will affect costs, quality, access, individual choice, and professional integrity.

Not all reform bills proposed to Congress were based on principles of management and competition. Some were based on different systems of financial incentives and organization of care. A proposal to expand Medicare to everyone under age 65 simply built on part of the existing system (Stark 1993), whereas a plan based on the Canadian single-payer model proposed entirely new financing (Wellstone and Shaffer 1993). Neither of these proposals relied on competition to reform health care. Below, we describe some of the ramifications of these alternative approaches to reform.

We begin with a discussion of the priorities by which to evaluate various reform models. Next, we briefly describe the current mental health system and assess the need for reform. Third, we discuss the theory behind managed competition and identify its possible impact on mental health care. Fourth, we describe a single-payer approach to reform and its mental health care provisions. Fifth, we discuss the impact of recent power shifts in Washington on the possibility of health care reform. We conclude by discussing the impact of managed competition on currently evolving mental health systems.

Criteria for Evaluating Health Care Systems

To evaluate both past and future health care reform proposals, we ask whether each plan can ensure the traditional dimensions of public health: quality of care, access to care, and affordable cost. Access and quality are of utmost concern to consumers. Can all who need services obtain them, without regard to socioeconomic or health status? Are benefits comprehensive and equitable for all types of illness? With regard to quality, are available services effective? Effectiveness has an important bearing on cost control, but cost control should not undermine physicians' regard for their patients' well-being. The maintenance of professional integrity is an important criterion by which to judge reform proposals. Consumers should be empowered to choose treatments, health plans, and providers. To do this, consumers need adequate information that allows them to weigh treatment choices according to quality and individual preference. Sound research should provide the basis for determining the effectiveness of clinical treatment. Health benefits offered by insurers should be easily comprehensible to consumers and providers alike.

From the point of view of advocates for consumers of mental health care, we propose several criteria by which to evaluate health care proposals. Everyone with mental illness should have access to effective treatment. Persons disabled by severe mental disorders should not be excluded from health plans because of their illness, and they should not be denied treatment because they are unable to secure a job with health care benefits. We agree with several principles proposed by the Little Rock Group, an assembly of researchers hoping to influence national health reform (R. F. Smith and B. J. Burns, Recommendations of the Little Rock Working Group on Mental Health and Substance Abuse Disorders in Health Care Reform. Little Rock, University of Arkanasas for Medical Sciences, unpublished report, February 3–5, 1993). They recommended that health care plans should have incentives to provide care for persons with mental illness. They advised that benefits should cover appropriate treatment, not arbitrary amounts or levels of care. Technology assessment and research on outcomes and cost-effectiveness were recommended as essential to obtaining reform goals.

Is There a Need for Reform?

Upwardly spiraling costs in the United States health care sector reached 15% of the gross national product (GNP) and $1 trillion in 1994 (U.S. Commerce Department 1994). Direct costs of mental health and substance abuse treatment made up approximately 15% of this total, a figure that had held constant for many years (Rice et al. 1990). Some argued that spending so much on health care diverts funds from other societal needs. Another view was that existing high costs resulted from years of waste, greed, poor management, and unnecessary and ineffective treatments. Buyers of insurance, mainly the government and employers, responded to increased costs with new financing mechanisms that limited payments to providers and increased the cost-sharing responsibility of consumers; they alerted Americans to rising costs and to a perceived need for reform.

In the mental health care sector, questions about equity are particularly important. The existing mental health system consists of a multitude of insurers and other payers interacting with a multitiered system of public and private services (Sharfstein and Stoline 1992). The categories of insured and uninsured and private and public are overlapping as a result of underinsurance for mental illness, which is covered less completely than other medical care services. Catastrophic mental illness is rarely covered by insurance, so persons suffering from severe and persistent mental illness often must resort to the public system. The public system has several components, with funding from federal, state, county, and local sources. The public insurance plans, Medicaid and Medicare, provide often inadequate coverage for persons with mental disabilities. "Free care" for the uninsured or those who have exhausted their benefits may or may not be available in state hospitals, in community mental health centers, or local hospitals, where budgets usually limit the amount of such care. State hospitals are widely perceived as providers of last resort, but they operate with limited, politically vulnerable budgets and serve a very disabled and disenfranchised population.

Although approximately $150 billion was spent in 1994 for direct treatment costs of mental and substance abuse disorders, many of these expensive services were criticized as lacking value. Wide variations in treatment methods and deep theoretical divisions within the psychiatric profession contributed to those perceptions. The American Psychiatric Association, in response to such criticisms and to advance the credibility of the field in the national health care debate, began generating a series of practice guidelines based on sound epidemiologic evidence and professional consensus (see Chapter 4 Zarin et al. 1993). Outcomes studies clearly demonstrated the effectiveness of a wide range of therapies (Michels and Marzuk 1993a, 1993b). Psychiatric treatment was shown to lower overall health care costs for families with a mentally ill family member (Holder and Blose 1987).

Despite the large amount spent on health care, up to 50 million Americans, each year lacked the security of health insurance for at least some part of the year (Swartz 1989). This figure was widely publicized and was a major reason behind the call for system reform. In the existing system, access to mental health care was limited not only by a systematic lack of insurance coverage for many with mental illness but also by barriers to adequate care imposed by arbitrary service limits for the insured. Co-payments and deductibles, based on empirical economic evidence and designed to limit insurers' risk, limited access to care for many of the insured (Frank et al. 1992). Exclusions for preexisting conditions prevented many persons with serious and persistent mental illnesses from obtaining insurance coverage.

The ethical situation in mental health care is complex. Fee-for-service systems with volume-based compensation carry the risks and costs of unnecessary or inappropriate treatment (Roberts 1993). Managed care brings with it ethical dilemmas related to divided loyalties. As growing numbers of psychiatrists become employees of clinics, hospitals, and HMOs, their obligations to their patients may be affected by the demands of their employers. The nature of the physician-patient relationship is undergoing significant strains.

Primarily because of theoretical and political reasons, health care reform proposals varied in their emphasis and in the approach to access, quality, and cost control. Managed competition emphasized reform of the health care market. In its theoretically pure form, there was no guarantee of universal access. Costs were to be controlled and quality maintained through the forces of a regulated market, which was to lead providers and plans to compete on the strengths of low price and, supposedly, high quality. The Clinton version of managed competition mandated universal coverage and proposed using report cards to give consumers a way to judge provider quality. Cost containment was to be ensured through regulations. Supporters of single-payer approaches to reform emphasized the need for universal access. They contended that autonomous professional clinical judgments, unencumbered by third-party review, would maintain high quality. They aimed to control costs by imposing a global budget.

The call for health care reform was far from universal. On the issue of cost containment, health economist Joseph Newhouse (1993) argued that the crisis of increasing health costs was overstated. Richard Stelzer (1994) of the American Enterprise Institute believed that there was no need for reform. He argued that there was no reason to believe that 15% of the GNP is too much to allocate for health care in a wealthy country and that historical and international comparisons were not relevant to the modern, sophisticated medical system of the United States. He maintained that only a very small percentage of people were uninsured for significant amounts of time, and that even these people were not denied essential treatment. George Will (1994) argued that any mandated national plan would be an unnecessary government intrusion impinging on personal freedoms. These commentators were joined by countless advocacy and interest groups also resisting government-mandated reform.

Managed Competition

Managed competition as a scheme to reform health care was first promulgated by the Jackson Hole Group, most prominently represented by Alain Enthoven. He argued that only market forces could bring about the innovations necessary to improve quality and value in the U.S. health care system (Enthoven and Singer 1994). He asserted that the medical care industry was far too complex and dynamic for government regulation alone to make these improvements effectively.

Based on the theory that problems in the health care sector were rooted in market inefficiencies, managed competition sought to reform health care by creating better market conditions. Inadequate consumer knowledge and the lack of a homogeneous product were the essential missing conditions for an efficient health care market (Fielding and Rice 1993). According to the Jackson Hole theorists, managed competition would create a homogeneous product by mandating a standardized coverage plan. Consumer knowledge and bargaining power would be improved through the creation of regionally based health insurance purchasing cooperatives (HIPCs) that would act as brokers for individuals and groups seeking to buy health insurance. The HIPCs would pool resources, judge the quality and efficiency of competing accountable health plans (AHPs), and facilitate consumer choice among these plans. Enrollment in the plans would be made through the HIPCs to avoid selection of good risks by the insurers. Risk-adjusted premiums would eliminate a plan's financial incentive to avoid difficult cases. The AHPs would be required to offer a standardized benefit, so that comparison shopping by consumers would be possible and market segmentation would be limited. (One example of segmentation would exist if a plan sought to exclude people with mental illness by offering poor mental health benefits.) Plans were to be prohibited from excluding people because of preexisting conditions.

Managed competition was market oriented in that it promoted regulated competition among the AHPs, which were expected to be HMO-like prepaid systems of care, owned and run by insurance companies (Relman 1993). The AHPs would be accountable for quality, as measured by outcomes and costs (Enthoven 1993). Two key assumptions of managed competition were that market forces would generate competition between plans on the basis of price and quality and that competition would reduce the cost of care effectively. Enthoven (1993) supported a limit on the tax-free employer contribution to health insurance premiums set at or below the lowest-price plan, so that consumers would no longer be unaware of the true costs of increasingly expensive insurance plans. In the existing system, employees were largely insulated from the steadily rising costs of insurance coverage because employers provided health insurance as a tax-free benefit to the employee. Enthoven's intention was to induce employees to shop for value when choosing an insurance plan by making the employees pay the full cost of optional benefits. Employees would also have an incentive to avoid inefficient plans because they would have to pay any additional premium that such a plan might charge. Managed competition's proposed financing was employment based, primarily because this was seen as the least disruptive approach to reform.

Research on the rapid privatization of mental health services in the past decade has shown marked effects on institutional and provider behavior. Among institutions, the elimination of marginally profitable services was a highly prevalent trend when competition was perceived to be significant. For example, Medicaid payments made up a smaller proportion of hospital income as competition increased, suggesting that there was screening of patients on profitability and ability to pay (Dorwart et al. 1991). Stevens (1989) noted that competition among psychiatrists is associated with lower average fees, less solo practice, and more group or hospital-based work. Many predict the quick demise of fee-for-service practice under managed competition because plans offering this option are unlikely to control costs effectively (Enthoven and Singer 1994; Reinhardt 1994).

Increased competition raises the anxiety of psychiatrists for a number of reasons. Many still rely on solo private practice as their primary source of income. If fee-for-service practice is no longer possible, these psychiatrists fear they will be forced into managed care plans where their autonomy will be limited and where clinical decisions will be made by insurers intent on controlling costs by rationing services. They fear that they will be subject to "termination without cause," as is stipulated in some managed care contracts. Another fear is the arbitrary exclusion from plans because insurers have the right to limit the number of specialists in their plans. Furthermore, because managed care plans use primary care providers as gatekeepers and do not allow direct access to specialists, psychiatrists fear that they will not get an adequate volume of referrals.

Managed Competition Proposals in the 103rd Congress

The founding principle of the Clinton Health Security Act was managed competition, but under pressure from conflicting interest groups, the proposal changed rapidly and finally did not closely resemble the Jackson Hole Group's initial proposal (Enthoven and Singer 1994). The act was to be financed through a mandatory employer contribution. Universal coverage, without regard to preexisting conditions, was a central tenet of the proposal (White House Domestic Policy Council 1993). Quality determinations were to be facilitated through the use of provider report cards available to the public and through an emphasis on effective treatments as demonstrated by outcome measures. The proposal sought to promote consumer choice by requiring three basic coverage options, including a fee-for-service option. There was no "any willing provider" clause, meaning that some clinicians could have been "locked out" of plans. Independent fee-for-service practices were not expected to remain financially viable (Enthoven and Singer 1994; Lazarus 1994). The main method of cost control was expected to be inflation-indexed regulation of what providers could charge. The plan did not limit tax-free employer contributions for health benefits and thus failed to give consumers the full incentive to choose the health plan offering the best value (Enthoven and Singer 1994).

The Clinton plan proposed a mandatory, but limited, mental health benefit. Psychopharmacology visits were to be reimbursed more generously than psychotherapy sessions. Coverage for mental health services (except medication management) was not as generous as coverage for medical treatment. Co -payments and deductibles were set at a level intended to discourage discretionary use. Managed care techniques, with their imperfections, were prominent components of the Health Security Act. Because of limits to mental health coverage, a separate state-operated public system would have remained necessary.

Representative Jim Cooper (D-TN) proposed a health care reform plan that closely resembled "pure" managed competition and was endorsed by the Jackson Hole Group (Enthoven and Singer 1994). The plan relied on an employer mandate to generate revenues and limited the tax deductibility of this employer contribution to the cost of a basic benefits package. Cooper's plan mandated no mental health benefit and was unlikely to lead to improvements for persons with mental illness; the perpetuation of separate public and private systems was probable.

Senator John Chafee (R-RI) sponsored another managed competition–based plan that used an individual rather than an employer mandate to finance care. This financing method responded to objections to employer coverage made by small business owners and their threats of increased unemployment if they were forced to take on this expense. Significantly, this plan did mandate coverage for mental health services, at least for those with severe illness. Chafee's plan was otherwise similar to the Cooper proposal.

Alternative Plans: Medicare and Single Payer

Representative John Stark (D-CA) proposed to expand Medicare to everyone under age 65 years (Stark 1993). This model would have preserved most aspects of the existing Medicare system, including fee-for-service outpatient care, and limited inpatient mental health coverage. Managed care and competition were not integral to this plan, which proposed to use a global budget to contain costs. Increased taxes were likely to be required to finance such a plan. Distinctions in coverage for medical disorders and mental illnesses were expected to continue. In the existing Medicare system, psychiatric medical management in outpatient settings has the same co-payment structure as other medical care (20%), but psychotherapy has a much higher (50%) rate of cost sharing. There is a 190-day lifetime limit for inpatient services at freestanding psychiatric hospitals. This limit on hospital days was originally meant to ensure that Medicare would not finance long-term custodial care; if Medicare's existing rules were part of a reform plan, the limit would perpetuate the need for an alternative public system for severely mentally ill persons (Sharfstein et al. 1993).

Single-payer approaches to health care reform in the United States are based on the Canadian model, in which the government is responsible for financing and administration of the health system and sets regional budgets as a cost-control measure. Advocates of single-payer plans assert that the existing multiple systems of administration in the United States add considerable cost, but no benefit, to the health care system (Himmelstein and Woolhandler 1986). Single-payer proponents reject a market orientation as a means of distributing services efficiently and equitably.

"Health care is a right" was a central tenet of the single-payer plans proposed in Congress (H.R. 1200/S. 491) by psychiatrist and U.S. Representative Jim McDermott (D-WA), among others. Single-payer proposals *would have* guaranteed universal access to health care, with everyone getting a standardized benefit. Public and private systems would have been integrated into a single system. All caps on hospital days and outpatient visits, as well as deductibles and co-payments, would have been eliminated because these were seen to conflict with the principle of universal access. The creation of a range of cost-effective services was expected to enhance consumer choice and contain costs by decreasing use of the most expensive services. The system would have been funded through various taxes, and cost control would have taken place through global budgeting. Mental health and substance abuse care were to be provided on parity with all other benefits, based on a principle of nondiscrimination and on the assertion that treatment of mental illness is cost-effective. Although proponents of single-payer plans did not reject all managed care techniques, they favored keeping decisions about setting, duration, and intensity of treatment in the clinical rather than management domain. This, however, would have put the burden of deciding how the budget would be spent on clinicians, who may have needed to make unwelcome rationing choices. Respect for the physician-patient relationship was promoted as a quality enhancement. Single-payer plans accepted the notion of practice guidelines and promoted research on outcomes and treatment effectiveness (J. E. Sabin and the Working Group on Mental Health and Substance Abuse Care of the Physicians for a National Health Program: Mental health and substance abuse in a single payer system: affordable and nondiscriminatory care, unpublished paper, 1993; Wellstone and Shaffer 1993).

Power Shifts in Washington, D.C.

The 104th Congress, which came to power in 1995, was dominated by Republicans and claimed to have a mandate to implement a Contract with America, which promoted, among other things, reduced federal government spending and increased state autonomy. The change in congressional power followed an extended debate during 1993 and 1994 on health care reform. There were numerous failed proposals in the midst of the most extensive lobbying efforts ever seen in Washington, D.C. (Iglehart 1994). Some argued that voter frustration with the futile efforts of the 103rd Congress in the health care reform endeavor was an important factor in the overthrow of the Democratic majority. Others, including the new leadership, pointed to fear of a large federally mandated and regulated health care system as a reason for the election of a Congress dedicated to downsizing federal programs.

Key topics in the health care reform debate included universal coverage, the nature of financing, the extent of benefits (with considerable focus on mental health coverage), consumer choice, exclusions for preexisting conditions, and portability of coverage. Lobbyists representing small businesses successfully campaigned to defeat all proposals that would have financed reform through mandated employer contributions. Universal coverage was abandoned as unachievable and overly expensive, as President Clinton backed off his emphatic pledge to veto any bill falling short of this goal. Government-managed programs that would have clearly required increased taxes, such as single-payer and expanded Medicare plans, never neared approval. Instead, various plans that maximized continuity with the existing system and adhered to the wishes of powerful business lobbies gained considerable support, only to fall under the weight of opposition to employer-mandated financing. In the end, only health care reform that ensured the continuing profitability of large insurers gained meaningful congressional support.

There were only two components of reform that the 104th Congress seemed likely to consider. Portability, which would guarantee people with existing insurance continuing coverage when changing jobs or relocating, had little opposition. Representatives of the insurance industry agreed that people who faithfully pay their premiums should not have to go through a new underwriting cycle when relocating. Proposals to end exclusions for preexisting conditions were likely to meet opposition from the insurance industry, however. Insurance lobbyists alleged that these exclusions were necessary to prevent people from buying insurance only when they needed medical care ("Portability; Preexisting Condition Limits not as Easy to Draft as Many Suggest" 1995).

The Impact of Managed Competition on Mental Health Care

Managed competition in itself will not fulfill all the wishes of health care reformers nor solve all the problems of the current system. In many respects, it will represent only a subtle adjustment of the currently evolving system. Managed competition is a concept that can be adapted outside a federal mandate. For example, insurance purchasers (such as alliances of small businesses) already band together to increase their bargaining power in the insurance marketplace. In any form of managed competition, many existing trends related to increased privatization and competition will continue. Health plans competing for enrollees will continue to use managed care techniques to control costs. Employment-based insurance financing will be another stable trend (Enthoven and Singer 1994). Private insurance companies will remain powerful under managed competition. The political reality is that Congress will continue to respect the wishes of the interest groups who favor these aspects of the status quo.

Managed competition may strengthen the profession of psychiatry by increasing its accountability and credibility. Outcomes research and report cards on provider performance can strengthen a profession increasingly based on sound scientific method and with an expanding array of effective treatments. Managed competition will not, however, decrease the financial pressures on psychiatrists or relieve them of the difficult clinical burdens of the current mental health system.

For consumers, managed competition may facilitate increased knowledge about treatment options and provider quality. An expanded array of services, likely to become available as health plans compete, may lead to more appropriate and less restrictive treatment settings. Increased knowledge and an increased range of services are potentially empowering aspects of managed competition for consumers, but limited benefits will continue to disadvantage psychiatric patients. Managed competition will not eliminate the multitiered mental health system, and the sickest group of patients will quite likely continue to receive suboptimal treatment.

Aspects of health care that do not naturally follow from increased managed care and competition, such as mandatory universal coverage and insurance portability, would have more noticeable and dramatic effects on the United States health care system. Managed competition is a subtle adjustment to the status quo rather than a dramatic change.

On the other hand, a single-payer plan would clearly reorder system financing and care delivery. Because proponents of a single-payer plan are less concerned with minimizing potential disruptions and insist on positive change, their program design most comprehensively addresses the goals of health care reform. A single-payer system mandates nondiscrimination among consumers and explicitly attempts to keep financial micromanagement out of clinical decisions. A single-payer plan is most likely to have provisions favorable for those needing mental health care, but chances of passage of a single-payer bill in the near future are small. We conjecture that an initial phase of health care reform will be based largely on managed competition and managed care plans, with a second phase 5–10 years later more closely resembling a single-payer plan.

Conclusion

Managed competition, if it works as designed, can reform some aspects of mental health care, but trade-offs will abound. The influence of managed care will expand and with it the dilemmas outlined in this book. Costs may be lowered and that may in turn help facilitate access to insurance for many now without this security. Quality may improve as inappropriately restrictive settings and unnecessary treatments are avoided, but undertreatment and restricted access may also result. Consumer choices of providers and plans will be limited, and mental health professionals may have difficulty joining plans. A wider range of treatments and settings may be available, however. Improved consumer information may allow for better decision making about the available choices. Provider prerogatives will decrease as third parties become pervasive in making treatment decisions. Provider behavior will inevitably respond to competition, and treatment patterns will be influenced by financial incentives. More psychiatrists will be employed by others and will thus be subject to business decisions made in a competitive marketplace. There will be continued infringements on clinical autonomy. In the absence of comprehensive reform, there will be no parity for mental health services, no end to a two-tiered system, and thus little improvement for persons with severe mental illness.

Managed competition is not a panacea for the ills of the mental health care system, nor is it an ominous plague. It was a politically feasible component of many reform proposals that sought to emphasize continuity with the existing system, and its principles were incorporated into many incremental changes. Managed competition is an inevitable step in a much longer journey to comprehensive reform.

References

Dorwart RA, Epstein SS: Privatization and Mental Health Care: A Fragile Balance. Westport, CT, Auburn House, 1993

Dorwart RA, Schlesinger M, Davidson H, et al: A national study of psychiatric hospital care. Am J Psychiatry 148:204–210, 1991

Enthoven AC: The history and principles of managed competition. Health Aff 12 (suppl):24–48, 1993

Enthoven AC, Singer SJ: A single-payer system in Jackson Hole clothing. Health Aff 13(1):81–95, 1994

Fielding JE, Rice T: Can managed competition solve problems of market failure? Health Aff 12 (suppl):216–228, 1993

Frank RG, Goldman HH, McGuire TG: A model mental health benefit in private insurance. Health Aff 11(3):98–117, 1992

Himmelstein DU, Woolhandler S: Cost without benefit: administrative waste in U.S. health care. N Engl J Med 314:441–445, 1986

Holder HD, Blose JO: Changes in health care costs and utilization associated with mental health treatment. Hosp Community Psychiatry 38:1070–1075, 1987

Iglehart JK: Who spoke for the people? Health Aff 13(4):5–6, 1994

Lazarus A: Ten reasons why psychiatrists may dislike managed competition. Hosp Community Psychiatry 45:496–498, 1994

Michels R, Marzuk PM, Progress in psychiatry: part 1. N Engl J Med 329:552–560, 1993a

Michels R, Marzuk PM: Progress in psychiatry: part 2. N Engl J Med 329:628–638, 1993b

Newhouse J: An iconoclastic view of health cost containment. Health Aff 12 (suppl):152–171, 1993

Portability, preexisting condition limits not as easy to draft as many suggest. Inside Health Care Reform 3(2):1, 1995

Reinhardt UE: Reorganizing financial flows in U.S. health care. Health Aff 12 (suppl):172–193, 1993

Reinhardt UE: The Clinton Plan: A salute to pluralism. Health Aff 13(1):161–177, 1994

Relman AS: Medical practice under the Clinton reforms—avoiding domination by business. N Engl J Med 329:1574–1576, 1993

Rice DP, Kelman S, Miller LS, et al: The Economic Costs of Alcohol and Drug Abuse and Mental Illness, 1985 (DHHS Publ No ADM 90-1694). Washington, DC, U.S. Government Printing Office, 1990

Roberts MJ: Your Money or Your Life: The Health Care Crisis Explained. New York, Doubleday, 1993

Sharfstein SS, Stoline AM: Reform issues for insuring mental health care. Health Aff 11(3): 84-97, 1992

Sharfstein SS, Stoline AM, Goldman HH: Psychiatric care and health insurance reform. Am J Psychiatry 150:7–18, 1993

Stark JP: Mediplan Act of 1993. HR 2610. U.S. House of Representatives, 103rd Cong. 1st Session

Stelzer RM: What health-care crisis? Commentary 97(2):19–24, 1994

Stevens R: In Sickness and in Wealth: American Hospitals in the 20th Century. New York, Basic Books, 1989

Swartz K: The Medically Uninsured: Special Focus on Workers. Washington, DC, The Urban Institute Press, 1989

U.S. Commerce Department: Annual Report of the Secretary of Commerce. Washington, DC, Government Printing Ofiice, 1994

Wellstone PD, Shaffer ER: The American Health Security Act: a single-payer proposal. New Engl J Med 328:1489–1493, 1993

White House Domestic Policy Council: The President's Health Security Plan. New York, Times Books, 1993

Will G: The Clinton's lethal paternalism. Newsweek, February 7, 1994, p 64

Zarin DA, Pincus HA, McIntyre JS: Practice guidelines (editorial). Am J Psychiatry 150:175–177, 1993

Chapter 24

Does Consolidation in Health Care Mean That Bigger Is Better?

Anthony F. Buono, Ph.D.
Joseph S. Lombardi, Ph.D.

Strategic alliances between health care organizations—mergers, acquisitions, and joint ventures—are rapidly becoming a critical dimension of the industry's strategy and of many reform initiatives. As the expense associated with medical technologies and health care delivery continues to escalate, many observers view such alliances as crucial to retaining quality and containing costs as well as maintaining the ability to offer a sufficient variety of plans and services to meet the needs of an increasingly diverse population (Baker 1989; Gawande 1994; Major 1994; Meyer 1994). Similar to the trend within the business community (Gold and Sauvant 1990; Lynch 1993), during the course of the late 1990s there is likely to be a growing number of these alliances and an increase in their influence as more and more health care systems with a "go-it-alone" policy will be forced to reevaluate their position (Johnson 1993). It is estimated, for example, that by the year 2000, 50% of all hospitals in the United States will be involved

We would like to thank Mary Cuniff, our graduate research assistant, for her help in collecting data for this chapter.

in some form of alliance (Kalzuny and Zukerman 1993). Our premise is that all organizational alliances—whether between hospitals, banks, or computer firms—involve systems, processes, and interactions between internal and external stakeholders that must be analyzed, understood, and effectively integrated if the combination is to realize its full potential.

Comparable to the consolidation taking place within the banking, computer, and information technologies industries, health care providers, looking at alliances as a solution to their problems, are gradually altering their organizational structures in an attempt to create integrated delivery systems. As current and projected industry trends indicate, we are entering a shakeout period in health care during which a growing number of hospitals and medical practices will close beds or shut down altogether, merge and ally with one another, and cut staff. Indeed, instead of a multitude of separate, autonomous groups offering different aspects of health care, the emerging vision for most metropolitan areas is a small number of large health networks that will include both teaching and community hospitals (Carpenter and Peters 1990; Stein 1994a). Such consolidation is especially evident with respect to mental health care, where the trend has been toward significantly increased vertical and horizontal integration to the point that it is becoming increasingly difficult for smaller and solo practice vendors to compete (Edlin 1994; Saeman 1994; Sardella 1994). The question that lingers is whether this level of concentration will actually lead to better health care. As critics of our business system have emphasized, bigness, in and of itself, does not necessarily translate into effectiveness and efficiency (Adams and Brock 1986).

Strategic Alliances: Promises and Pitfalls

Interfirm partnerships offer organizations the opportunity to expand their project and service options beyond existing capabilities or current product-market domains (Buono 1991; Lynch 1993). A common objective is to avoid the disadvantages and limitations faced by single organizations (e.g., resource scarcity, restricted economies of scale, undue risk) by drawing on the capacity and potential of multiple, autonomous firms (Borys and Jemison 1989). Thus, within the corporate sector, interfirm alliances have emerged as a way of raising complementary resources and attaining important attributes from partner firms: marketing, technological, financial, managerial, and raw materials (Alster 1986; Blank 1987; Harrigan 1986; Schillaci 1987). As we have learned from our experience with the business community, however, there is an inherent fragility in these interfirm agreements that makes them quite complex to manage (Buono 1991; Buono et al. 1989; Harrigan 1986; Waddock 1988).

A basic problem associated with strategic alliances in general, and health care alliances in particular, is that many, if not most, managers and administrators are unfamiliar or uncomfortable with the problems and difficulties of managing in these interorganizational arrangements (Buono 1991; Carpenter and Peters 1990; Gulati et al. 1994; Lynch 1993). Although these types of alliances are not new, they are unique in both a strategic and an organizational sense. Most assessments of management emphasize fairly conventional contexts, for example, unitary, freestanding companies, small businesses, and entrepreneurial activities in larger organizations (intrapreneurship). Strategic alliances, in contrast, are hybrid organizations with distinctive characteristics and problems: they have an "instant" presence and size; they face performance expectations that are immediate, substantial, and externally imposed; the partners often lack a common cultural domain or experience base; and their management and governance structures, which are based on cooperation and collaboration, are generally untested (Borys and Jemison 1989). Despite these dynamics, far more time and effort tend to be spent on developing alliance plans and drafting legal documents than are spent on those considerations and processes involved with the day-to-day running and management of the alliance (Buono and Bowditch 1989; Cody 1990; Levine and Byrne 1986; Schweiger and Ivancevich 1985). As Gulati et al. (1994) argued, even if different stages of an alliance require different time commitments by managers, the paucity of time devoted to actually managing its daily affairs is startling.

This reality is especially true for health care alliances. Indeed, one of the key problems concerns how to organize and manage an integrated system of health care. Problems range from signing people up for health coverage and collecting insurance premiums to prevention, inpatient care, and rehabilitation. Although alliance-based approaches are attractive, such interorganizational endeavors must still be sufficiently linked to ensure seamless care and meet the needs of a broad range of stakeholders. As recent experience is beginning to indicate, developing truly integrated health care delivery services can be a daunting challenge (Baker 1989; Breisch 1994; Carpenter and Peters 1990; Gosselin 1994a; Lambrew et al. 1993; Lazarus 1995; Porter et al. 1994). Problems range from the coordination of services delivered across different practices to disagreement on goals and what constitutes fair sharing of risk and reward, resultant political maneuvering and outright hostilities between alliance members, the danger of creating a civil service mentality among physicians, and the potential overextension of full-service provider networks.

Finally, it is also important to realize that an alliance that might look good on paper does not necessarily translate into success in the marketplace (Buono 1991). To draw an example from the business community, one need only look at one of the most talked about United States–European joint ventures of the 1980s—the partnership between AT&T and Olivetti (the Italian office equipment manufacturer)—for an illustration of how promising ventures can collapse. Similarly, mergers that appeared to make good strategic sense in the recent past are now being viewed as disastrous mistakes, and many of the most promising joint ventures have either failed outright or have not fulfilled their promise. In fact, in far too many instances, the actual performance of these alliances simply falls short of the operational, strategic, and financial goals envisioned during preformation feasibility studies and assessments. The reality is that despite the growing number of such alliances, a disproportionately large percentage end prematurely and in failure (Alster 1986; Buono 1990, 1991; Buono and Bowditch 1989; Levine and Byrne 1986; Lynch 1993; Murphy 1991; Shenkar and Zeira 1987).

Despite these concerns, it appears that a range of interorganizational managed care endeavors will continue to grow in both number and influence. Indeed, current and emerging pressures and forces in the health care industry literally demand greater collaboration among hospitals, medical centers, physicians, insurers, health maintenance organizations (HMOs), and related members and organizations in existing and yet to be developed alliances (Carpenter and Peters 1990; Cody 1990). In this chapter we examine some of the fundamental organizational and human resource concerns associated with typical consolidation strategies: *mergers,* the total consolidation of two or more organizations into a single entity; *acquisitions,* the purchase of one firm by another such that the acquiring organization takes control of the target; and *joint ventures,* cooperative agreements between two or more organizations that want to achieve similar objectives (Borys and Jemison 1989; Buono 1991). The chapter concludes with a discussion of some of the general guidelines for facilitating successful health care alliances.

Management and Organizational Issues in Strategic Alliances

As our experience with alliances in the business community underscores, individual strategic alliances are unique entities because of the myriad ways in which different firms might interact with one another as well as the potential diversity of the partners themselves (Buono and Bowditch 1989; Gulati et al. 1994; Nevaer et al. 1990; Shenkar and Zeira 1987). Thus, efforts to make one alliance work may very well result in quite different outcomes in another. Moreover, much of the evaluation of alliance effectiveness depends on the strategic intent of the partnership (Finnerty et al. 1986; McConnell and Nantell 1985). A related problem is that health care alliances are relatively new and, as such, they will require at least a few more years until the problems and difficulties associated with them can be fully dissected and explored (Baker 1989; Carpenter and Peters 1990). Nevertheless, because of the growing attractiveness of these strategic alliances and the myriad questions that remain about coalition dynamics, it is important to draw lessons from existing ventures to serve as a guide for thinking about managing other such partnerships and dealing with the disparate managerial and organizational considerations involved (see Buono 1991). To suggest that the health care industry learn from business alliances is, of course, not to imply that manufacturing goods or rendering services are the same as caring for patients (Kaufman 1994). Obviously, there are differences. At the same time, all business alliances, health care or otherwise, face similar organizational challenges. These challenges must be managed strategically and operationally, as well as effectively and efficiently, if new alliances are to succeed.

Mergers and Acquisitions

Despite the avalanche of corporate merger and acquisition activity in the past two decades, a growing body of research indicates that these combinations do not reliably yield the desired financial, operational, or strategic returns suggested by precombination feasibility assessments (Halpern 1983; Jensen and Ruback 1983; Lefkoe 1987; Lubatkin 1983; Lubatkin and O'Neil 1987; Michel and Shaked 1985; Mueller 1985). Studies indicate that acquiring firms have less than a 50–50 chance of achieving their acquisition goals (Louis 1982; Pritchett 1985). In fact, as *Business Week* ("Do Mergers Really Work?" 1985) has estimated, one of every three mergers and acquisitions is later undone. Given the difficulties that the business community has had with making mergers and acquisitions successful, it is clear that the health care industry is facing a significant challenge.

Mergers and acquisitions seldom fail because one or both parties did an inadequate job of due diligence. As experts in this area have argued, the technical issues involved in health care consolidations—such as understanding financial performance, debt, market share, patient origin, physician type and reputation, program or service fit, and physical plant—are typically addressed with a high level of intensity and expertise (Cody 1990; Kazemek 1989). The behavioral and cultural dimensions involved in the combination of previously autonomous organizations, in contrast, rarely receive the same focus and attention. As agents for their organizations, however, managers and administrators need to know much more than the investments and input conditions required for an interfirm relationship. There must also be careful and systematic attention given to the underlying processes through which individuals and groups from the organizations involved interact with each other (Ring and Van de Ven 1994).

When two companies physically combine with each other, organizational instability increases as a cloud of uncertainty and ambiguity permeates the firms. As the individuals involved share their perceptions of what will take place, they often discover that what they each thought initially were relatively clear images of merger or acquisition outcomes vary considerably from person to person. Although organizational members are generally cooperative at first, goodwill can quickly erode as cultural and role uncertainties increase as a result of shifts in norms and expectations. The actual or potential loss of organizational identity, new or ambiguous job responsibilities and work routines, and separation from valued co-workers are just a few of the factors that may create anxiety and disruption for organization members.

The uncertainties and concerns that follow the formal combination of two organizations are often compounded by a we versus they mentality between the different groups. During this period, there is a danger of "merger standstill" or "postmerger drift" (Ivancevich et al. 1987; Pritchett 1985) as managers struggle with the actual integration and consolidation of the two firms. This process can take years to resolve and is typically manifested in lowered productivity and operating effectiveness. At this stage, many business mergers fail, resulting in spinoff or divestment decisions.

The reactions that individuals report when going through a merger or acquisition are part of a fairly predictable syndrome of merger-related stresses and tensions (Buono and Bowditch 1989; Marks and Mirvis 1985). During the transformations that occur in a merger or acquisition, the stresses and tensions of everyday organizational life are greatly intensified. Although people do vary in their ability to cope with such stressful situations, the sheer magnitude of the uncertainties and ambiguities that organization members must endure typically leads to anxiety, feelings of grief and loss, preoccupation with the combination, eroded trust levels, and self-centered activities. These psychological manifestations are often translated into a breakdown in communication, productivity, and commitment as well as a rise in interfirm tensions, power struggles, and employee "bailouts."

The degree of interfirm consolidation in a merger or acquisition is much greater than in a joint venture. Although the actual level of consolidation and related dynamics are influenced by the strategic intent of the combination and the degree of integration desired between the firms (Buono and Bowditch 1989; Mirvis and Marks 1992), merger or acquisition partners do not retain the level of autonomy that they once had or that joint venture members maintain. To bring about this level of consolidation, integration efforts tend to be highly normative in nature, relying on culture change efforts and group socialization processes (Borys and Jemison 1989). As a result, the direct effects on the individuals involved tend to be much more extreme than in other forms of alliance. Although there is a range of cultural integration possibilities, from cultural pluralism to cultural blending (American Bankers Association and Ernst & Whinney 1985), in any merger or acquisition the degree of threat perceived by the organizations' employees tends to be high. Especially in horizontal mergers and acquisitions, organizational members expect reductions in force as overlapping job responsibilities create a certain degree of organizational redundancy (Buono et al. 1988; Cody 1990). It is estimated, for example, that in the next 3–5 years in Massachusetts alone hospital-based job losses could range from 6,500 to 30,000 depending on how tightly the industry is squeezed financially (Stein 1994b). Moreover, these staff cuts will fall heavily on nurses and lower-skilled service workers. The potential for such job losses as well as shifts in organizational culture and practices contribute to a perception of threat among managers and employees (Buono and Nurick 1992; Marks and Mirvis 1985; Schweiger and Walsh 1990). As such, the potential for turnover of key organizational members and resistance to the combination tend to be high.

Hospital mergers are attractive primarily because the anticipated synergies (e.g., consolidating computer systems and support, shared space in medical facilities) will reduce costs and expenses. Although a merger can ensure that two colocated hospitals are not duplicating a particular specialty service, the question remains which of the hospitals will stop performing that service. The recently announced merger between Massachusetts General Hospital (MGH) and Brigham and Women's Hospital in Boston, for example, was expected to save millions of dollars and ensure their continued strength as premier academic medical centers. During the negotiations, however, MGH chose to continue to launch a new obstetrics program despite a decline in occupancy in the same program at Brigham and Women's (Davidson and Maxwell 1994; Knox 1994b). Although the two hospitals were talking cooperation, many of those involved were skeptical about the competitive realities of developing and maintaining similar services (Knox 1994a). As an analyst from Coopers & Lybrand observed, the controversy over the plan to open the new obstetric unit is "a microcosm of every decision these hospitals will make in the merger. This starts to tell us how difficult it will be to pull together these institutions to act as one" (Knox 1994a, p. 16). Less than 4 months after the initial announcement, the "merger" was turned into an affiliation, with far less planned integration, a growing number of partners, and less optimistic outcomes. At the same time, the potential power and influence that such consolidated systems could conceivably yield have led to a grassroots backlash among consumer groups about possible "merger mania" leading to decreased quality, reduced choice, and diminished competition among specialty-care providers (Page 1994; Porter et al. 1994; Reichard 1994; Stein 1994a).

Not only must hospital and other health care administrators deal with each other in an open and effective manner, they must also attempt to quell the fears of a growing number of internal and external stakeholders. Thus, in mergers and acquisitions, upper-level administrators must emphasize interventions that can ameliorate some of the tension, strain, and discontent associated with the postcombination integration of two previously autonomous organizations (Buono and Bowditch 1989; Marks 1988; Mirvis and Marks 1992; Schweiger and DeNisi 1991):

- Two-way communication channels with internal and external stakeholders
- Community outreach efforts
- Realistic merger previews that provide organizational members with a sense of impending changes
- Combination-related workshops and counseling efforts that help members deal with the resultant uncertainty and stress
- Focus groups and survey feedback that allow for an exchange of information
- Interfirm mirroring and team building that bring to the surface and deal with cultural and operational differences
- Transition teams and parallel organization structures that oversee and guide the combination
- Organizational symbols and rituals that support the integration
- Humanistic approaches to employee retention and dismissal when necessary
- Joint evaluation and integration review.

It is important to realize that although such efforts can minimize employees' fears and anxieties, research has indicated that members of acquired organizations still maintain feelings of suspicion and, at least during the immediate postmerger period, never feel fully informed or comfortable in the combined organization (Bastien 1987; Buono et al. 1985; Marks and Mirvis 1985). Especially with respect to health care consolidations, the same is true about key stakeholder groups in the surrounding communities. Two years after the consolidation of the Framingham Union and Leonard Morse hospitals in the west suburban area of Boston, for example, physicians and nurses are still at odds with the administration (two "no-confidence" votes), and area residents are still contemplating legal action in an attempt to terminate the combination (Small and Mont 1994).

Joint Ventures

Because of the underlying difficulties involved with mergers and acquisitions, many health care operations are turning instead to joint ventures. This type of alliance can provide hospitals, medical centers, physicians, and related organizations with the advantages of being part of a multimedical system, while still allowing them to exist as freestanding, self-governing units (Kalzuny and Zukerman 1993). A joint venture arrangement also allows providers to pool available capital without the restrictions of a merger (Peters 1991). Yet, although these interfirm alliances appear to sidestep many of the difficulties associated with mergers and acquisitions, studies have suggested that the failure rate of joint ventures is even higher than that in mergers and acquisitions—as high as 80% (Levine and Byrne 1986).

Joint ventures do not typically involve the same level of threat to the firms' employees as do mergers and acquisitions. Rarely, if ever, are these alliances associated with reductions in force or major organizational culture change efforts. They do, however, face a host of managerial and organizational difficulties. Conflicts over which partner has the most control, changes in partners' objectives, different management styles and organizational customs, a lack of trust between partners, and declining interest from either partner can easily contribute to failure (Buono 1990). Moreover, because of competing pressures and work demands, managers and employees often direct their attention toward other job responsibilities and away from the venture itself. Accordingly, one of the keys to joint venture success is the degree of fit between the venture's strategic purpose and the actual activities of the venture partners (Borys and Jemison 1989). However, as research has indicated, the stated purposes of a joint venture are often much broader than the actual efforts and activities of the venture partners (Pekar 1986).

Although the need for consolidation in joint ventures is not as high as in a horizontal merger or acquisition, it is critical that member roles are clearly defined and sufficient motivation exists to ensure cooperation. Some normative control and related socialization efforts are important, but joint ventures typically rely on more explicit contractual and structural agreements between member firms. An underlying problem, however, is that even apparently clear agreements are often interpreted quite differently by venture partners. In the past decade, for instance, one of the most common forms of health care joint venture has been the hospital-physician ancillary service venture, in which a hospital and group of physicians form a partnership that operates as a service facility (e.g., as an imaging center, ambulatory surgery center, urgent care clinic) or leases equipment to a service provider. Although the goals of such ancillary service alliances are to pool capital, improve market share, combine skills and expertise, and develop favorable hospital-physician relationships, many of these ventures have fallen far short of those objectives, damaging hospital-physician relationships in the process (Peters 1991). Management disputes; disagreement over goals, mission, and even philosophy; value clashes; and conflicts about performance and evaluation standards tend to be major contributing factors toward failure (Baker 1989; Breisch 1994).

Health care joint ventures face the basic challenge of attracting and retaining physicians. Virtually all the successful vertically integrated health care ventures today are staffed by physicians who have chosen to work in large organizations, essentially operating as salaried employees with guidelines and incentives created in a collaborative environment. Although an increasing number of physicians are becoming dissatisfied with the risks and inconveniences of private practice, the simplicity and security provided by alternative delivery systems are particularly attractive to recent medical school graduates with high education debt (Peters 1991). As experience has shown, however, it can take years for such collegial cultures to develop and work in a capitation and managed care environment (Johnson 1993). Moreover, many physicians do not necessarily see themselves as employees or team players (Tremonti and Manning 1983), and once the initial euphoria that accompanies a new undertaking wears off, the loss of autonomy that comes with becoming an employee of an alliance can be profound (Breisch 1994). No matter how carefully joint ventures are planned and initiated, they create stress and strain between members and, in many instances, only the promise of a potentially high payoff keeps the partners working together (Baker 1989).

More complex ventures, of course, readily complicate the managerial and organizational challenges involved. For example, integrated health networks comprising family medical care, hospital care, nursing home care, mental health care, and long-term care may be in the best position to compete for employers' health plans if and when a managed competition–based reform package becomes law (Findlay 1993), but there are many difficulties and obstacles associated with bringing together such an array of services. Thus, in joint ventures it is important that planning and subsequent interactions be viewed as part of an iterative process. Realizing the probability of cultural differences between organizations, clearly spelling out the goals and obligations of the partners, attempting to create and maintain a vision of the partnership, using appropriate parallel structures and transition teams to oversee and support the venture, and building and mobilizing coalitions of key organizational members and external stakeholders provide a basic foundation so that many of the internal pitfalls undermining joint ventures can be dealt with in an effective and constructive manner (Buono 1990). The key is to make such health care endeavors as collaborative, empowering, and self-governing as possible as well as intellectually tolerable and financially acceptable (Johnson 1993).

Facilitating Health Care Alliances

The success of any interorganizational venture depends in large part on what has been referred to as the *coalition game* (Kang 1990). Simply stated, an alliance will be effective only as long as the benefits of membership or group activity are greater than the costs of participation for individual members. An underlying problem, however, is that each alliance partner often fears that the other(s) will receive a larger payoff by acting in an opportunistic manner while it cooperates in good faith. As a result, the partners do not fully cooperate with each other, leading, in many instances, to a situation where they are worse off than if they had cooperated (Gulati et al. 1994; Murphy 1991). Thus, although integrated networks—whether through merger, acquisition, or joint venture—appear to be a solution for hospitals and other health care providers trying to gain market share, fend off competition, contain costs, and ensure continued quality, the providers that will be successful are those who have learned how to cooperate with each other and their key stakeholders, achieving a balance between clinical competence and cost and realizing that adversarial approaches to relationships among hospitals, physicians, and payers are outdated (Carpenter and Peters 1990).

Observers have noted that the politics of health care have been substantially more complex than the Clinton administration and its supporters have expected (Coats 1994; Gawande 1994; Gosselin 1994b; Reichard 1994). Similar to these political dynamics at the macro level, political maneuvering and confrontations also must be dealt with at the individual alliance level. As noted earlier, alliances between hospitals and physicians are often problematic because of the negative ways in which the parties view each other. Because hospital administrators tend to be focused on concerns such as building patient flow, economizing operations, and ensuring a profit, physicians often view administrators as overly "bureaucratic, amateurish and risk adverse" (Baker 1989, p. 71). In contrast, physicians usually emphasize preserving autonomous medical decision making and upholding their ability to extend the best possible care regardless of cost. Thus, hospitals often perceive physicians as "selfish, emotional, and egotistical" (Baker 1989, p. 71). These different orientations can readily undermine the most well-intentioned alliances (Breisch 1994; Rosenfield 1985).

If interfirm health care endeavors are to be successful, it is critical that top managers and administrators utilize cultural and structural supports to ensure that appropriate levels of consultation and collaboration are developed. In the health care industry in general, and the mental health industry in particular, this process will take time. Mental health providers typically have unique personality characteristics, entering solo or small group practices to exert their independence and control their own destiny. Any alliance effort that ignores this reality will have limited success.

The development of strategic alliances in the health care industry is rapidly becoming a major force contributing to the further politicalization of the health administrator's role. Instead of simply controlling a set of subordinates or even mobilizing a coalition of supporters within the organization, administrators must be increasingly adept at juggling a shifting set of stakeholders—internal and external to the venture—over which they have no direct control. As management experts point out, this idea is not new, going back to the early work of management theorists who recognized that an important dimension of management is to develop and mobilize a network of cooperative relationships across people, groups, departments, and divisions (Kanter 1988). Indeed, the underlying theme of agenda setting, network building, and agenda implementation through that network is reflected in a growing number of depictions of the general manager's role (Kotter 1982). The emergence of a broad array of strategic alliances, however, has essentially multiplied the complexity of this reality.

Although interorganizational partnerships require a level of consultation and collaboration that goes well beyond typical patterns of management and organization (Buono 1991; Kanter 1988), mobilizing such support will not be an easy process. Mental health and substance abuse providers in particular, for example, tend to be relational in their orientations. The current pressure to form integrated groups may therefore cause undue stress and lead to the creation of ill-conceived alliances. For these providers, relationship building is an important dimension of successful practice, and it takes time to know and trust the other individuals, groups, and organizations one is joining. Creating alliances in a rushed manner, which many practitioners are now faced with, will lead to discouragement, resentment, and, possibly, a decrease in the quality of treatment. Moreover, once in a network, providers will also be faced with the possibility of a decreased income level caused by lower reimbursement profiles and capitation plans. There is also the threat of termination from a network based on the failure to meet certain, potentially vague, criteria. All of these issues contribute to the reality that bigger may not necessarily translate into better care; instead, it may raise many more conflicts and pressures for providers and consumers alike.

Another concern in health care alliances focuses on whether providers will administer care to serve patients or employers (Gawande 1994). One of the objectives in managed care is to manage the needs of a variety of stakeholders, including health care reform advocates, providers, insurers, employers, and consumers (Findlay 1993). Yet, although the needs of insurers and employers may be to cut costs, consumers and providers have needs that go well beyond cost cutting. Patients, for example, tend to be concerned about things such as access to a physician or therapist of their choice, minimizing the potential embarrassment and stress associated with giving personal information to an unknown screener, referrals based on provider-client trust, and especially with respect to mental health care, confidentiality. Providers in managed care networks tend to focus on maintaining control over diagnosis and treatment, preserving confidentiality about their patients, and having the emotional and financial security that allows them to treat their patients. At the same time, mental health providers will have to become more sensitive to issues of prevention and brief treatment (e.g., pharmacological "tune-ups"), despite the fact that their training often contributes to negative attitudes toward these methods (Lombardi 1974). It is naive to think that balancing these disparate needs and goals will be an easy process, especially given the rather arbitrary and unrefined processes often used in selecting providers for particular networks.

As a way of coping with these changes and emergent structures, managers need to focus on ways to mobilize and bring order to such alliances. Yet, although traditional organization development-related interventions have focused on what may be referred to as *overorganized* systems, strategic alliances are more appropriately conceptualized as *underorganized* systems (Brown 1980). As suggested in this chapter, alliances are loosely coupled systems that vary across a number of important organizational and human resource dimensions, with leadership and power dispersed among autonomous organizations and sporadic member commitment to interfirm collaboration efforts. Thus, efforts to facilitate such links should be guided by a transorganizational perspective, focusing on the dynamics associated with this higher level of social system, identifying and convening members of the relevant organizations, and designing structures and mechanisms for regulating collaborative efforts (Cummings 1984).

Compared with the typical phases of planned change—entry, diagnosis, intervention, and evaluation—the process of change in strategic alliances assumes the need to create new systems and assimilate those involved: identification of relevant stakeholders, systems, and appropriate representatives; convention of those members and initiation of linkage processes; and organization of the system to regularize behaviors (Brown 1980). A problem, however, is that we are just beginning to fully comprehend and understand the nature of and underlying dilemmas involved in interfirm interactions. For instance, although reactive change is largely viewed in negative terms (especially when contrasted to proactive management efforts), given the uncertain nature of strategic alliances significant questions linger as to whether managers can accurately predict exactly what is going to happen in such linkages (Buono 1991). Moreover, the nature of the relationship between alliance members should model the change process. Accordingly, it seems that being prepared to cope with the resultant changes and dynamics appears to be a more realistic posture than one of directly managing and controlling such dynamics (Buono and Nurick 1992).

Within this context, it is also important that a broad-based, long-term time frame be used to assess alliance effectiveness and contribution. Instead of simply using traditional profitability and cash flow measures, it is important to move toward longer-term measures that reflect the true state of the alliance (e.g., adaptiveness, innovativeness, quality of care, productivity appraisals, the level of morale and harmony between the partners). Although such an approach may be cumbersome and highly subjective, it holds greater promise than financial resource indicators alone (Anderson 1990). This broad-based view, of course, does not mean that alliances should be given unlimited time to prove their worth. It does, however, reflect the reality that the value that such health care alliances are intended to create is wide ranging and requires corresponding input and output measures.

Conclusion

It is becoming increasingly clear that many of the key problems and barriers in health care alliances are as much organizational and behavioral as they are strategic and financial. Given the consolidation taking place in the health care industry today, it is critical that we develop an appropriate understanding and appreciation of the interpersonal, intergroup, interorganizational, and interstakeholder processes and dynamics inherent in interfirm endeavors if hospital and health center administrators are to help health care alliances fulfill our expectations of them. Consolidation of the health care industry does indeed have the *potential* to facilitate improved care. No health care alliance will result in better or less expensive care, however, unless administrators, physicians, and other key parties succeed in meeting this challenge.

References

Adams W, Brock JW: The Bigness Complex: Industry, Labor and Government in the American Economy. New York, Pantheon Books, 1986

Alster N: Dealbusters: why partnerships fail. Electronic Business 12 (April): 70–75, 1986

American Bankers Association, Ernst & Whinney: Implementing Mergers and Acquisitions in the Financial Services Industry. Washington, DC, American Bankers Association, 1985

Anderson R: Two firms, one frontier: on assessing joint venture performance. Sloan Management Review 31(2):9–30, 1990

Baker MK: The joint venture: a solution or another problem? Health Care Supervisor 7(2):65–75, 1989

Bastien DT: Common patterns of behavior and communication in corporate mergers and acquisitions. Human Resource Management 26(1):7–33, 1987

Blank AH: The growth of joint venture marketing. The Bankers Magazine 170(2):60–63, 1987

Borys B, Jemison DB: Hybrid arrangements as strategic alliances: theoretical issues in organizational combinations. Academy of Management Review 14(2):234–249, 1989

Breisch SL: Look out for landmines: hospital purchases of physician practices can be fraught with peril. Am Med News, February 14, 1994, pp 23–25

Brown LD: Planned change in underorganized systems, in Systems Theory for Organization Development. Edited by Cummings TG. New York, Wiley, 1980 pp. 239–257

Buono AF: Managing joint ventures: interfirm tensions and pitfalls. SAM Advanced Management Journal 55(2):28–32, 1990

Buono AF: Managing strategic alliances: organizational and human resource considerations. Business in the Contemporary World 3(4):92–101, 1991

Buono AF, Bowditch JL: The Human Side of Mergers and Acquisitions: Managing Collisions Between People, Cultures, and Organizations. San Francisco, CA, Jossey-Bass, 1989

Buono AF, Nurick AJ: Intervening in the middle: coping strategies in mergers and acquisitions. Human Resource Planning 15(2):19–33, 1992

Buono AF, Bowditch JL, Lewis JW: When cultures collide: the anatomy of a merger. Human Relations 38(5):477–500, 1985

Buono AF, Bowditch JL, Lewis JW: The cultural dynamics of transformation: the case of a bank merger, in Corporate Transformation. Edited by Kilmann RH, Covin TJ, Associates. San Francisco, CA, Jossey-Bass, 1988, pp 497–522

Buono AF, Weiss, JW, Bowditch JL: Paradoxes in merger and acquisition consulting: thoughts and recommendations. Consultation 8(3):145–159, 1989

Carpenter RB, Peters GR: Joint ventures in the next decade: four approaches. Healthc Forum J 33(1):43–46, 1990

Coats D: Kennedy health plan: a bureaucrat's dream. Boston Globe, May 18, 1994, p 17

Cody TG: Strategy of a Megamerger: An Insider's Account of the Baxter Travenol-American Hospital Supply Combination. Westport, CT, Quorum Books, 1990

Cummings TG: Transorganizational development, in Research in Organizational Behavior, Vol. 6. Edited by Staw B, Cummings TG. Greenwich, CT, Jai Press, 1984 pp. 367–422

Davidson SM, Maxwell J: Major hospital merger not so major after all. Boston Globe, March 30, 1994, p 25

Do mergers really work? Business Week, June 3, 1985, pp 88–100

Edlin M: The bigger the better: mental health care companies consolidate to survive tough market competition. Managed Health Care February, 1994, 43–44

Findlay S: Networks of care may serve as a model for health reform. Business and Health 11(2):26–31, 1993

Finnerty JE, Owers JE, Rogers RC: The valuation impact of joint ventures. Management International Review 26:14–27, 1986

Gawande A: Don't dump health alliances. Boston Globe, May 4, 1994, p 21

Gold D, Sauvant KP: The future role of transnational corporations in the world economy. Business in the Contemporary World 2(3):55–62, 1990

Gosselin PG: Health alliance plans become focus of fears. Boston Globe, April 17, 1994a, pp 1, 27

Gosselin PG: Health: a sense of Clinton setbacks. Boston Globe, May 8, 1994b, p 14

Gulati R, Khanna T, Nohria N: Unilateral commitments and the importance of process in alliances. Sloan Management Review 35(3):61–69, 1994

Halpern P: Corporate acquisitions: a theory of special cases? A review of event study cases applied to acquisitions. Journal of Finance 2:297–318, 1983

Harrigan KR: Managing for Joint Venture Success. Lexington, MA, Lexington Books, 1986

Ivancevich JM, Schweiger DM, Power FR: Strategies for managing human resources during mergers and acquisitions. Human Resource Planning 10(1):19–35, 1987

Jensen M, Ruback R: The mark for corporate control: the scientific evidence. Journal of Financial Economics 11(1):5–50, 1983

Johnson DE: Reforms offer rare strategic opportunities to providers. Health Care Strateg Manage 11(5):2–3, 1993

Kalzuny A, Zukerman H: Strategic alliances ensure TQM's full potential. Healthc Exec 8(3):33–35, 1993

Kang TW: Gaishi: The Foreign Company in Japan. New York, Basic Books, 1990

Kanter RM: The new alliances: how strategic partnerships are reshaping American business, in Business in the Contemporary World. Edited by Sawyer HL. Lanham, MD, University Press of America, 1988 pp. 59–82

Kaufman DA: Achieving quality health care. Boston Globe, April 12, 1994, p 42

Kazemek EA: Why mergers and acquisitions fail. Healthc Financ Manage 43(1):94, 97, 1989

Knox RA: Merger or no, 2 hospitals may compete in obstetrics. Boston Globe, February 11, 1994a, pp 1, 16

Knox RA: New name, new slant on hospital 'merger.' Boston Globe, March 22, 1994b, pp 21, 29

Kotter JP: The General Manager. New York, Free Press, 1982

Lambrew JM, Ricketts TC, Morrissey JP: Case study of the integration of a local health department and a community health center. Public Health Rep 108(1):19–29, 1993

Lazarus A: The effect of mergers and acquisitions on behavioral health care. Med Interface 8(1):103–106, 1995

Lefkoe M: Why so many mergers fail. Fortune, July 20, 1987, pp 113–114

Levine JB, Byrne JA: Corporate odd couples: joint ventures are the rage, but the matches often don't work out. Business Week, July 21, 1986, pp 100–105

Lombardi JS: The college counseling center and preventive mental activities. Journal of College Student Personnel, November 1974, pp. 435–438

Louis AM: The bottom line on 10 big mergers. Fortune, May 3, 1982, pp 84–89

Lubatkin M: Mergers and the performance of the acquiring firm. Academy of Management Review 8(2):218–225, 1983

Lubatkin M, O'Neil HM: Merger strategies and capital market risk. Academy of Management Journal 30(4):665–684, 1987

Lynch RP: Business Alliance Guide: The Hidden Competitive Weapon. New York, Wiley, 1993

Major MJ: Managed care is credited for breaking the boom-bust cycle of premium costs. Managed Healthcare, February 1994, pp. 44, 46

Marks ML: How to treat the merger syndrome. Journal of Management Consulting 4(3):42–51, 1988

Marks ML, Mirvis PH: The merger syndrome: stress and uncertainty. Mergers & Acquisitions 20(2):50–55, 1985

Meyer H: Alliances in jeopardy. Am Med News, March 7, 1994, pp 38–39

McConnell JJ, Nantell TJ: Corporate combinations and common stock returns: The case of joint ventures. Journal of Finance 40(2):519–536, 1985

Michel A, Shaked I: Evaluating merger performance. California Management Review 27(3):109–118, 1985

Mirvis PH, Marks ML: Managing the Merger. Englewood Cliffs, NJ, Prentice-Hall, 1992

Mueller DC: Mergers and market share. Review of Economics and Statistics 67:259–267, 1985

Murphy WJ: R&D Cooperation Among Marketplace Competitors. Westport, CT, Quorum Books, 1991

Nevaer LE, Louis EV, Deck SA: Strategic Corporate Alliances: A Study of the Present, A Model for the Future. Westport, CT, Quorum Books, 1990

Page L: Will too many mergers stifle competition? Am Med News, July 11, 1994, pp 1, 8–9

Pekar P: Joint Venture. Planning Review, July 1986, pp. 15–19

Peters GR: Revamped, joint ventures make a comeback. Healthc Finan Manage 45(8):62–74, 1991

Porter M, Teisberg E, Brown G: Innovation: medicine's best cost-cutter. New York Times, February 27, 1994, p F11

Pritchett P: After the Merger: Managing the Shockwaves. Homewood, IL, Dow Jones-Irwin, 1985

Reichard J: Backlash beginning to develop against merger mania. Health Alliance Alert 9(5):1, 1994

Ring PS, Van de Ven AH: Developmental processes of cooperative interorganizational relationships. Academy of Management Review 19(1):90–118, 1994

Rosenfield R: Joint venture organizational models. Topics in Health Care Financing 12(2):38–45, 1985

Saeman H: Psychology's health reform priorities 'off track,' Cummings says. The National Psychologist, January–February 1994, p. 10

Sardella S: Alliances are key to practitioner survival. Monitor March, 1994, p. 32

Schillaci CE: Designing Successful Joint Ventures. The Journal of Business Strategy 8(2):59–63, 1987

Schweiger DL, DeNisi A: Communication with employees following a merger: a longitudinal field experiment. Academy of Management Journal 34(1):110–135, 1991

Schweiger DL, Ivancevich JM: Human resources: the forgotten factor in mergers and acquisitions. Personnel Administrator 30(11):47–54, 58-61, 1985

Schweiger DL, Walsh JP: Mergers and acquisitions: an interdisciplinary view. Research in Personnel and Human Resource Management 8:41–107, 1990

Shenkar O, Zeira Y: International joint ventures: implications for organization development. Personnel Review 16(1):30–37, 1987

Small K, Mont J: Fractured hospital: Metrowest medical staff say distrust carves deep rift. The Tab, February 15, 1994, pp 9–12

Stein C: A mixed bag for Mass. health insurers. Boston Globe, February 17, 1994a, pp 1, 45

Stein C: Mass. hospitals face job loss. Boston Globe May 8, 1994b, pp 1, 18

Tremonti L, Manning MR: Merging hospitals and physician support. JAMA 250:2628–2632, 1983

Waddock S: Building successful social partnerships. Sloan Management Review, Summer 1988, pp. 17–23

Chapter 25

Will the Transition Into Integrated Networks Appear Seamless?

Michael J. Bennett, M.D.

Among the many changes that have rocked the health care industry, none has produced more profound effects than the reconfiguration of the last of the great medical cottage industries—private mental health practice. Under pressure to reduce costs as a result of unregulated excesses of the past decade, the introduction of managed care has begun to reshape long-entrenched practice patterns in the mental health field. How has this come about? Why are reactions in the professional community so negative? What is the current status of mental health practice and how will it change in the future? In this chapter I explore the trend toward the regionalization of health care and the integration of mental health provider networks. I identify specific challenges that lie ahead and suggest ways to make the upcoming transition into integrated networks as smooth as possible.

The Birth of Managed Care

Managed care has its roots in the 1960s. With the passage of legislation related to Medicare and Medicaid, there was a dramatic increase in the public funding of health care. Associated with a broadened public health responsibility was the notion of public scrutiny. Amendments to the Social

Security Act in 1972 led to the creation of professional standards review organizations, which were charged with monitoring the utilization of health care services. The Peer Review Improvement Act of 1982 established a precedent for external review of treatment with reimbursement at stake. The principle of accountability was thus clearly established with regard to public sector programs (Goodman et al. 1992).

Additional federal initiatives broadened the scope of accountability to include the private sector and prompted a pervasive reconfiguration of the medical landscape. In the early 1970s the Nixon administration adopted a health care policy that favored the establishment of prepaid group practices, dubbed by Paul Ellwood as "health maintenance organizations" (HMOs) (Mayer and Mayer 1985, p. 593). The interest in prepaid group practices culminated in the HMO Act of 1973. Two features of the act significantly modified the concept of the HMO, which until then had been regarded as an idealistic movement of limited scope. First, there was the inclusion of for-profit organizations in the national strategy to contain health care spending. Second, there was a broadening of the definition of HMO to include open, community-based systems of care (independent practice associations) as well as traditional staff- and group-model prototypes. These actions set in motion a variety of experiments related to the structure, financing, and management of medical services that have continued at an ever-accelerating pace (Bennett 1988, 1993a).

Ironically, despite concerns about cost, the 1980s saw a dramatic increase in the number of psychiatric inpatient programs. Under pressure to fill beds, many facilities developed inpatient substance abuse programs and programs for adolescents. Development was facilitated by a climate of deregulation, growing public acceptance of psychiatric treatment, aggressive advertising, a proliferation of for-profit hospital chains, a shrinkage of the number of acute medical and surgical beds, and a third-party system that, in its inflexibility, often favored inpatient treatment over outpatient alternatives. As mental health costs became the most rapidly expanding sector of health care in general, payers revolted. Managed care, in its present form, was born and came to symbolize additional regulatory mechanisms in private sector health care.

The Evolution of Managed Behavioral Health Care

Characteristically, a payer who seeks to bring mental health care costs under control proceeds in a sequence that recapitulates the history of managed care itself. The least intense form of management, *managed indemnity*, employs utilization management procedures to influence patient care decisions (see Chapter 13). Utilization management usually requires a reviewer who operates at a site remote from the actual care and uses a protocol to assess the necessity for treatment. Historically, great emphasis has been placed on reviewing inpatient treatment, but this is changing to include all levels of treatment. The introduction of utilization management alone can lead to significant cost savings through reduced hospitalization; however, the limitations of inpatient utilization review are well known. Cost savings may not be sustainable, relationships between peer reviewers and attending physicians tend to be adversarial, and review often focuses on contingencies to treatment rather than treatment itself. Utilization review carries little potential to remedy issues of quality that have become an increasing concern to consumers and payers.

To ensure quality, a manager must monitor treatment. This involves a fundamental shift from managing benefits (demand for service) to managing care (supply). In closed systems, such as staff-model HMOs, such monitoring may be performed directly through supervision, because the HMO typically owns the delivery system and employs the provider. In open systems, which are composed of independent practitioners loosely affiliated with each other and with the HMO, such oversight must be accomplished indirectly, through quality assurance mechanisms.

Within the past few years, independent practice associations have evolved into networks: organized systems of care. An early emphasis on cost containment, which assigned preferential provider status on the basis of unit (hourly) discounts, has given way to methods of selection and performance assessment that emphasize access, efficiency, patient satisfaction, clinical outcome, and the quality of the working relationship between the provider and the managed care organization. With performance as the yardstick of preferential status, providers have increasingly been asked to share in the financial risk. Risk sharing tends to create partnerships between the managed care organization and its providers and thus replaces compliance with alliance. Most contracts that ask providers to share risk have been developed within the context of the behavioral health care *carve-out.*

The Carve-Out

In its simplest form, the mental health and substance abuse carve-out is a system of care that is structured, financed, and accessed differently from other medical care. Mental health carve-outs are typically administered by specialty companies contracted to HMOs and self-insured businesses. There are several advantages to the carve-out configuration. Services may be priced and provided according to the mental health and substance abuse needs of a specific population; treatment may be given in decentralized, office-based settings with low overhead and capital investment; available resources are likely to reflect modern treatment methods; and quality, cost, and consumer satisfaction are generally more readily identified and measured in carve-out programs. The popularity of the carve-out also reflects the fact that payers are anxious about escalating mental health and substance abuse costs and view them as separate from overall health care costs, best left in the hands of experts who will assume the risk and manage it. There is a definite appeal to isolating behavioral health care to control it.

Capitalizing on the popularity of mental health carve-outs, behavioral health care vendors have proliferated rapidly in recent years. Along with this growth, the concept of the preferred provider network has further evolved. It has been estimated that as much as 95% of all insured care now involves some form of management (Zaldivar 1993), yet only about 50% of insurance plans actively limit the patient's choice of a provider. This limitation may take one of two forms. In the first form, known as an exclusive provider organization, to be reimbursed the subscriber must see a clinician from the designated provider pool. In the second form, known as a point-of-service plan, greater choice of provider is available, but at a lower rate of reimbursement. Point-of-service plans presume that less costly service can be provided within a designated network of providers because the network can be tightly managed. They also implicitly assume that the quality of care provided within the network will be at least equal to that in the general community. Increasing demands from insurance regulators, payers, and the public have pressured managed care organizations to demonstrate that they meet quality expectations. This pressure has led to renewed efforts in the management and enhancement of quality of care. Questions fundamental to health care are once again being asked: Who needs treatment? What type and how much treatment is needed? How can care best be provided and how can good treatment outcomes be identified and achieved? In search of answers to these questions, managed care vendors have moved beyond unidimensional monitoring of single episodes of care to multidimensional planning for the needs of defined populations.

The shift to monitoring populations rather than individuals has raised significant questions about the activities of providers within managed care systems. There is greater demand for clinicians to offer cost-effective treatment by eliminating unnecessary hospitalization, shortening the treatment episode of care, and confining therapeutic interventions to modifying observable behavior. Implicit in this requirement is a refinement of the goals of practice and the methods used to achieve them: choice of method should be based on objectives and on knowledge of what works rather than on intuition. More than ever, clinicians are being asked to intervene rapidly, set realistic goals, and terminate treatment when the goals have been achieved. Pragmatism and eclecticism are prized, as is the coordination of multiple providers who may operate at various levels of care. The overall quality of treatment in managed systems depends on the effectiveness of interventions at any level or intensity of care as well as a smooth transition between or among levels. Such systems are therefore integrated both horizontally, embracing treatment alternatives, and vertically, linking various levels of service.

Solo practice is likely to be eclipsed by practice within groups as the modular infrastructure of the integrated network. This preference is based on the premise that groups offer more flexibility, providing a range of service options rather than a narrower choice limited by the theoretical orientation, personal preference, knowledge, and skills of the clinician who works alone. Group structure underscores the importance of coordinated systems at both the micro and macro level. The emphasis on systems rather than individual providers is associated with a concomitant shift in quality management from quality assurance to continuous quality improvement. Quality assurance involves inspection of the episode of care performed by an individual clinician. The problematic pattern is either modified or the "bad apple" removed. Continuous quality improvement, by contrast, places emphasis on the way the system functions and seeks to progressively improve it. Within a group practice, and among the various components of an integrated network, care managers seek to facilitate patient flow and promote an integrated, seamless system of care.

A number of factors create seams in the system. The individuals and institutions involved are often historical competitors rather than collaborators (Bennett 1994). Furthermore, the carve-out is structurally aloof from many of the systems required for an integrated continuum, including medical caregivers. Despite these limitations, carve-outs may be regarded as the building blocks of integrated systems of care.

Carved-In Or Carved-Out?

A trend to consider at this point is the move away from carve-outs to carve-ins. The term *carve-in* has several meanings. First, it refers to a close working relationship between the managed care vendor and medical caregivers and institutions. Second, the term *carve-in* refers to the ability of the mental health program to operate as a component of larger systems of care while maintaining a degree of fiscal, administrative, and clinical autonomy. Finally, a carve-in suggests a closer working relationship between the managed care organization and the behavioral health care delivery system. It is not uncommon for managed care companies to own and operate components of a service delivery system rather than solely manage providers from a distance. Alliances among managed care organizations, hospitals, provider groups, HMOs, and community mental health centers represent expanded arrangements within the carve-in. Pomerantz and associates (1994) described a carve-in involving an HMO owned by several hospitals that created its own small behavioral health care network as an alternative to carving out treatment to a national managed care company. In this instance, the managed care organization was viewed as a competitive adversary.

A second trend affecting the future of the carve-out is related to the problem of surplus providers, which makes it necessary to consolidate networks or at least reduce the provider pool (Freeman 1992; Savitz 1991). Elimination of providers, however, generally raises havoc within professional communities because it threatens the livelihood of nonparticipants. Fink (1994) and others have suggested that all "willing providers" should have an opportunity to participate in provider networks. However, a willing provider is not necessarily an able provider because not all clinicians are prepared to operate effectively as part of an organized system (Bennett 1993b). Still, a number of states have enacted legislation to ensure that all qualified providers will be eligible to join networks. This legislation places considerable pressure on managed care organizations to develop precise criteria for the inclusion of providers in their networks and to make these criteria public.

Finally, carve-out vendors face stiff competition from other integrated delivery systems such as physician-hospital organizations (PHOs). Reaching outward into the community from a tertiary care base, PHOs may compete directly with managed care vendors by developing their own networks. Rather than form partnerships with managed care organizations, PHOs may operate their management systems internally, posing a threat to the viability of managed care vendors. One can only speculate that in an era dominated by "mega-networks," the single-specialty carve-out organizations must adapt and evolve to survive.

Integration Under Health Care Reform

Discussions about health care reform have inspired significant debate at both the national and state levels. It seems likely that the insurance base will be broadened to include all or most individuals currently uninsured. The fate of behavioral health care under health care reform remains uncertain. Clearly the concept of managed competition calls for managed care, and thus the experience gained in the present phase of managed care will be invaluable. It has not been determined, however, how current managed care systems will be incorporated in future systems of care.

Accountable health plans, as envisioned in the Clinton reform proposals, would have been composed of providers and facilities operating as integrated service units. The state of Vermont, a leader in the early phases of the debate over reform, proposes integration based on direct contracting between insurers and providers. Financing mechanisms must be worked out, and funding shortfalls may limit action at either the federal or state level. Still, the reality of managed competition has fueled activity within the professional community. This activity has taken two major forms: a spate of mergers and acquisitions by the major managed care vendors and their parent organizations and the development of joint ventures between managed care vendors and institutions. This activity will most likely continue and accelerate rapidly during the next few years.

Integrated treatment systems will involve not only individual providers and hospitals but also residential treatment facilities, home care services, suppliers of medication, and others. Network development may be either centrifugal or centripetal, proceeding from disparate, community-based centers of service toward regional tertiary care centers, or the reverse, from the hospitals toward the periphery. The PHO is an example of the latter type of movement. It is likely that hospitals will attempt to accomplish in the behavioral health care arena what they have been aggressively achieving in the medical and surgical arenas, namely, positioning themselves to operate as total health care systems by developing or purchasing ambulatory and community-based services.

Academic institutions are actively developing "hub and spoke" arrangements (Adelman 1994). The medical school and its primary teaching hospital serve as the hub, and connections to outlying practices and facilities are the spokes. This type of configuration may include purchased existing practices, management or shared-services agreements, or new practices established in strategic areas by the university. The spoke sites typically employ nurse-practitioners and physician assistants in addition to physicians.

Integration may take other forms as well. For example, combined employee assistance programs and behavioral health care contracts are increasingly common. Links with employers may extend to cover services not traditionally associated with managed care networks (e.g., disability and workers' compensation programs). These new arrangements inevitably will require resolution of a major shortcoming of the carve-out: its separation from the mainstream of medical care. Bridges must be built to primary caregivers if integrated care is to be delivered. No mental health and substance abuse program can be considered integrated without paying attention to the medical needs of patients, the practice needs of primary care physicians, and the "boundary" areas where mental health and medical practice overlap.

It is important to note that integrated systems of care must include a mix of public and private resources. The public-private pairing appears to be well under way as evidenced by the privatization of programs in the public sector and the contracting of behavioral health care for Medicaid populations to national managed care vendors. Partnerships between public sector resources and managed care vendors appear to be logical given that many of the strategies used by managed care companies to control costs resemble those developed by the public sector (Shore 1992). An interesting experiment in pairing public and private systems into a unified funding stream that "follows the patient" is taking place in Minnesota, where the Consolidated Fund has expanded services to underserved populations and has brought effective substance abuse treatment to many persons who had previously had difficulty accessing the traditional health care system (Turnure 1994).

Problems and Prospects

National debate surrounding the organizing and financing of health care services has paralleled discussions in the behavioral health care arena. For example, the concept of regional purchasing alliances contracting with accountable health plans invokes contracting strategies related to the development of behavioral health care networks. It is not known, however, whether behavioral health care will be accorded significant status in accountable health plans. Will the emphasis on primary care and gatekeepers undermine the carve-out? Will staff- and group-model HMOs regain their market share with respect to behavioral health care? The answers to those questions may depend on the capacity of the managed care industry to advance beyond its current status by integrating existing networks.

Most market transitions, however, are disruptive to working relationships. In the health care industry, transition threatens the economic viability of providers, the relationship between clinicians and patients, and customary patterns of patient referral (Lazarus 1994). Transition is painful and it involves risks, but changes in the delivery of mental health care are clearly necessary. Two large epidemiological studies (Kessler et al. 1994; Regier et al. 1993) have documented that only a small percentage of individuals who need mental health treatment actually receive it. This is a national tragedy that must be addressed.

Behavioral caregivers must be acknowledged by primary caregivers, who continue to see the majority of patients with mental health and substance abuse disorders yet struggle to manage their care. As with all treatment, the hospital can no longer be a common meeting ground. Outpatient consultation coupled with increased education of medical caregivers in behavioral health care must be attained. As an example, Medco Containment Services, a manager of pharmaceutical products has undertaken a major initiative to educate primary caregivers in drug-prescribing practices. Other methods must be found as well.

Established clinicians and those in training must be educated about the goals of properly managed care (Bennett 1993b). Information systems must be developed to provide feedback to clinicians about patient outcomes and patient satisfaction. In some areas, community standards must be improved, for example, by the use of practice guidelines and practice parameters. Patients who enter managed care programs must be educated about limitations of their insurance policies and their role in primary and secondary prevention of illnesses. Ultimately, managers of care must evolve into managers of health.

Shortell (1993) underscored three dimensions of effective organized delivery systems: breadth, depth, and geographical concentration of resources. The latter two dimensions may be especially elusive, even when resources are plentiful; when they are not plentiful, such as in rural areas, significant challenges exist (Christianson and Moscovice 1993). A major impediment to organizing health care is the difficulty in bridging disparate cultures, especially when the "prime mover" is a hospital. The roles of hospitals in organized delivery systems must be modified so that hospitals are no longer the crucible of care. In addition, physicians must be linked more closely to hospitals and to each other with regard to sharing strategies to reduce health care spending. Networks of the future must be conceptualized in terms of partnership rather than "rentership" as is common in many health care systems today.

Partnerships must be supported by fiscal incentives to share accountability. Case-based reimbursement carries a potential for building partnerships while attempting to keep the population healthy, as do capitated contracts. Capitation, however, may involve a degree of risk sharing that is unacceptable for any but a large group of providers. Fee-for-service reimbursement creates perverse incentives to treat illness rather than promote health; therefore, it encourages overtreatment. Utilization review procedures guard against such excess but are disliked by providers. Prospective payment, with safeguards against undertreatment, offers the best hope of moving from external review to internal accountability as a guiding principle. Conrad (1993) suggested that the more global the unit of payment, the stronger is the incentive to coordinate care.

Fiscal realities may help shape the behavior of clinicians, but other strategies will be needed as well to modify practice behavior. Some guidance will be supplied in the form of practice parameters and standards as monitored through quality assurance efforts. Technological advances such as electronic data systems, telemedicine, and videoconferencing will also contribute to the practice development of providers, not only in terms of disseminating information but also in terms of providing feedback about a provider's performance. Aggregate and individual provider feedback can be introduced into group practices by the manager. If properly processed, such information may enhance quality while reinforcing collaborative practice patterns.

Integrated networks will function optimally if all components are linked through a common culture and set of values. Clinical protocols and standards will be most acceptable if participation in them is voluntary. Continuous quality improvement initiatives may supply a common ground for clinicians to bond through practice. Quality improvement processes must be carefully implemented and managed to gain credibility, however. A major concern of participants in organized systems of care will be how to achieve excellence. Endeavors that further that aim will improve integration by lessening undesirable variation and by engaging providers in shared responsibilities for improvements to the system. Eventually, the formal accreditation of health care provider networks may become a federal requirement.

Conclusion

The mental health professions are in the midst of turbulence and on the threshold of significant change. At no other time has the security of the professionals involved been more threatened. It seems clear that any reform measure that includes behavioral health care will be highly managed. Building on the accomplishments of managed care carve-out programs in the past decade, the continued development of networks will be a prominent part of reform efforts. Networks, as they currently exist, represent a core piece of a future integrated delivery system. Using improved technology, network managers will move beyond inspection and problem identification and establish a common identity with institutions and clinicians. They will monitor treatment outcome and seek to improve the results of treatments. Education, information sharing, and alliance building will be seen as essential activities leading to the integration of provider networks. The development of reimbursement mechanisms that support the formation of alliances rather than foster passive compliance with a set of expectations will be crucial. Perhaps a major force driving the expansion of networks will be the continued evolution of managed care vendors into system owners and operators who actually deliver treatment. Alternatively, managed care organizations may become less important as integrated delivery systems develop their own capacity to manage care.

The transition into integrated networks will not appear seamless. The profound transformation required will produce scars as would any attempt to blend discrete cultures. Providers will be pressured to change the nature of their practices, and care systems may be significantly disrupted during such massive realignment. Networks will not appear seamless insofar as they are likely to contain gaps in the treatment continuum, especially in underserved and rural areas. There will continue to be a role for care managers, at least for high-risk patients and for those with serious mental illness who utilize multiple sources of help, both within and outside an organized system. The coordination of emergency care poses similar problems and calls for a level of cooperation between clinicians and administrators that is frequently lacking. Patients who leave existing care systems and enter new networks may require help dealing with the impact of forced change, and provisions must be made for their safe transition. Similarly, clinicians who enter networks ill prepared, especially through "any willing provider" provisions, will need to be accommodated and educated.

Integration cannot be seen as a structural phenomenon alone. It must be viewed as an end toward which quality improvement is largely dedicated and toward which the system as a whole continues to move. This end is entirely consistent with the transcendent value of any health care professional: commitment to the well-being of patients. It is they, after all, who stand to lose most by becoming lost in the seams.

References

Adelman SH: Academic physicians are caught up in changes too. American Medical News, May 2, 1994, pp 23–24

Bennett MJ: The greening of the HMO: implications for prepaid psychiatry. Am J Psychiatry 145:1544–1549, 1988

Bennett MJ: View from the bridge: reflections of a recovering staff model HMO psychiatrist. Psychiatr Q 64:45–75, 1993a

Bennett MJ: The importance in teaching the principles of managed care. Behavioral Healthcare Tomorrow 2(3):28–32, 1993b

Bennett MJ: Are competing psychotherapists manageable? Manag Care Q 2(2):36–42, 1994

Christianson J, Moscovice I: Health care reform and rural health networks. Health Aff 12(3):58–75, 1993

Conrad DA: Coordinating patient care services in regional health systems: the challenge of clinical integration. Hosp Health Serv Adm 38:491–508, 1993

Fink P: Any willing provider. Psychiatric News, January 21, 1994, p 25

Freeman M: Perspectives on the future of network-based managed behavioral health care systems. American Association of Preferred Provider Organizations Journal 2:17–22, 1992

Goodman M, Brown J, Dietz P: Managing Managed Care. Washington, DC, American Psychiatric Press, 1992

Kessler R, McGonagle K, Zhao S, et al: Lifetime and 12-month prevalence of DSM-III-R psychiatric disorders in the United States. Arch Gen Psychiatry 51:8–19, 1994

Lazarus A: Transferring psychiatric patients into managed care networks. Annals of Clinical Psychiatry 6:141–142, 1994

Mayer TR, Mayer CG: HMOs: origins and development. NEJM 312:590–594, 1985

Peer Review Improvement Act (Tax Equity and Fiscal Responsibility Act of 1982, Title I, Subtitle C, 2142)

Pomerantz JM, Liptzin B, Carter AH, et al: The professional affiliation group: a new model for managed mental health care. Hosp Community Psychiatry 45:308–310, 1994

Regier D, Narrow M, Rae D, et al: The de facto US mental health and addictive disorders service system. Arch Gen Psychiatry 50:85–94, 1993

Savitz S: Networks in mental health and substance abuse. J Ambulatory Care Management 14:27–29, 1991

Shore M: Managed care: reinventing the wheel. Hosp Community Psychiatry 43:205, 1992

Shortell SM: Creating organized delivery systems: the barriers and facilitators. Hosp Health Serv Admin 38:447–466, 1993

Social Security Amendments of 1972, Pub L No 92-603

Social Security Amendments of 1983, Pub L No 98-21

Tax Equity and Fiscal Responsibility Act of 1982, Pub L No 97-248

Turnure C: Implications of the State of Minnesota's Consolidated Chemical Dependency Treatment Fund for Substance Abuse Coverage Under Health Care Reform. Presented to U.S. Senate Labor and Human Resources Committee, Washington, DC, March 8, 1994

Zaldivar R: Managed health care: a cure or terminal mayhem? Tuesday Worklife, January 5, 1993, p F1.

Chapter 26

Who Will Manage the Managers?

Stephen J. O'Connor, Ph.D.

> The . . . managers with patronizing smile tell the poor doctor that he is no business man; the doctor admits it, and with hat in hand begs for an opportunity to give his services free. ("A lack of professional business" 1896)

> The ability to make cheap bargains, should not be compared to the ability to restore to health the sick and injured. (Biddle 1904)

> By definition, managed care introduces elements of management control into the arena of health care delivery, management that clearly reduces the physician's autonomy. (Kongstvedt 1993)

> While many physicians fall prey to an illusion of omnicompetence and believe that their medical training has endowed them with superior management judgment, most are incapable of submitting to the authority of anyone, even a fellow physician. (Goldsmith 1993)

In the past decade, a great deal of attention has centered on how to improve relations between physicians and health care managers. More recently, these relations have sharply deteriorated as the amount, complexity, and pace of change in our health care environment have threatened to unravel the fragile working relationships that have existed between physicians and health care managers. Improving these relations is critical, not only for the survival of any one health care organization or profession, but for the overall performance of the United States health care delivery system. Undoubtedly, it is in the best interest of managers and physicians to reexamine and modify the nature of their relationships so that they can prepare themselves to take advantage of the opportunities, as well as to avoid the hazards, a changing health system will bring.

In this chapter I examine the relationship between physicians and managers and ultimately attempt to answer the question, "Who will manage the managers?" In doing so, I first consider how this tempestuous and conflict-ridden association has evolved and speculate where it may be heading in the future. Next, I examine the many obvious and not so obvious differences that exist between physicians and managers that have a bearing on this relationship. Finally, suggestions are put forth for improving manager-physician relations.

Evolution of the Relationship

Although the management-medicine relationship has always been rife with tension and conflict (Starr 1982; Stevens 1989), it only recently has provoked an outpouring of anxiety and interest. Much of the current fascination with this relationship is a consequence of the apparent transfer of control and authority of medical affairs to nonphysician administrators and the potential effects of this movement on health care costs, quality, and professional autonomy. To help put the current situation in perspective, what follows is a brief examination of the management-medicine interface from an evolutionary point of view.

The Preeminence of Hospital Governing Bodies

During the latter half of the 19th century, long before there were any managed care organizations, managed competition–based health reform plans, or any holders of the master of business administration (M.B.A.) degree, physicians who wanted a hospital-based clinical education and the secure and lucrative employment prospects of holding hospital privileges generally were compelled to acquiesce to a hospital's board of managers or governing body. These boards were typically composed of prominent citizens who contributed both money and social legitimacy—possessions physicians had little of, but greatly desired. It was the governing body that held final decision-making authority in most hospitals. The governing body's range of authority included the usual organizational decisions, such as how money would be raised and spent, but also extended to clinical matters such as whether a patient would be admitted, when a patient would be discharged, and how satisfied a patient was with a given physician. Physicians were clearly at a relative disadvantage, but this situation would change.

Doctors' Workshops and the Bestowal of Professional Autonomy

By about 1910, a unique confluence of social, technological, scientific, political, and legal forces served to confer occupational autonomy on physicians in the United States. At the same time, physicians also began to experience greater exposure to organizations and management as they spent more of their time training and practicing in hospitals. However, because they were primarily engaged in solo, independent, fee-for-service practice they were not considered organizational employees and thus were not under the direct supervisory control of the hospital administration. It was during this time that hospitals came to be known as *doctors' workshops* and where the classical dual lines of authority emerged—one medical, the other administrative. The reason for this peculiar arrangement was that, by this time, only physicians had the authority and autonomy to practice medicine and to make clinical decisions; administrators and governing boards existed solely to garner resources and support from the environment and to manage the nonmedical hospital bureaucratic structure. The role of managers in these doctors' workshops was essentially limited to serving the nursing, equipment, and other resource needs of physicians so high-quality medicine could be practiced as the physician saw fit.

Thus, the nature of the management-physician relationship changed considerably during the early part of the 20th century, with physicians enjoying unparalleled professional authority and unfettered freedom from management in medical decision making. However, because their practices were becoming increasingly dependent on formal organizational settings (i.e., community hospitals), they were unable to break completely away from the influence of managers, even though it was advocated by some that all lay managers should be replaced by physicians. It was envisioned that these physicians would specialize in administration, in much the same way other physicians specialized in surgery or internal medicine.

Nevertheless, the hospitals' separate dual lines of authority turned the classical management precept of *unity-of-command* upside down, and resulted in an awkward marriage of medicine and management. The adage "We can't live with them, but we can't live without them" would surely have been considered a truism by both parties in this uneasy union.

The Tilt Toward Management

In the years following World War II, the management side of the relationship began to slowly but inexorably reassert itself vis-à-vis physicians. This change was caused by a variety of factors that included

- having to meet hospitalwide standards of accreditation as specified by the Joint Commission on Accreditation of Hospitals;

- the landmark legal case of *Darling v. Charleston Community Memorial Hospital*, which established that not only physicians, but also hospitals, are accountable for the quality of care delivered (this decision encouraged hospital managers and governing bodies to take steps to ensure that physicians were providing high-quality care and that the medical staff was taking its quality assurance responsibilities seriously);
- the passage of Medicare and Medicaid legislation and their subsequent demands for utilization and quality control in the form of Professional Standards Review Organizations and later Peer Review Organizations; and
- the growth of for-profit multihospital systems and extensive hospital diversification into non–health-related businesses during the 1970s and 1980s, coupled with the introduction of Medicare's prospective payment system based on diagnosis-related groups in 1983. All of these elements were influential and helped to further infuse management into medical practice.

Abundant Resources and the Masking of Conflict

A popular assumption of the 1960s and early 1970s was that, given enough resources, ever higher levels of health and health care could be achieved by the population. For that reason, society tended to be less concerned with issues such as clinical appropriateness and efficiency. A belief in "more equals more" prevailed. More physician visits, more surgeries, more X rays, more hospital inpatient admissions, more facilities, more funding, and so on, were desired by not only physicians and administrators, but by society as well. Physicians could keep busy and make more money by doing more tests and procedures, and administrators saw hospital revenues increase proportionately with hospital use. In fact, a proverbial saying of the time was "A full hospital is a happy hospital!"

Tensions between managers and physicians continued, however. Although they became more serious during the 1980s, these tensions were not generally viewed as intolerable because the seemingly disparate goals of physicians and managers were usually accommodated by the incredibly abundant financial resources that flowed from third-party payers, who reimbursed most services retrospectively on the basis of costs or charges. Hospitals, medical schools, clinics, and physicians flourished in this generous environment. Because of the surplus of resources, managers and physicians were not obliged to make the really hard decisions that scarcer resources would have required (e.g., make meaningful trade-offs among various components such as growth, access, quality, cost, and professional autonomy and authority).

Both managers and physicians gained from the surfeit of fiscal resources that fueled the growth and demand for health care services; however, the conflict, tension, and mistrust that traditionally characterized the relationship were never diminished. Instead, they were suppressed by slack economic resources, a relative symmetry of power among administrators and various physician specialties, as well as by their growing incomes, prestige, and pleasing privileges and perquisites (Rosenberg 1987).

Employers, Health Reform, and the Rush to Managed Care

By the mid-1980s, relations between physicians and managers were severely strained as society became increasingly concerned with containing health care costs and as the autonomy of the medical profession came under attack on a number of fronts. These assaults were numerous and included decreased control over physician training and licensing, a deteriorating sense of professional cohesiveness brought on by physician oversupply, heightened competition, increased malpractice litigation, discrepancy in the rewards received by different physicians, and the extreme fragmentation of medicine through specialization (O'Connor and Lanning 1992). Moreover, there was a growing awareness that physicians were not always certain of what worked and what did not work. In addition, research on small area variations in practice patterns demonstrated that extreme variability existed in the application of what they did know. This knowledge and practice gap, combined with a rising consumerism and general suspicion that some physician decisions were determined more by personal economic incentives than by a pure service orientation, tended to jeopardize society's faith in the medical profession and confidence in its authority.

Currently, the principal assault on physician autonomy comes from employers and the growth of the managed care sector. Although managed care has existed in the United States for decades, first in the form of prepaid group practice, it slowly began to grow during the 1970s following the passage of the Federal HMO Act (Raffel and Raffel 1989), and in recent years it has virtually exploded in popularity. Likewise, United States business, for the most part, has provided health care benefits to employees since World War II. As long as these benefits remained popular with employees, the premiums remained tax free, and businesses felt they were getting value for their money, businesses tended to limit their involvement in health care to sending a premium check to the insurance company.

Employers appeared to be happy in their check-writing role while the percentage of the American gross national product spent on health care remained less than 10%. However, since 1980, health care expenditures have risen dramatically, currently costing the United States well over $900 billion annually and constituting more than 13% of the gross national product. Recently, private businesses have found themselves spending as much on health care as they have earned, after taxes, in profit. Accordingly, employers have been painfully aware of the financial toll these skyrocketing costs have had on their businesses and have tried everything to contain costs and maintain quality for their beneficiaries—beneficiaries that include not only the productive employee, but his or her spouse and dependents. There are also millions of retired employees who receive some sort of health care benefit from former employers.

Many businesses have claimed that the net effect of these substantial and ballooning health care expenses is an impaired competitive position in the national and global marketplace. To stay competitive, they have become extremely aggressive in managing health care costs, with many choosing to become self-insured and continuing to embrace managed care as an alternative or as a requirement for their workers. Many other businesses have decided not to provide health care because the cost is so great. Additionally, employers in many cities have joined purchaser coalitions to provide them with more clout and information vis-à-vis physicians and hospitals, further restructuring the customary roles of health care purchasers and providers.

Like their private business counterparts, federal and state governments have also been severely challenged as they attempt to pay for the health care services of Medicare and Medicaid beneficiaries as well as government employees. Here too, managed care plays an increasingly prominent role in the solution.

Finally, many of the current state and national health reform proposals that appear to have the greatest appeal are those based on the concept of managed competition. Very simply, managed competition is nothing more than regulated competition among various managed care plans (Relman 1993). To the extent that these proposals become mandated by law, managed care will become even more prevalent.

As health care costs have grown dramatically, so too has the movement toward managed care. Thus, managed care has become a thriving and principal feature of the United States health care landscape. Although it resists a standard definition, one generally thinks of managed care as incorporating elements such as primary care gatekeepers, shared financial risk and incentives, utilization management, and comprehensive prepaid service. It is an alternative to the traditional, but decidedly inflationary, fee-for-service payment systems and indemnity insurance schemes that helped permit the remarkable autonomy of the United States medical profession in the first place. A consequence of the managed care movement, and its desire to manage utilization and costs, is that payers and health plans have been speedily expropriating control of the practice of medicine as they exercise greater influence over health care resources and dollars.

A Growing Mutual Dependency

Medical education instills in physicians the desire and ability to act as the autonomous expert and arbiter of clinical practice. Because the issue of professional autonomy carries so much emotional freight, it is relinquished to nonphysicians only with great difficulty and resentment. Ironically, although the many assaults on physician autonomy, especially the rise of managed care, have done much to thwart the relationship of physicians and managers, they have also served to emphasize the growing dependency of physicians and managers on one another. Health care managers and their organizations can't provide high-quality medical services without the commitment and direction of dedicated physicians. Alternatively, fewer and fewer physicians are able to provide high-quality services in the absence of the specialized support an organizational setting can provide (Schulz and Detmer 1994). Thus, despite a turbulent and hostile health care environment, which has sorely tested and endangered the physician and management relationship, sheer survival in this environment is requiring that they band together as allies, pushing both toward an ever-growing mutual dependency (O'Connor and Shewchuk 1993).

True collaboration between managers and physicians, although increasingly necessary, is still not a natural state of affairs, and most of the initial attempts to achieve it are driven by fear. The ingrained mutual skepticism and disaffection have not dissipated; instead, they have persisted and intensified. Many physicians chafe with anger and exasperation as they observe the erosion of their professional autonomy and may seek a cooperative relationship with managers only as a last ditch effort to survive. Many lay managers, especially hospital administrators, harbor deep animosity toward physicians. They have long resented not only their substantial earnings and astuteness but especially their characteristically imperious forays into organizational management (Goldsmith 1993).

The current state of mutual resentment notwithstanding, the present health care environment continues to demand greater interdependency between the roles of physicians and management. Physicians are being required to take on more responsibility for administrative obligations such as problem solving, negotiation, and leadership (Shortell 1991) and have been forced to better accommodate their services to available organizational resources (Ashley 1989). At the same time, as managers come under greater pressure to ensure the appropriate, efficient, and effective delivery of patient care services, they have become much more involved in clinical areas. Thus, the traditionally separate and distinct domains of physicians and managers have become blurred as physicians take on greater managerial roles (Romeo 1988) and as managers become more involved in patient care (Rohrer 1989).

The Differences: Cultural and Psychological

The responsibility for further cultivating relationships between physicians and managers, and for encouraging the continued consolidation of their respective roles, dictates that both parties seek a better comprehension of who their counterparts are and why they think and act as they do. How well each is able to understand the other's unique culture, values, and goals is an important first step in getting physicians and managers to work with each other more effectively. Because strong dissimilarities exist between the professions of medicine and management, in both cultural and psychological attributes, it is helpful for both parties to recognize these dissimilarities and make an honest attempt to understand each others' perspectives.

Cultural Differences

Numerous differences do exist, most of which can be attributed to unique educational and socialization processes that impart different bases of knowledge, professional values and cultures, and world views. According to Shortell (1991), the attributes in which the major cultural distinctions are observed include the underlying basis of knowledge, the pertinent exposure to patients and other health professionals during training, a broad versus narrow patient focus, the time frame for action, how "rules of evidence" are viewed, beliefs regarding resources, and professional identity. These differences are summarized in Table 26–1. However, even more central to these cultural differences is the strong probability that the groups differ with respect to fundamental and enduring psychological attributes.

Psychological Differences

Recently, the enduring psychological attributes of physicians and managers have been measured and contrasted through the use of the Myers-Briggs Type Indicator (MBTI). Managers and physicians who are aware of such information have the capacity to improve their relationships by seeking to develop their less preferred psychological processes or by building on the similar or dissimilar background of the other. The theory undergirding the MBTI is very useful in this regard, because it can allow the physician and manager to view each other as dissimilar individuals, as

Table 26–1. Cultural differences between health care executives and physicians

Attribute	Health care executives	Physicians
Basis of knowledge	Primarily social and management sciences	Primarily biomedical sciences
Exposure to relevant others while in training	Relatively little exposure to physicians, nurses, other health care professionals, or patients	Great deal of exposure to nurses, other health care professionals, and patients; little exposure to broader business/economic world of health care
Patient focus	Broad: all patients in the organization and the larger community	Narrow: own individual patients
Time frame of action	Middle to long run; emphasis on positioning the organization for the future	Generally short run; meet immediate needs of patients
Rules of evidence	Understand the need to act on "soft" qualitative information; loose-linked cause-effect relationships that may not be well understood	"Soft" qualitative information viewed with skepticism; prefer "hard" facts; tightly linked cause-effect relationships that are well understood
View of resources	Always limited; challenge lies in allocating scarce resources efficiently and effectively	Resources essentially unlimited or at least should be unlimited: resources should be available to maximize the quality of care
Professional identity	Less cohesive; less well developed	More cohesive; highly developed

Source. Shortell SM: *Effective Hospital–Physician Relationships.* Ann Arbor, MI, Health Administration Press, 1991. Reprinted with permission from the Hospital Research and Educational Trust.

"someone you don't quite understand, but someone you can, with a sense of puzzlement perhaps, gradually come to appreciate" (Kiersey and Bates 1984, p. 4). The theory put forth by the MBTI is relatively easy to understand. The MBTI measures the mental processes preferred among four bipolar dimensions:

1. extroversion/introversion (E/I)
2. sensing/intuition (S/N)
3. thinking/feeling (T/F)
4. judging/perceiving (J/P)

These dimensions are described extensively in other sources (Kiersey and Bates 1984; Myers and McCaulley 1989; Myers and Myers 1988). Extroversion/introversion is an attitude that indicates how people are oriented to the world around them. Very simply, extroverts (E) are oriented to an external world of people and situations. Introverts (I) prefer an internal world of thoughts and ideas.

The function of sensing/intuition depicts how an individual prefers to absorb stimuli from his or her environment. Sensors (S) favor concrete information that can be assimilated through the five senses. Alternatively, intuitors (N) favor more theoretical and abstract information.

The function of thinking/feeling indicates how an individual prefers to make decisions once information has been received. Thinkers (T) prefer to make impersonal judgments based on logic, whereas feelers (F) prefer to make decisions based more on their own system of values and how the outcome of their decisions might affect others.

Judging/perceiving indicates whether an individual prefers to take in more information or act on information that has already been received. The perceiver (P) prefers to focus attention on new information and decision alternatives and is less concerned with making a final decision or choice. Judgers (J), on the other hand, prefer closure and therefore tend to be more decisive.

The MBTI indicates which of the four bipolar processes are preferred through 1 of 16 four-letter codes called *types* (e.g., ESTJ, INTP, ENFJ, ISTP). These relatively enduring type configurations provide characteristic details that offer insights into how individuals might think and behave.

Physicians

Since the 1950s, physician samples have exhibited modest increases in intuitive, feeling, and judging types. More recently, substantial increases in the numbers of intuitive-feeling (NF) types have been observed. These have been described as "humanistic . . . types who are motivated more by idealism and who are interested in the psychosocial aspects of medicine" (McCaulley 1978, p. 6). It is important to note that, among those desiring to become physicians, the INFP types are approximately four times more likely to pursue a medical school education than the opposite ESTJ types (Myers and Myers 1988).

Health Care Managers

The type pattern of health care managers is similar to that of their counterparts in the public and private sectors. According to type theory, the decision-making roles of management should be especially attractive to thinker/judgers (TJ). Type tables of both health- and non–health-related management samples typically exhibit high numbers of thinker/judger types that reside in the four outer corners of a type table, resulting in what has come to be known as the classic four-corner type table.

The single most commonly occurring type among managers is the extroverted-sensing-thinking-judging (ESTJ). ESTJs have been characterized as in control of situations; making decisions; getting the work completed (Myers and McCaulley 1989); and appearing to be sensible, methodical, and productive. Although the ESTJ is regarded as the quintessential "business type," it is also the type least likely to be attracted to a career in medicine (Myers and Myers 1988).

O'Connor and Shewchuk (1993) compared a sample of 1,881 physicians with a sample of 522 health care managers. The comparison contrasted the respective type tables from each sample through the use of a statistical program known as the Selection Ratio Type Table. For each comparison, an index known as the self-selection ratio (I) was derived. A clarification of how those ratios should be interpreted is provided in Table 26–2.

The most remarkable feature of the type table comparison can be observed between the two outer and inner columns. Specifically, when compared with physicians, managers are more likely to be depicted as thinking types (two outer columns) and less likely to be feeling types (two inner columns). Additionally, managers were significantly more likely to prefer extroversion, sensing, and judging than physicians, who collectively tended to hold greater preferences for introversion, intuition, and perceiving.

Suggestions for Improving the Relationship

The results of the type table comparison described above have two important implications for helping to improve the relationship of managers and physicians. First, in addition to the influence of well-known cultural and socialization differences, the continuing tensions can also be partially attributed to substantial differences at the unseen psychological level. Second, because people tend to better understand those communications

Table 26–2. Type table of health administrators as contrasted with physicians

Sensing types: With thinking	Sensing types: With feeling	Intuitive types: With feeling	Intuitive types: With thinking	
ISTJ*	ISFJ**	INFJ**	INTJ	INTROVERTS / JUDGING
N = 94	N = 14	N = 7	N = 44	
% = 18.01	% = 2.68	% = 1.34	% = 8.43	
I = 1.27	I = 0.27	I = 0.17	I = 1.21	
ISTP	ISFP*	INFP**	INTP	INTROVERTS / PERCEPTIVES
N = 18	N = 3	N = 13	N = 34	
% = 3.45	% = 0.57	% = 2.49	% = 6.51	
I = 1.20	I = 0.24	I = 0.27	I = 1.32	
ESTP	ESFP*	ENFP**	ENTP**	EXTRAVERTS / PERCEPTIVES
N = 10	N = 3	N = 19	N = 42	
% = 1.92	% = 0.57	% = 3.64	% = 8.05	
I = 1.16	I = 0.31	I = 0.46	I = 2.44	
ESTJ**	ESFJ*	ENFJ***	ENTJ**	EXTRAVERTS / JUDGING
N = 112	N = 18	N = 14	N = 77	
% = 21.46	% = 3.45	% = 2.68	% = 14.75	
I = 2.73	I = 0.56	I = 0.42	I = 2.27	

	N	%	I
E	295	56.51	1.36**
I	227	43.49	0.74**
S	272	52.11	1.11*
N	250	47.89	0.90*
T	431	82.57	1.71**
F	91	17.43	0.34**
J	380	72.80	1.10***
P	142	27.20	0.80***

Note. The type table displayed here reveals the patterns of psychological type among health administrators as compared to physicians. I is the self-selection ratio. Numbers > 1.0 indicate a higher likelihood of health administrators selecting a particular type than physicians. Differences evaluated with the chi-square test (or Fisher's exact probability test where there were fewer than five cases to a cell). The sidebar shows the frequency (N), percentage (%), and self-selection ratio (I) for the health administrators' preferred psychological process in each of the four bipolar personality dimensions: extraversion-introversion (E/I), sensing-intuition (S/N), thinking-feeling (T/F), and judging-perceiving (J/P).

*$P < .05$; **$P < .001$; ***$P < .01$.

Source. Reprinted from O'Connor SJ, Shewchuk RM: "Enhancing Administrator-Clinician Relationships: The Role of Psychological Type." *Health Care Management Review* 18(2)57–65, 1993, with permission of Aspen Publishers, Inc., © 1993.

agreeable with their psychological preferences (Barr and Barr 1989; Myers and McCaulley 1989), one can begin to realize how those findings can be used to improve communication between physicians and managers. As Shortell (1991) has stated; "Communication is at the center of all relationships" (p. 252), and improved communication is at the heart of developing the trust, understanding, and respect required for creating better and effective relationships.

Table 26–3 contains prescriptive strategies that can be used by health administrators to improve communication with physicians. Obviously, because an individual can hold preferences for any one of the 16 types, these strategies will not be suitable for every circumstance; however, because they reflect the general and dominant preferences of physicians and managers, they should be suitable in many cases.

The thinking/feeling (T/F) dimension probably has the greatest impact on communications between physicians and managers. Whereas managers harbor very strong preferences for thinking, physicians tend to prefer feeling. As such, the communication style most often used by managers has been characterized as *reasoned logic.* When taken to an extreme, continual reliance on reasoned logic can become problematic because thinkers tend to "believe their opinions are based upon valid reasoning; therefore, anyone who disagrees must be incorrect, unreasonable, or not quite smart enough to think clearly" (Barr and Barr 1989, p. 128). To the feeling physician, managers who tend to rely most heavily on a reasoned-logic communication style may be viewed as being deficient in emotional content and, consequently, artificial. There are two ways administrators can overcome or avoid this pejorative perception. First, because feelers have such a strong people orientation, communications with them should certainly emphasize how a course of action will serve people. Communiqués couched in human terms will be much better received by feelers. Second, before raising disagreeable matters, communication with physicians should readily express those areas where harmony exists.

In addition to communication, there are several other important suggestions managers should consider when seeking to improve their relationship with physicians. These include improving utilization review (UR) systems, educating physicians on market dynamics, involving them in the process of governance and strategic planning, and creating organizational designs that emphasize collaboration and the development of leadership potential.

Even though managers are increasingly being exhorted to serve as patient advocates, UR remains a hotly contentious area for physicians. Thus, any way in which these systems can be made more palatable will be helpful. Some organizations have begun using more trained clinicians in the UR process. Others have actually stated their abandonment of traditional UR,

Table 26–3. Using psychological type differences to prescribe strategies for improving communication between physicians and health care managers

1. Finding:	Managers are significantly more extroverted (E) than physicians, who tend to be more introverted (I).
Communication strategies:	
A.	Managers can defer to the physician's greater needs for privacy by not becoming too personal in conversations or by asking questions that assault psychological space.
B.	Physicians need to be provided with adequate warning regarding topics to be discussed in group situations.
C.	Physicians need to be clear about whether a conversation is for the purpose of deliberating ideas and possibilities or announcing firm decisions.
D.	Any new courses of action to be undertaken need to be conveyed to physicians with reasoned justification and free of the social chatter that may be confusing (Barr and Barr 1989).
2. Finding:	Managers are significantly more sensing (S) than physicians, who tend to exhibit preferences for intuition (N).
Communication strategies:	
A.	Because physicians tend to be more abstract thinkers than managers, they prefer communication that includes illustration, narrative, figures, and personal examples (Shortell 1991).
B.	As physicians are often quick to detect where a discussion is heading, they may be apt to draw hasty conclusions and miss the essential message being conveyed. Managers need to be sure their communications are very focused, but also slightly open-ended. This allows physicians to draw their own conclusions from a narrower range of possibilities.
3. Finding:	Managers are significantly more thinking (T) than physicians, who tend to be more feeling (F).
Communication strategies:	
A.	Physicians tend to be more people oriented; thus communication with them should indicate how a decision alternative will benefit people.
B.	Before raising contentious issues, recognize those areas where consensus already exists.

choosing instead to focus on selecting efficient and high-quality physician practitioners. Others have begun focusing less on UR and more on the overall pattern of expenses incurred.

Physicians also need to be made aware of changing health care market dynamics and the trends associated with a managed care environment.

This information is probably best conveyed not through a health administrator's shrill warnings of impending doom, but through objective education. Berger and Sudman (1994) suggested that a senior executive from a major local employer can be brought in to inform physicians how the company deals with suppliers and how it intends to purchase health care in the future. The changes in the relative power and influence between administrators and physicians, as well as friction between the two, are as much related to a shift in the control of resources and dollars as differences in personality.

Involving physicians in governance and policy making is often suggested as a sure way to build understanding of mutual interests and goals, as well as to impress on physicians the realities of a changing health care environment. Appointing physicians to meaningful roles on governing boards and strategic planning committees is one way that this can be accomplished.

Finally, the importance of organizational structures and cultures that incorporate physicians into managerial roles and that emphasize collaboration and teamwork in seeking common goals cannot be emphasized enough. A primary indicator of how well physicians are being incorporated as decision makers is the extent of their inclusion in such roles within the organizational and committee structure. Likewise, a culture that seeks to develop physician leadership and managerial skills, that involves physicians in administrative decisions, that encourages teamwork, that mandates respect for physicians, and that encourages trust and a desire to collaborate is generally considered necessary.

Will Physicians Manage the Managers?

There exists a belief that managers will eventually control the entire American health care delivery system, with physicians being little more than labor automatons for the system. The fear is that, absent a degree of oversight and control, these managers will operate unchecked, focusing only on making profits, cutting services, and, in general, making life miserable for physicians.

This fear is harbored by many in the medical profession and was made explicit in a recent public relations piece from the American Medical Association that appeared nationally in a number of magazines and newspapers. The advertisement featured the hands of a physician touching a patient's shoulder. The caption read; "This is the moment of truth. Would you rather trust your life to an MD or an MBA?" It went on to state that "these bureaucrats may have good intentions. But they don't have the scientific knowledge and training to make such decisions. After all, most studied business. Not medicine."

Alternatively, one might argue that most physicians have very good intentions but don't have the management knowledge to design and run a revamped health care system. Most physicians don't have training in the management sciences: organizational theory and behavior, strategic planning, finance, total quality management, health care administration, and human resources management, nor extensive training in epidemiology, actuarial science, public health, or the legislative process.

In a sense, the American Medical Association's public appeal is somewhat reminiscent of the Luddite's reactionary response to the development and diffusion of the power loom and other cost-saving machinery during the English Industrial Revolution. Correctly anticipating that their own jobs would eventually be replaced by the power loom, the Luddites went on a rampage, trying to burn and destroy the new technology in an attempt to save their jobs. Eventually the power loom won. Many textile workers did lose their jobs, but the economy and the public benefited greatly. Textile-related productivity and quality rose sharply, and prices dropped dramatically. Similarly, during the North American Free Trade Agreement (NAFTA) debates, opponents painted a grim, but unfounded, picture of what would happen to the United States economy as a result of expanding trade with Mexico.

Extensive change occurred during the English Industrial Revolution and with the passage of NAFTA. Those changes diminished the economic well-being of some but helped improve it for most. Because health care reform will undoubtedly be the grandest scale experiment in organizational change that has ever occurred, physicians will feel more threatened than ever.

The rapid pace of change in the United States health care environment will only escalate. To achieve success in this brave new environment requires, not a wistful hope for the return of the "good old days," but the ability of managers and physicians to function as members of a team. The integrated delivery networks of today are generally viewed as harbingers of the future (see Chapter 23). Increasingly, one observes the management of these networks to be distributed through teams that include managers, physicians, nurses, epidemiologists, and others. However, it is essential that physicians play an even greater role in the management and leadership of these teams. In fact, a recent study concludes that "successful integration suggests there is no exception to this finding" (Coddington et al., 1994 p. 115). This is especially true because physician manager input is required to help contain costs, support and oversee ancillary practitioners, size clinical services appropriately, implement patient-focused care (Heydt and Sherer 1993), evaluate new technology, and institute critical pathways and practice parameters to best allocate available resources (Kongstvedt 1993). However, additional interpersonal and strategic management skills will be needed.

The interpersonal skills include facility with leading groups, building relationships, negotiating, and empowering others. The strategic management skills require an understanding of strategy formulation and how an integrated organization should best be structured to properly fit its increasingly competitive and capitated external environment.

To the extent that lay and physician managers are able to develop and carry out these skills, especially the interpersonal and relationship-building ones, they will maintain a degree of real power and control over their destiny. However, continued poor interpersonal skills and unstable relationships will create high-conflict markets that, by default, will allow management control to flow to diverse arrangements such as for-profit managed care organizations, insurance firms, or business coalitions (Goldsmith 1993).

Unfortunately, there is a fairly good probability that the latter situation will occur unless adequate preventive measures are taken (Relman 1993). Disturbingly, recent research appears to indicate that collaborative attempts to integrate physicians into organizational management actually increase conflict (Burns et al.1993) and do not necessarily result in cost-effectiveness (Alexander and Morrisey 1988). Moreover, as a result of their collectively strong needs for autonomy and personal achievement, many physicians cannot function collaboratively even if they want to. In fact, Goldsmith (1993) stated that many physicians "lack the interpersonal skills or civility to function as part of a larger enterprise" (p. 163).

Conclusion

For years, physicians in the United States have held remarkable autonomy over their profession and have had enormous influence on the delivery and structure of health care. As systems of managed care continue to proliferate, and as power accrues to those paying for health care, physicians will increasingly play key roles as members of health care provider teams. In the future, concern will be increasingly directed toward the cost of, appropriateness of, effectiveness of, and satisfaction with health care delivery, while the issue of physician autonomy will be less frequently debated and ultimately not considered at all.

As patients and payers continue to gain access to more and better clinical and cost information, they will eventually begin to drive the system. Physicians, instead of mourning their loss of autonomy to nonphysicians, can regain some control by making proactive attempts to collaborate meaningfully with managers, other clinicians, purchasers, and communities. Ultimately, decisions will most likely be made by teams of clinically oriented administrators who will be advised by seasoned physicians representing all specialties and who will be able to place patient welfare in its proper context on the basis of good data acquired from well-designed outcome studies. This may be pie in the sky, but it would be a logical solution to the question, "Who will manage the managers?"

References

A lack of professional business (editorial). Medical Record 49:730, 1896

Alexander JA, Morrisey MA: Hospital–physician integration and hospital costs. Inquiry 25:388–401, 1988

Ashley JT: Physicians in administration: working at the medicine management interface, in A Future of Consequence: The Manager's Role in Health Services. Edited by Filerman GL. Arlington, VA, Association of University Programs in Health Administration, 1989, pp 291–300

Barr L, Barr N: The Leadership Equation: Leadership, Management, and the Myers-Briggs. Austin, TX, Eakin Press, 1989

Berger S, Sudman SK: M.D./hospital integration: staying on course. Healthc Exec 9:9–11, 1994

Biddle JC: The physician as a hospital superintendent. Transactions of the American Hospital Association 6:48–53, 1904

Burns LR, Andersen RM, Shortell SM: Trends in hospital/physician relationships. Health Aff 12:213–223, 1993.

Coddington DC, Moore KD, Fischer, EA: Integrative Health Care: Reorganizing the Physician, Hospital, and Health Plan Relationship. Englewood, CO, Center for Research in Ambulatory Health Care Administration, 1994

Goldsmith J: Hospital/physician relationships: a constraint to health reform. Health Aff 12:160–169, 1993

Heydt S, in Sherer JL: Structure follows strategy: Now that you've formed a network, who will make up your new executive team? Hosp Health Netw 67:22–28, 1993

Kiersey D, Bates M: Please Understand Me: Character and Temperament Types. Del Mar, CA, Prometheus Nemesis Book, 1984

Kongstvedt PR: Changing provider behavior in managed care plans, in The Managed Health Care Handbook, 2nd Edition. Edited by Kongstvedt PR. Gaithersburg, MD, Aspen Publishers, 1993, pp 91–101

McCaulley MH: Application of the Myers-Briggs Type Indicator to Medicine and Other Health Professions (Monograph I). Gainesville, FL, Center for Applications of Psychological Type, 1978

Myers IB, McCaulley MH: Manual: A Guide to the Development and Use of the Myers-Briggs Type Indicator. Palo Alto, CA, Consulting Psychologists Press, 1989

Myers IB, Myers PB: Gifts Differing. Palo Alto, CA, Consulting Psychologists Press, 1988

O'Connor SJ, Lanning JA: The end of autonomy? Reflections on the post-professional physician. Health Care Manage Rev 17:63–72, 1992

O'Connor SJ, Shewchuk RM: Enhancing administrator-clinician relationships: The role of psychological type. Health Care Manage Rev 18:57–65, 1993

Raffel MW, Raffel NK: The U.S. Health System: Origins and Functions. Albany, NY, Delmar, 1989

Relman, AS: Medical practice under the Clinton reforms—avoiding domination by business. New Engl J Med 329:1574–1576, 1993

Rohrer JE: The secret of medical management. Health Care Manage Rev 14:7–13, 1989

Romeo SJW: The challenges of medical management. Med Group Manage J 35:14–18, 1988

Rosenberg CE: The Care of Strangers: The Rise of America's Hospital System. New York, Basic Books, 1987

Schulz R, Detmer DE: Physician organization and management, in The AUPHA Manual of Health Services Management. Edited by Taylor RJ, Taylor SB. Gaithersburg, MD, Aspen Publishers, 1994, pp 182–203

Shortell SM: Effective Hospital-Physician Relationships. Ann Arbor, MI, Health Administration Press, 1991

Starr P: The Social Transformation of American Medicine; The Rise of a Sovereign Profession and the Making of a Vast Industry. New York, Basic Books, 1982

Stevens R: In Sickness and in Wealth: American Hospital in the Twentieth Century. New York, Basic Books, 1989

Afterword

Is Managed Care Psychiatry's Internecine War?

Arthur Lazarus, M.D.

The *American Heritage Dictionary* (1994) defines *internecine* as "mutually destructive," (p. 438) often involving conflict within a group. Examples of issues that have divided psychiatrists are legion: biological versus psychodynamic orientation, long-term versus short-term therapy, and eclecticism versus specialization. Perhaps it is healthy that psychiatrists are a heterogeneous group. On the other hand, internal differences may create an external appearance of weakness and vulnerability. Disputes among psychiatrists, it seems, invariably become public knowledge. As I discussed in Chapter 8 and elsewhere (Lazarus 1994), and as many contributors to this book have observed, there seems to be no aspect of practice more fraught with rancor and contentiousness than that of managed care.

Proliferation of Therapists

A few years ago at a workshop sponsored by the American Psychiatric Association (APA) I suggested that one reason APA opposed managed care was that endorsing it could cause further division within the ranks of psychiatry by fusing the identity of psychiatrists with that of allied mental health professionals. However, my idea was lightly dismissed. More credibility was given to other disturbing aspects of managed care such as the loss of professional autonomy, the intrusivenesss of utilization review, and increased administrative demands. However, I maintain that also at issue is whether psychiatrists are willing to accord nonmedical therapists greater responsibility in treating patients and the polarization of psychiatrists that is likely to occur if parity is effected.

Managed mental health care has expanded the roles and responsibilities of nonpsychiatric providers—primarily psychologists and social workers—while the scope of psychiatric practice has been narrowed. Competition has intensified. Reimbursement has been ratcheted down. Long-term psychotherapy has been virtually eliminated for all but private-pay patients. Psychiatrists are being forced into new practice arrangements, including consulting for multidisciplinary groups, with a heavier concentration on psychopharmacology and critical care.

As a result of these changes, psychiatrists will basically have two choices: adapt or fight back and risk being left out in the cold (see Chapter 20). To avoid the latter fate, it will be important for psychiatrists to know when to assert their strengths and when to relinquish psychiatrically nonessential functions to other providers. Not the least consideration is the fact that psychiatrists are outnumbered by allied mental health professionals by more than three to one (DeWitt 1992). Moreover, psychiatrists appear to be less responsive than psychologists to changes in market conditions (Knesper et al. 1989).

Roles of Psychiatrists

In my opinion, psychiatrists must put forward the qualities of their profession that make their contributions incontrovertible. These qualities are essentially derived from medical school and residency and form the backbone of the medical profession. Among mental health providers, only psychiatrists can lay claim to a program of education that requires nearly a decade of study, provides such a rich and diversified curriculum, and encompasses a wide range of patient care responsibilities. Psychiatrists offer a truly comprehensive health care perspective, possess special expertise in the neurosciences, and retain nearly exclusive competence in combining psychotherapy and pharmacotherapy. Psychiatrists are well grounded in the biopsychosocial model of treatment.

I believe that health maintenance organizations (HMOs) and other managed care delivery systems will value these attributes, placing psychiatrists in the critical role of treating severely mentally ill and other complex patients. Our therapeutic armamentarium is comprehensive, comprising a broad array of psychopharmacological agents. Psychiatrists working in managed care programs will practice brief, symptom-focused supportive psychotherapy; coordinate treatment with nonmedical therapists and primary care physicians; and provide supervision and consultation. There will, however, still be room for nonpsychiatric practitioners and for those psychiatrists who wish to do more.

The position that psychiatrists cannot give ground to other mental health professionals will surely be self-defeating. Managed care programs value outpatient therapy, community-based care, and inexpensive treatment, which gives an edge to psychologists and social workers. Psychologists have also made significant contributions to the fields of marital and family therapy, behavior therapy, and psychosocial rehabilitation (Geezy and Sultenfuss 1994). If psychologists are granted prescribing privileges, the distinction between them and psychiatrists will fade considerably.

The ongoing debate between psychiatrists and psychologists over prescribing privileges clearly speaks to the issue of managed care and division of labor. Former APA president John McIntyre (1994) observed, "It is unfortunate that this ill-conceived plan for psychologists prescribing privileges and other such initiatives detract from our legitimate and effective collaboration with the other mental health disciplines"(p. 3). Psychiatrist Thomas M. Duffy (1994) offered this perspective: "We psychiatrists can hardly blame psychologists for wanting to intrude on our turf by prescribing medication; we've been intruding on their turf—psychotherapy—for decades. . . . If we stuck to treating only those disorders that require medical treatment—those with a true biological basis such as schizophrenia, bipolar disorder, panic disorder, OCD, organic brain disorders—and referred the rest to our nonphysician colleagues, the turf wars would quickly end"(p. 5).

Every Living Provider

Managed care systems will rewrite traditional job descriptions throughout the health care industry. Many nonmedical practitioners will be given greater responsibility for patient care. The tension observed between psychiatrists and nonmedical therapists also exists between various physicians and professional groups whose practice and skills overlap, for example, physicians' assistants, nurse-practitioners, and chiropractors.

My concern is that if the psychiatric profession decides to wage battle—whether a civil war or an interdisciplinary attack—the ideals and principles that ultimately shape health reform will be developed in absentia. What a shame this would be if we—divided into several factions—discover that the moment has passed us by, without our input or endorsement of the new system.

We must not let ourselves be led into a nonproductive battle. Instead, we should seek ways to work for the common good of the patient and cooperate with the managed care industry and with each other. The following outline summarizes how we can prepare for the challenges ahead (Lazarus 1995).

Preparing for Managed Care

Restore Professional Balance

APA should promote managed care in a more favorable light and with greater balance. Commentaries that allege managed care "abuses" or that appear to denigrate the value of managed care should be tempered by the reporting of positive outcomes. APA-sponsored periodicals should reconsider publishing overwrought distortions of managed care that portray the industry as "Gestapo-like" (Sharma 1993) simply based on anecdotes. Unfair characterizations of managed care, as well as an apparent failure of APA to represent the interests of HMO psychiatrists and psychiatrists who conduct utilization review, have alienated many APA members.

APA and its disenfranchised members must strive to heal previous wounds and work together proactively. APA's committee on managed care, which represents psychiatrists in various settings including managed care, is a good example of such collaboration. Changing the name of the managed care hotline to the managed care "helpline" is also a positive move. Despite its attacks on managed care, APA has apparently endorsed it in an effort to convince Congress that nondiscriminatory health coverage is feasible (Barlas 1994).

Ensure Representation Through Unity

According to Fink ("APA to increase help to members as they adapt to managed care" 1994), professional disunity "allows psychiatry to be in the same position it's been for the last 20 years, which is essentially a pox on all of you" (p. 2). Dissension among psychiatrists is costly for a number of reasons, but perhaps most important, a show of unity is critical in achieving the goal of nondiscriminatory health coverage.

Psychiatrists must be united not only with each other but also with the rest of organized medicine. Dividing into political interest groups will only strengthen the lobbying efforts of legislators interested in exploiting the diversity of physicians' interests (Inglehart 1994).

Steps must be taken to ensure that physicians benefit from contributing to political action committees and that their contributions do not belie important public health issues (Sharfstein and Sharfstein 1994). Physicians must be given a greater voice in management and have adequate representation at the national policy level.

Improve Relations Between Providers and Payers

Ensuring cooperation between providers and payers of services is important. The development of networks through selective contracts with mental health providers should be based on quality and compatibility, not only on costs.

Managed care companies should clearly state their policies, procedures, and clinical orientation so providers will know what is expected of them. Providers who have expressed satisfaction with the business and clinical changes that have resulted from managed care requirements have cited more precise admissions and assessment criteria and more individualized treatment plans as among the positive changes (Creager 1993).

Provide Training in Managed Care

Psychiatrists and other mental health specialists work as a team. A study by Olfson and colleagues (1993) revealed that of 1.29 million outpatients treated in United States mental health organizations for at least 1 month, the majority (56.0%) were treated at multiservice mental health organizations and nearly one-half (48.2%) of the outpatients were treated by psychiatrists. Olfson et al. (1993) concluded that "the high prevalence of interdisciplinary treatment in mental health clinics and the expanding role of clinics in the nation's mental health care system suggest that psychiatrists will be increasingly engaged in interdisciplinary clinical work" (p. 629).

Dual treatment, that is, pharmacotherapy provided by a psychiatrist and psychotherapy provided by a nonpsychiatric therapist, requires great skill on the part of both clinicians. If it is handled improperly, the arrangement can lead to intertherapist conflict and patient mismanagement (Chiles et al. 1991). Training programs in psychiatry should provide residents with extensive experience in coordinated interdisciplinary treatment, not only in managed care but also in other settings, so their entry into the marketplace is not a traumatic one (Gabbard 1992).

Managed health care organizations need to become more involved with academic health centers and help provide a framework for teaching the principles of managed care. Training and education should extend beyond the basic operations of managed care companies.

Make Utilization Review Equitable

It seems ironic that professionals who specialize in resolving conflict have become adversaries. Yet the breakdown of collegial relations surrounding peer review has become a grave concern. In some regions, relationships between reviewing psychiatrists and attending psychiatrists have deteriorated to a crisis level. Relationships may be restored, however, if both parties adhere to certain ground rules.

Attending psychiatrists must learn to communicate effectively by offering objective, measurable goals of therapy in language free of jargon. They should not be defensive or feel compelled to distort information for the purpose of certifying care. Attending psychiatrists should not be verbally abusive to their peers during telephonic review. Psychiatrists must refrain from leading patients and their families into assaults against managed care companies and their employees before appealing insurance disputes.

In return, managed care organizations must offer an equitable process in which attending psychiatrists can appeal their treatment to a panel of peers, if necessary. Managed care firms must unlock the secrets of medical review and share their criteria with providers and the public. They should participate with organized psychiatry and lobby for comprehensive, flexible benefits that would allow coverage for catastrophic illnesses and conditions that have been refractory to treatment.

Follow Guidelines

All psychiatrists must become familiar with and follow practice guidelines. If used properly, guidelines will promote the standardization of care and enhance quality (Sturm and Wells 1995). Guidelines should not be perceived as a threat to practice or a reduction in autonomy, even though they could become weapons for plaintiffs in malpractice cases (Felsenthal 1994).

APA has published numerous clinical and practice guidelines (see Chapter 4); guidelines for psychiatrists practicing in staff-model HMOs have been in existence since 1989 (American Psychiatric Association 1989). Psychiatrists should become familiar with these guidelines and incorporate them in everyday practice when applicable.

Participate in Quality Improvement

Psychiatrists must provide uniformly good treatment and measure the efficacy of their work. They must be willing to become active in quality assurance programs and strive for continuous quality improvement (Berwick 1989). Participation in outcome studies is a vital component of this activity.

It has taken decades for the psychiatric profession to start taking outcome measurements seriously. Psychiatrists were known for using untested treatments and arguing that outcome measurements were meaningless. It is very difficult to argue that nonmedication therapies psychiatrists use are well tested and carry clear agreement within the profession as to their effectiveness. Our losing control of something that we did not do very well is not surprising. The question is whether those gaining control will do any better than we have done.

Future health care delivery will be measured on the basis of quality, and psychiatrists will quite likely compete with each other and with nonmedical therapists on that basis. Outcome studies will serve as a measure of quality and help determine value in selecting health care providers. Outcome studies will also provide data to help decide whether the guidelines in use are correct. Psychiatrists must prove to themselves and to a nonphysician-controlled corporate system that their treatment is scientifically based and cost-effective.

Conclusion

Managed care is probably the most divisive issue ever to confront the psychiatric profession. I have identified several objectives to help psychiatrists prepare for the era of managed care and to minimize polarization with respect to each other and to allied mental health professionals. These objectives include 1) promoting managed care practice positively and with greater balance, 2) giving physicians a voice in management and ensuring physician representation in developing national policies, 3) increasing cooperation between providers and payers of mental health services, 4) providing skills training for the delivery of coordinated interdisciplinary care, 5) improving relations between reviewing psychiatrists and attending psychiatrists, and 6) following practice guidelines and participating in outcome studies and other quality improvement activities. Attainment of those objectives should position psychiatrists favorably in a new economic climate—a goal we all agree is important.

References

American Heritage Dictionary, 3rd edition. New York, Dell Publishing, 1994

American Psychiatric Association: Guidelines for Psychiatric Practice in Staff Model Health Maintenance Organizations. Washington, DC, American Psychiatric Association, 1989

APA to increase help to members as they adapt to managed care. Psychiatric News, January 7, 1994, p 2, 16

Barlas S: APA study reveals that nondiscriminatory mental health care can pass actuarial muster. Psychiatric Times, July 1994, p 21

Berwick DM: Continuous improvement as an ideal in health care. N Engl J Med 330:53–56, 1989

Chiles JA, Carlin AS, Benjamin GAH, et al: A physician, a nonmedical psychotherapist, and a patient: the pharmacotherapy-psychotherapy triangle, in Integrating Pharmacotherapy and Psychotherapy. Edited by Beitman BD, Klerman GL. Washington, DC, American Psychiatric Press, 1991, pp 105–118

Creager C: Managed care: hope amid the horror. Professional Counselor, February 1993, pp 24–27

DeWitt PM: The psyche market. American Demographics, September 1992, pp 62–65

Duffy TM: Decades of intrusion. Psychiatric Times, July 1994, p 5

Felsenthal E: Doctors' own guidelines hurt them in court. The Wall Street Journal, October 19, 1994, pp B1, B16

Gabbard GO: The big chill: the transition from residency to managed care nightmare. Academic Psychiatry 16:119–126, 1992

Geezy B, Sultenfuss JF: Contributions of psychologists to inpatient care of persons with chronic mental illness. Hosp Community Psychiatry 45:54–57, 1994

Inglehart JK: Health care reform: the role of physicians. N Engl J Med 330:728–731, 1994

Knesper DJ, Belcher BE, Cross JG: A market analysis comparing the practices of psychiatrists and psychologists. Arch Gen Psychiatry 46:305–314, 1989

Lazarus A: Ten reasons why psychiatrists may dislike managed competition. Hosp Community Psychiatry 45:496–498, 1994

Lazarus A: Preparing for practice in an era of managed competition. Psychiatr Serv 46:184–185, 1995.

McIntyre J: Changes in health care, medical education. Psychiatric News, September 3, 1994, p 3

Olfson M, Klerman GL, Pincus HA: The roles of psychiatrists in organized outpatient mental health settings. Am J Psychiatry 150:625–631, 1993

Sharfstein JM, Sharfstein SS: Campaign contributions from the American Medical Political Action Committee to members of Congress: for or against the public health? N Engl J Med 330:32–37, 1994

Sharma TL: Medication and managed care. Psychiatric News, February 19, 1993, p 40

Sturm R, Wells KB: How can care for depression become more cost-effective? JAMA 273:51–58, 1995

Index